Caring for Women Through the Lifecycle

By
Elaine Weil, BA, RN, FPNP

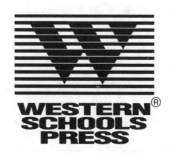

WESTERN®
SCHOOLS
PRESS

21 Bristol Drive
South Easton, MA 02375
1-800-618-1670

ABOUT THE AUTHOR

Elaine Weil, BA, RN, FPNP, received her bachelor's degree in human biology from Stanford University (Palo Alto, CA), her RN after completion of the basic curriculum for professional nursing at Santa Rosa Junior College (Santa Rosa, CA), and her certification as a Family Planning Nurse Practitioner from Educational Programs Associates (Campbell, CA). She received certification as a Clinical Nutritional Consultant from the Institute for Educational Therapy (Cotati, CA) and served on its faculty, teaching courses in women's health. Elaine has studied Western herbology with David Hoffman, Kathi Keville, and Lois Johnson, MD. She has worked for many years as a clinician and health educator at Commonwoman's Health Project (Santa Rosa, CA), a nonprofit clinic serving women of low income. Elaine has written health education materials, facilitated support groups, and conducted workshops on a variety of health topics.

Subject Matter Expert: Vivian Haack, RN, FPNP

Copy Editor: Janice Jerrells, RN, BA, ELS

Indexer: Sylvia Coates

Typesetter: Kathy Johnson

Western Schools' courses are designed to provide nursing professionals with the educational information they need to enhance their career development. The information provided within these course materials is the result of research and consultation with prominent nursing and medical authorities and is, to the best of our knowledge, current and accurate. However, the courses and course materials are provided with the understanding that Western Schools is not engaged in offering legal, nursing, medical, or other professional advice.

Western Schools' courses and course materials are not meant to act as a substitute for seeking out professional advice or conducting individual research. When the information provided in the courses and course materials is applied to individual circumstances, all recommendations must be considered in light of the uniqueness pertaining to each situation.

Western Schools' course materials are intended solely for *your* use and *not* for the benefit of providing advice or recommendations to third parties. Western Schools devoids itself of any responsibility for adverse consequences resulting from the failure to seek nursing, medical, or other professional advice. Western Schools further devoids itself of any responsibility for updating or revising any programs or publications presented, published, distributed, or sponsored by Western Schools unless otherwise agreed to as part of an individual purchase contract.

ISBN: 1-57801-030-6

COPYRIGHT© 1999—Western Schools, Inc. All Rights Reserved. No part(s) of this material may be reprinted, reproduced, transmitted, stored in a retrieval system, or otherwise utilized, in any form or by any means electronic or mechanical, including photocopying or recording, now existing or hereinafter invented, nor may any part of this course be used for teaching without the written permission from the publisher and author.
P1102

IMPORTANT: Read these instructions *BEFORE* proceeding!

Enclosed with your course book you will find the FasTrax® answer sheet. Use this form to answer all the final exam questions that appear in this course book. If you are completing more than one course, be sure to write your answers on the appropriate answer sheet. Full instructions and complete grading details are printed on the FasTrax instruction sheet, also enclosed with your order. Please review them before starting. *If you are mailing your answer sheet(s) to Western Schools, we recommend you make a copy as a backup.*

ABOUT THIS COURSE

A "Pretest" is provided with each course to test your current knowledge base regarding the subject matter contained within this course. Your "Final Exam" is a multiple choice examination. **You will find the exam questions at the end of each chapter.** Some smaller hour courses include the exam at the end of the book.

In the event the course has less than 100 questions, mark your answers to the questions in the course book and leave the remaining answer boxes on the FasTrax answer sheet blank. **Use a <u>black pen</u> to fill in your answer sheet.**

A PASSING SCORE

You must score 70% or better in order to pass this course and receive your Certificate of Completion. Should you fail to achieve the required score, we will send you an additional FasTrax answer sheet so that you may make a second attempt to pass the course. Western Schools will allow you three chances to pass the same course...*at no extra charge!* After three failed attempts to pass the same course, your file will be closed.

RECORDING YOUR HOURS

Please monitor the time it takes to complete this course using the handy log sheet on the other side of this page. See below for transferring study hours to the course evaluation.

COURSE EVALUATIONS

In this course book you will find a short evaluation about the course you are soon to complete. This information is vital to providing the school with feedback on this course. The course evaluation answer section is in the lower right hand corner of the FasTrax answer sheet marked "Evaluation" with answers marked 1–25. Your answers are important to us, please take five minutes to complete the evaluation.

On the back of the FasTrax instruction sheet there is additional space to make any comments about the course, the school, and suggested new curriculum. Please mail the FasTrax instruction sheet, with your comments, back to Western Schools in the envelope provided with your course order.

TRANSFERRING STUDY TIME

Upon completion of the course, transfer the total study time from your log sheet to question #25 in the Course Evaluation. The answers will be in ranges, please choose the proper hour range that best represents your study time. You MUST log your study time under question #25 on the course evaluation.

EXTENSIONS

You have 2 years from the date of enrollment to complete this course. A six (6) month extension may be purchased. If after 30 months from the original enrollment date you do not complete the course, *your file will be closed and no certificate can be issued.*

CHANGE OF ADDRESS?

In the event you have moved during the completion of this course please call our student services department at 1-800-618-1670 and we will update your file.

A GUARANTEE YOU'LL GIVE HIGH HONORS TO

If any continuing education course fails to meet your expectations or if you are not satisfied in any manner, for any reason, you may return it for an exchange or a refund (less shipping and handling) within 30 days. Software, video and audio courses must be returned unopened.

Thank you for enrolling at Western Schools!

WESTERN SCHOOLS
P.O. Box 1930
Brockton, MA 02303
(800) 618-1670

Caring for Women
Through the Lifecycle

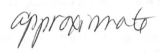

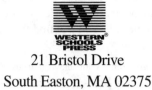

WESTERN®
SCHOOLS
PRESS

21 Bristol Drive

South Easton, MA 02375

Please use this log to total the number of hours you spend reading the text and taking the final examination (use 50-min hours).

Date	Hours Spent
3-3-03	1½ h
3-5-03	1
4-03	1
4-03	1½
4-03	2
4-03	1
7-03	1
7-03	1½
7-03	1
7-03	2
8-03	1
8-03	1½
8-03	1
8-03	1½
8-03	2
TOTAL	

Please log your study hours with submission of your final exam. To log your study time, fill in the appropriate circle under question 25 of the FasTrax® answer sheet under the "Evaluation" section.

PLEASE LOG YOUR STUDY HOURS WITH SUBMISSION OF YOUR FINAL EXAM. Please choose which best represents the total study hours it took to complete this 30 hour course.

A. less than 25 hours

B. 25–28 hours

C. 29–32 hours

D. greater than 32 hours

Caring for Women Through the Lifecycle

WESTERN SCHOOLS
CONTINUING EDUCATION EVALUATION

Instructions: Mark your answers to the following questions with a black pen on the "Evaluation" section of your FasTrax® answer sheet provided with this course. You should not return this sheet. Please use the scale below to rate the following statements:

A	Agree Strongly	C	Disagree Somewhat
B	Agree Somewhat	D	Disagree Strongly

The course content met the following education objectives

1. Identifies some of the forces and trends that have shaped the lives of women in the United States during the past century, as well as how these forces and trends have affected the field of women's health.

2. Identifies the basic events that occur in the menstrual cycle, and describes the complex orchestration of hormonal communications between the brain and the reproductive organs.

3. Recognizes the diversity of human sexual expression, and describes normal sexual function.

4. Recognizes the events that occur during the process of sexual maturation.

5. Identifies current methods of birth control, as well as ways to counsel women in choosing a method of contraception that best suits their needs.

6. Identifies trends in fertility among women and men, as well as the process involved in infertility evaluation, and recognizes currently available tests and procedures, as well as new technologies, for infertility.

7. Recognizes the most common sexually transmitted infections, as well as modes of transmission, treatment options, prevention, self-care, and the practicing of safer sex in relation to these infections.

8. Recognizes how views about premenstrual syndrome have changed in recent years, and identifies the theories that have been put forth regarding possible causes of this syndrome.

9. Identifies the components of health maintenance and good preventive health care for women.

10. Specifies problems associated with Pap smears, particularly related to quality of smear preparation and accuracy of results, and recognizes the link between the presence of certain strains of human papillomavirus and cervical cancer.

11. Recognizes common gynecologic problems and treatments, including self-care and prevention.

12. Recalls the anatomy of the breast, and selects breast self-examination techniques and teaching points.

13. Recognizes the special health care needs of women growing older, with particular focus on the transition of menopause.

14. Recognizes the prevalence in the environment of chemicals and pollutants called estrogen "mimics," as well as the obsession in American culture with a very narrow and confining standard of beauty that is giving rise to an epidemic of low self-esteem among women of all ages.

15. This offering met my professional education needs.

16. The objectives met the overall purpose/goal of the course.

17. The course was generally well written and the subject matter explained thoroughly. (If no please explain on the back of the FasTrax instruction sheet.)

18. The content of this course was appropriate for home study.

19. The final examination was well written and at an appropriate level for the content of the course.

Please complete the following research questions in order to help us better meet your educational needs. Pick the ONE answer which is most appropriate.

20. What nursing shift do you most commonly work?
    A. Morning Shift (Any shift starting after 3:00am or before 11:00am)
    B. Day/Afternoon Shift (Any shift starting after 11:00am or before 7:00pm)
    C. Night Shift (Any shift starting after 7:00pm or before 3:00am)
    D. I work rotating shifts

21. What was the SINGLE most important reason you chose this course?
    A. Low price
    B. New or newly revised course
    C. High interest/Required course topic
    D. Number of contact hours needed

22. Where do you work? (If your place of employment is not listed below, please leave this question blank.)
    A. Hospital
    B. Medical clinic/Group practice/ HMO/Office setting
    C. Long term care/Rehabilitation facility/Nursing home
    D. Home health care agency

23. Which field do you specialize in?
    A. Medical/Surgical
    B. Geriatrics
    C. Pediatrics/Neonatal
    D. Other

24. For your last renewal, how many months BEFORE your license expiration date did you order your course materials?
    A. 1–3 months
    B. 4–6 months
    C. 7–12 months
    D. Greater than 12 months

25. **PLEASE LOG YOUR STUDY HOURS WITH SUBMISSION OF YOUR FINAL EXAM.** Please choose which best represents the total study hours it took to complete this 30 hour course.
    A. less than 25 hours
    B. 25–28 hours
    C. 29–32 hours
    D. greater than 32 hours

CONTENTS

PRETEST

Begin by taking the pretest. Compare your answers on the pretest to the answer key (located in the back of the book). Circle those test items that you missed. The pretest answer key indicates the course chapters in which the content of the respective question is discussed.

Next, read each chapter. Focus special attention on the chapters for which you made incorrect answer choices. Examination questions are provided at the end of each chapter, so that you can assess your progress and understanding of the material.

1. Infant mortality is higher in the United States than in _____ other developed countries.

    a. 5

    b. 2

    c. 21

    d. 12

2. Estrogen is produced by the

    a. pituitary gland.

    b. hypothalamus.

    c. uterus.

    d. ovaries.

3. The first half of the menstrual cycle is called the

    a. luteal phase.

    b. follicular phase.

    c. ovulatory phase.

    d. menstrual phase.

4. Fertile cervical mucus is produced in response to

    a. progesterone.

    b. follicle-stimulating hormone.

    c. estrogen.

    d. gonadotropin releasing hormone.

5. Dyspareunia is the term for

    a. pain with urination.

    b. pain with intercourse.

    c. muscle spasms of the vaginal opening.

    d. painful menstruation.

6. Which Lesbians need to be concerned about sexually transmitted infection?

    a. Lesbians who have previously had sex with men.

    b. Lesbians who have had sex only with women.

    c. Lesbians who are former intravenous drug users.

    d. All sexually active Lesbians.

7. Anorexia nervosa involves

    a. binging and vomiting.

    b. distortion of body image.

    c. excessive exercise.

    d. pain syndromes.

8. In women, sexually transmitted infections

   a. usually produce some symptoms.

   b. always produce symptoms.

   c. are often asymptomatic.

   d. usually result in vaginal discharge.

9. As a birth control method, the minipill is

   a. less effective than combination pills.

   b. as effective as combination pills.

   c. more effective than combination pills.

   d. the pill of choice for most women.

10. If pregnancy occurs with the intrauterine device in place, there is a high risk of

    a. perforation.

    b. dysmenorrhea.

    c. ectopic pregnancy.

    d. expulsion of the device.

11. Results of studies (Lichtman & Papera, 1990) have shown that generally women who have had abortions

    a. experience few long-term psychologic problems.

    b. experience many long-term psychologic problems.

    c. always have psychologic problems.

    d. never have psychologic problems.

12. Zygote intrafallopian transfer (ZIFT) involves placing

    a. an unfertilized egg into the uterus.

    b. an unfertilized egg into the fallopian tube.

    c. a fertilized egg into the uterus.

    d. a fertilized egg into the fallopian tube.

13. The recording of measurements of basal body temperature can tell a woman

    a. whether ovulation has occurred.

    b. when ovulation will occur.

    c. when fertilization has occurred.

    d. whether she is fertile.

14. One of the most serious long-term consequences of untreated chlamydial infection is

    a. infertility.

    b. increased risk of miscarriage.

    c. chronic vaginal discharge.

    d. abnormal Pap smear findings.

15. Estrogen replacement therapy alone has been shown to decrease the risk of all but which of the following conditions or diseases:

    a. Alzheimer's disease.

    b. Heart disease.

    c. Uterine cancer.

    d. Osteoporosis.

16. Hepatitis B is

    a. a sexually transmitted infection.

    b. not considered to be transmitted sexually.

    c. contracted by eating contaminated food.

    d. contracted only through shared needles during intravenous drug use.

17. A good nondairy source of calcium in the diet is

    a. brown rice.

    b. whole grain breads.

    c. tofu.

    d. citrus fruits.

18. An herb that is good for premenstrual syndrome because it has an especially high mineral content is

    a. cramp bark.

    b. wild yam.

    c. nettle.

    d. black cohosh.

19. In addition to a pelvic examination, all women older than age 40 years should have a

    a. complete blood cell count.

    b. rectal examination and stool test for blood.

    c. sigmoidoscopy.

    d. check for sexually transmitted infections.

20. The transformation zone of the cervix is the term for the area in which the

    a. cells of the vaginal wall meet the cells of the cervix.

    b. columnar cells of the cervix meet the cells of the uterine lining inside the cervical canal.

    c. columnar cells of the cervix meet the cells of the vaginal wall.

    d. squamous cells of the cervix meet the columnar cervical cells.

21. Fibroids are

    a. precancerous growths of the uterus.

    b. benign growths of the uterus.

    c. misplaced endometrial tissue.

    d. growths that could lead to cancer if not treated.

22. Breast cancer is the second leading cause of cancer death in women, exceeded only by

    a. lung cancer.

    b. uterine cancer.

    c. colorectal cancer.

    d. ovarian cancer.

23. Most breast cancer occurs in women with

    a. known risk factors.

    b. no known risk factors, except being female and advancing age.

    c. a family history of breast cancer.

    d. early menarche and late menopause.

24. Menopause is defined as

    a. the gradual shutting down of the ovaries, leading to frequent cycles without ovulation.

    b. the absence of menstrual bleeding for at least 1 year.

    c. irregular periods, leading to lengthy intervals with no bleeding.

    d. a disease syndrome of estrogen deficiency.

25. Women who have gone through menopause may experience vaginal dryness due to lack of which hormone?

    a. Estrogen

    b. Progesterone

    c. Testosterone

    d. Luteinizing hormone

INTRODUCTION

The field of women's health is coming into its own. It is an exciting time for women and health care professionals who work with women. Links are forming worldwide, and as a more global perspective is taken, it becomes clear that the health of women is integrally tied to the social, economic, political, and religious forces shaping cultures and societies. For women's health to improve, society has to change. Education is one of the keys to this change. As women educate themselves, they are empowered to make better decisions about their health and that of their families. Health care providers play an important role in this educational process.

Caring for Women Through the Lifecycle is an introduction to the field of women's health for health professionals who work with women in any of a variety of roles and settings. It is intended to provide information that will help you increase your knowledge base and ability to work with various female client populations. I hope that your interest will be piqued to continue to investigate in more depth areas of special interest to you.

You will find in your reading that there are often more questions than answers in the field of women's health. This course is intended to expand your understanding of the controversies, as well as to enhance your ability to think through these issues yourself and thereby help your clients sort out their confusion.

You will find a "Key Words" section at the beginning of most chapters. These are words that are being introduced into the course, some of which you may find unfamiliar. All these words can be found in the glossary. You will also find an extensive resource guide at the end of the course to assist you in finding more information.

I hope you find this course enjoyable and useful.

CHAPTER 1

WOMEN'S HEALTH TODAY

CHAPTER OBJECTIVE

After completing this chapter, the reader will be able to discuss some of the forces and trends that have shaped the lives of women in the United States during the past century, as well as how these forces and trends have affected the field of women's health. The reader will also be able to discuss new developments that promise to impact on women's lives and give women cause for both hope and concern.

LEARNING OBJECTIVES

After studying this chapter, the reader will be able to

1. identify the reasons for major improvements in health in the past century.

2. describe the shift in major causes of illness that has occurred in the United States in the past two decades.

3. discuss some of the threats to women's health.

4. describe new developments occurring in health care for women.

5. describe some of the challenges nurses face related to women's health in the current health care system.

INTRODUCTION

Women's lives and health are shaped by vast forces as well as personal choices. This is both a challenge and a source of empowerment. As individuals, women can to a large degree change their personal environment, eating habits, and exercise patterns. However, individuals are connected integrally to all the forces that move society—social, economic, cultural, religious, and political. The most dramatic change occurring in the past century in the United States, and to some degree worldwide, is that women's voices are being heard. Growing numbers of women are speaking out about a greater diversity of issues and being heard more than ever before. The issues are basic, and they do not require a high degree of sophistication in education or training to be apparent. Because more women are walking in the higher echelons of politics, culture, religion, and economics, their voices are being heard and accepted. In addition, women of every ethnic group, socioeconomic position, and sexual preference are organizing and thereby finding a voice in both their communities and the larger structure of society.

THE PAST

It is difficult for women in the 1990s to recognize that it was only 70 years ago, in the 1920s, that the right to vote was granted after a long and courageous struggle by women's suffragette predecessors. In earlier times, women were accused of witchcraft and burned at the stake by the thousands for practicing healing arts in their communities (Boston Women's Health Book Collective, 1992). Looking at the past is sobering for women, but it is an important reminder to take on the seriousness required to continue to work for change.

Since the 18th century there has been a dramatic improvement in the health and life span of Americans, largely attributable to improvements in nutrition and economic status and broadscale advances in sanitation practices. Improvements in the water supplies, sewage disposal, milk pasteurization, and other community sanitation measures resulted in a reduced exposure to infectious diseases, the greatest causes of morbidity and mortality, especially for women and children. Infant and maternal deaths decreased dramatically as a result of these measures alone. Improvements in medical care itself had relatively little impact on these trends (Lee, Estes & Close, 1997). In the 1930s the first antibiotics were developed, beginning the era of modern medicine. In the 1960s the government initiated broad public health programs such as Medicaid and WIC (Women, Infants, and Children Program), improving health care and nutrition for pregnant women and children. (The WIC program provides essential food items for mothers and children in need.) This resulted in another dramatic increase in well-being for mother and child (Lee et al., 1997).

In the past three decades a shift has been occurring in patterns of health and disease. Currently emerging as major causes of diminished health and death in the general population, for both men and women, are the chronic cardiovascular diseases and cancer. For the young population, AIDS is one of the greatest threats. Management for these emerging health problems requires an entirely new approach. One cannot rely only on the cures of modern medicine. These must be combined with broader considerations: socioeconomic factors, education, income, work, environment, and access to health care—all of which are important factors and influence health-related behaviors. Preventive services and health education must become available to all (Lee et al., 1997).

LOOKING FROM THE PRESENT TO THE FUTURE

As health care providers stand on the verge of the 21st century, in spite of all the progress that has been made, the nation faces serious health issues. The number of uninsured individuals has increased to more than 60 million (Lee et al., 1997). Health care costs are rising rapidly. There is a proliferation of costly technology, which offers great hope for a few, coupled with depleting funds for broad basic health care services for all. Consider the following confounding factors (Lee et al., 1997):

- Expenditures for health care have exceeded $1 trillion and are expected to rise to $1.7 trillion by the year 2000, a figure greater than 18% of the gross national product.

- Americans spend more than twice as much per person for health care as people in most other industrial countries.

- Infant mortality is higher in the United States than in 21 other developed countries.

- Ethnic minority groups and those of low income suffer the highest rates of infant mortality.

In addition, violence, substance abuse, HIV/AIDS, homelessness, and unintended pregnancy have reached epidemic proportions.

Most experts agree that there is a need for a fundamental change and restructuring of the health care system. Defining what form this will take is the great challenge of the coming decade.

PROGRESS IN WOMEN'S HEALTH

In the past 5 years, unprecedented progress has taken place in the field of women's health in this country (Lee et al., 1997). However, a long-neglected and substantial agenda remains to be addressed. According to Lee and colleagues (1997), in 1995 the Fourth Worldwide Conference on Women, sponsored by the United Nations, was held in Beijing, China. A women's health agenda was considered in great detail from an international perspective, and "The Beijing Declaration and The Platform of Action" was adopted by 189 countries, representing a new international commitment to health for all women. Health is recognized as an integral part of the goal of equality and peace for all women. Lee and colleagues (1997) noted that the Platform developed a comprehensive definition of women's health and the rights of women worldwide to affordable, accessible, gender-sensitive, and nondiscriminatory health care and education. It also placed the subject of women's health in the context of the broader social, economic, and political forces that determine it. Steps were outlined for the achievement of these goals.

In the United States, researchers have long neglected women's health issues, and many studies have excluded women. Consequently, medication dosages and regimens for women with chronic diseases such as cardiovascular illnesses are based on results of studies with men (Lee et al., 1997). Currently, several large-scale investigations to study and clarify women's health issues are in progress, including the following three noted by Lee and colleagues (1997):

1. Study of Women's Health Across the Nation

Study of the experience of menopause in women age 42–52 years, comparing a broad range of physiologic, psychologic, psychosocial, and lifestyle influences among different ethnic groups.

2. Nurses' Health Study

Initiated in 1976 with 120,000 women age 30–55 years, a broad study of lifestyle influences on women's health. Data is being reported as the study continues.

3. Women's Health Initiative

Study of 63,000 postmenopausal women, age 50–79 years, in 40 centers around the country regarding postmenopausal health concerns. Three specific interventions are being studied: (a) the role of a low-fat diet in prevention of breast and colorectal cancer, (b) the impact of hormone replacement therapy on prevention of cardiovascular disease and osteoporotic fractures, and (c) the impact of calcium and vitamin D supplementation on the prevention of colorectal cancer and osteoporotic fractures.

Lee and colleagues (1997) have noted that in the past two decades the U. S. government has developed broad national goals for health. A process was begun to establish national health objectives progressing to the year 2000. Healthy People 2000 National Health Promotion and Disease Prevention Objectives were launched in 1990, involving government and private organizations. Three goals were outlined:

1. To increase the span of healthy life for all Americans

2. To reduce health disparities among Americans

3. To achieve access to preventive health care services for all Americans

According to Lee and colleagues (1997), to accomplish these goals Healthy People 2000 set forth 300 objectives, including broad public health measures; plans for improved health care access; preventive services, including education, nutrition, screening for sexually transmitted infections, family planning services, smoking cessation, and family violence and abuse prevention; and means for gathering data and monitoring progress.

This recent attention to women's health issues is largely the result of hard work by women who have organized and lobbied extensively at all levels of government for recognition of the need to allocate funds for women's health.

CONCLUSION

It is evident that the subject of women's health, perhaps more than any other health care arena, is all encompassing. Health care providers are faced with issues that strike at the very root of what it means to be human, that stretch caregivers' hearts as well as minds in seeking solutions. Health has become a planetary issue.

EXAM QUESTIONS

CHAPTER 1
Questions 1–3

1. Historically the most significant factor in improving the health of the American population was

   a. the development of birth control methods.

   b. the introduction of antibiotics.

   c. the sanitation measures.

   d. the Women, Infants, and Children Program (WIC).

2. Americans spend _____ per person for health care as people in most other industrial nations.

   a. half as much

   b. more than twice as much

   c. four times as much

   d. one third as much

3. Most of the research studies, in the first 20 years, on chronic diseases

   a. included women

   b. included both men and women.

   c. excluded women.

   d. included only post-menopausal women.

CHAPTER 2

THE MENSTRUAL CYCLE

CHAPTER OBJECTIVE

After completing this chapter, the reader will be able to discuss the basic events that occur in the menstrual cycle and describe the complex orchestration of hormonal communications between the brain and the reproductive organs. The reader will also be able to discuss how external events, such as stress, diet, and exercise, can affect the normal pattern of the menstrual cycle and how many women's health issues are not well understood, but seem to be related to an imbalance that occurs in the complex hormonal dance.

LEARNING OBJECTIVES

After studying this chapter, the reader will be able to

1. define the term hormone.

2. identify the major hormones involved in the menstrual cycle.

3. identify where these hormones are produced and which organs they affect.

4. indicate where in the menstrual cycle different hormones predominate.

5. describe the effects of the different hormones on their target organs.

6. describe normal parameters for the menstrual cycle.

Key Words

- Endometrium
- FSH
- Gn-RH
- HCG
- Hypothalamus
- LH
- Oocyte
- Ovarian follicle
- Pituitary gland
- Steroid

INTRODUCTION

Throughout the history of human civilization, the female menses has been viewed with awe, fear, and reverence. Laws, taboos, and beliefs about this cycle have been an inherent part of the social and religious structure of all societies. Whether viewed positively or negatively, it is evident that the menstrual cycle is a powerful aspect of women's lives, both personally and within the society in which women live. In modern times in American culture women have lost touch with much of this wisdom. Women expect themselves to function, think, and feel the same every day, without regard for the cyclic fluctuations and therefore without regard to the gifts that tuning into this cycle bring (Northrup, 1994). A scientific investigation of the menstrual cycle—describing the complex interactions of brain, organs, and hormones—only clarifies and enhances respect for the complex organization and functioning of women's bodies.

A grasp of the fundamentals of the menstrual cycle is primary to the ability to understand and educate patients about the whole range of women's health issues: birth control methods, premenstrual syndrome, infertility, and other gynecologic problems. The remainder of the course will build on this knowledge. Please refer to the glossary if you are unfamiliar with any of the terms listed in the "Key Words" section.

Notes to the reader: This chapter contains a lot of detail. For some of you it will be review; for others, perhaps a lot of new material. Please bear with me. The amount of detail is not without a purpose. With a good foundation in understanding the menstrual cycle, you will be well equipped to answer many of your patient's questions about women's health. For example, a patient might ask you, "Why do I spot midcycle? Is this normal?" or "My libido is wild around midcycle and zilch before my period. Am I the only one?" or "What's all this discharge about? I'm not even sexually active. Do I have an infection or what?"

A Word About Hormones

The word hormone describes a group of chemicals that may be quite diverse in both their makeup and their effects in the body. What hormones have in common is that they are produced by organs or tissues in the body and secreted internally, released into the blood stream to travel to target organs. A target organ has receptor sites for the particular hormone, a kind of lock-and-key effect in which the hormone shape fits cozily into the receptor site. This activates the effect of the hormone in the particular target organ.

Traditionally, major target organs have been identified for particular hormones. As research has progressed, however, receptor sites for the known major hormones have been found in unexpected places. For example, estrogen receptors have been found in the brain (Lichtman & Papera, 1990). Further, study findings have shown that communication is not only two way, but multileveled, with multiple feedback loops connecting numbers of tissues and organs (Lichtman & Papera, 1990). There is a complex form of intelligence and communication occurring within the body that women are not usually aware of unless something goes wrong.

THE MENSTRUAL CYCLE

The menstrual cycle occurs as a coordinated communication among the hypothalamus, the pituitary gland, the ovaries, and the uterus *(Figure 2-1)*. If any part of the system malfunctions, the normal cycle is interrupted.

Because the menstrual cycle is a circle that has no beginning, nor end, it has become standard to view the first day of menses, or bleeding, as the first day of the cycle (Hatcher et al., 1994). Of course, this has been preceded by a series of events leading to this shedding of the inner lining of the uterus. This lining has been building during the previous cycle, in response first to estrogen and then to progesterone. When fertilization of the egg does not occur, the levels of these hormones decline. Without the stimulation and support of hormones, the lining breaks down and is shed as menstrual blood.

Normal Cycle

The normal menstrual cycle has the following pattern and characteristics (Lichtman & Papera, 1990):

- 28-day interval, with a normal range of 21–35 days

- 4½ days of flow, with a range of 2–8 days

FIGURE 2-1
Coordinated Events of the Hypothalamus, Pituitary, and Ovarian and Uterine Systems

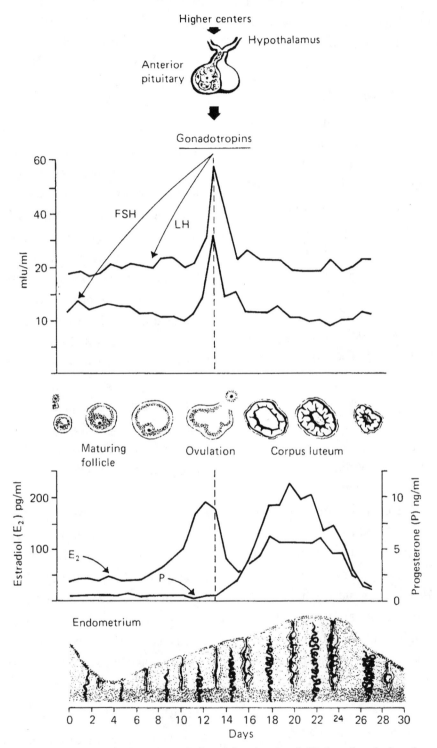

Notice that plasma estradiol peaks around day 12, plasma follicle-stimulating hormone (FSH) and luteinizing hormone (LH) around day 13, and ovulation around day 14.

Source: Scott, J. R., Disaia, P. J., Hammond, C. B. & Spellacy, W. N. (Eds). (1994). *Danforth's obstetrics and gynecology* (7th ed.). Philadelphia: J. B. Lippincott.

• 35 ml of blood loss, with a range of 20–60 ml

Please refer to the diagrams and illustrations in this chapter *(Figures 2-1, 2-2, and 2-3)* as you read the description of the changing hormones and their effects. It will help you visualize the whole process.

Hypothalamus and Pituitary Gland

The hypothalamus, which lies at the base of the brain, performs a variety of important regulatory functions. It is a processing center that receives messages from outside the body by means of higher brain centers and information from inside the body by means of the blood stream and the central nervous system. This allows the hypothalamus to perform several functions, such as regulation of body temperature and fat and carbohydrate metabolism; water balance; and the hormone balances that control the menstrual cycle and other hormone systems in the body. The hypothalamus may also influence sleep, sexual activity, and emotional control (Crouch, 1978).

The hypothalamus produces releasing factors, which stimulate the pituitary gland to release hormones that travel to a number of different organs—including the thyroid gland, the adrenal glands, and the ovaries—stimulating or inhibiting their function. The releasing factor produced by the hypothalamus that is involved in the menstrual cycle is called gonadotropin releasing hormone or Gn-RH. This hormone stimulates the pituitary gland to produce follicle-stimulating hormone (FSH) and luteinizing hormone (LH), which regulate the menstrual cycle. These hormones are further controlled by complex feedback loops from the ovary (Lichtman & Papera, 1990).

First Half of the Cycle—Follicular or Proliferative Phase

The menstrual cycle is divided into two phases, with ovulation (the release of an egg from the ovary) at midcycle. The first half of the cycle is termed the follicular phase, and it is marked by development of the egg follicle in the ovary. Another common term for this first half of the cycle is the proliferative phase, describing the growth of the uterine lining in response to the steroid hormone estrogen (Hatcher et al., 1994).

At puberty each ovary contains between 300,000 and 500,000 primitive egg follicles. During the first few days of the cycle, while menstrual bleeding is occurring, levels of estrogen and progesterone in the blood are very low. In response to this low hormone level, the hypothalamus is triggered to produce its hormone Gn-RH which acts directly on the anterior pituitary gland, stimulating the pituitary to release FSH (follicle stimulating hormone). FSH goes via the bloodstream to the ovaries and is the primary hormone responsible for stimulating the development of egg follicles within the ovary. The follicle itself is a structure which contains both an egg, or oocyte, and supportive cells which produce estrogen and other hormones. During each menstrual cycle, approximately 1,000 eggs begin to develop, but usually only one becomes dominant (by mechanisms not fully understood), and will go on to be released during ovulation. The other follicles are eventually reabsorbed. As the follicle grows it produces ever increasing quantities of estrogen. Estrogen has a stimulating effect on the lining of the uterus. The cells of the uterine lining multiply, the lining thickens and produces glycogen, a form of sugar. The cervix also responds to estrogen by producing a fertile cervical mucus, which is clear, slippery, and stretchy and thus conductive to the transport and survival of sperm (Hatcher et al., 1994).

Ovulation

As the egg follicle in the ovary continues its development, it produces increasing levels of estrogen. As estrogen enters the bloodstream and flows throughout the body, it reaches the brain, where the level is monitored by the pituitary gland. This

FIGURE 2-2
Lateral View of the Pelvic Viscera

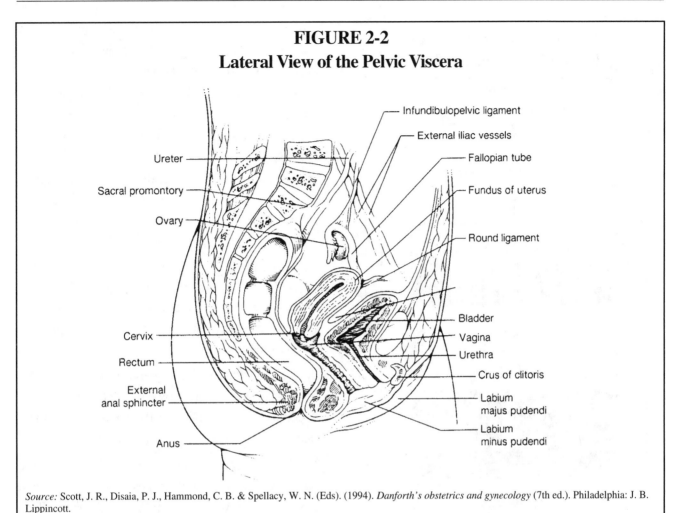

Source: Scott, J. R., Disaia, P. J., Hammond, C. B. & Spellacy, W. N. (Eds). (1994). *Danforth's obstetrics and gynecology* (7th ed.). Philadelphia: J. B. Lippincott.

increasing estrogen level stimulates the pituitary gland to release LH (luteinizing hormone). LH in turn stimulates the ovaries to continue to increase estrogen production. LH also stimulates the ovaries to produce progesterone and androgens. When estrogen production reaches a peak, it stimulates the pituitary to release a surge of LH. This is a critical point in the menstrual cycle. The surge of LH completes the maturation of the dominant egg follicle. It is this LH surge that is necessary for ovulation to occur. Ovulation, or the rupture of the mature egg from the ovary, occurs 10–12 hours after the LH peak (Lichtman & Papera, 1990).

When the follicle containing the egg ruptures and releases the egg from the ovary, a small amount of follicular fluid is released along with the barely visible egg. Some bleeding may occur as well. This accounts for the reported lower abdomi-nal discomfort often associated with ovulation. In addition, a slight drop in estrogen levels around ovulation may cause some spotting from the uterine lining. The rise in male hormones, including testosterone, just before ovulation may explain an increase in libido around this time (Lichtman & Papera, 1990).

Second Half of the Cycle—Luteal or Secretory Phase

After ovulation occurs, the remaining cells of the ruptured follicle reorganize. The cell walls take up lipids (fats), giving them a yellow appearance. This structure is called the corpus luteum or "yellow body," and it is the director of the next phase of the cycle.

The corpus luteum secretes some estrogen but mainly progesterone. Eighty percent of all the

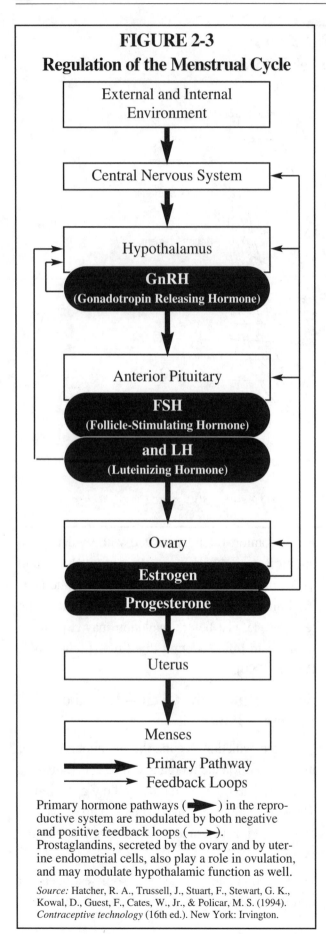

FIGURE 2-3
Regulation of the Menstrual Cycle

External and Internal Environment

Central Nervous System

Hypothalamus
GnRH
(Gonadotropin Releasing Hormone)

Anterior Pituitary
FSH
(Follicle-Stimulating Hormone)
and LH
(Luteinizing Hormone)

Ovary
Estrogen
Progesterone

Uterus

Menses

⟶ Primary Pathway
→ Feedback Loops

Primary hormone pathways (⟶) in the reproductive system are modulated by both negative and positive feedback loops (→).
Prostaglandins, secreted by the ovary and by uterine endometrial cells, also play a role in ovulation, and may modulate hypothalamic function as well.

Source: Hatcher, R. A., Trussell, J., Stuart, F., Stewart, G. K., Kowal, D., Guest, F., Cates, W., Jr., & Policar, M. S. (1994). *Contraceptive technology* (16th ed.). New York: Irvington.

progesterone secreted during the entire menstrual cycle is secreted during the first 8 days after ovulation (Hatcher et al., 1994). The presence of progesterone causes a slight rise in body temperature, which is sustained throughout the second half of the menstrual cycle until progesterone levels fall and menstruation occurs. This is one of the signs that is measured in the fertility awareness method of birth control (described in chapter 5). Progesterone stimulates the uterine lining in its final preparations for conception. This velvety, sugary lining provides an inviting environment for the implantation of a free-floating embryo. This phase of the menstrual cycle is also known as the secretory phase because of the changes that take place in the uterine lining.

The mucus-producing glands of the cervix also respond to progesterone by causing the mucus produced to be scant, sticky, and thick and thus inhospitable to sperm (Hatcher et al., 1994).

The next important event in the menstrual cycle occurs as estrogen and progesterone levels reach their peak midway through the luteal phase. This peak causes a negative feedback loop to the brain, and FSH and LH levels decline (Lichtman & Papera, 1990). The corpus luteum begins to degrade, and estrogen and progesterone levels start to fall. At this point the cycle begins again as shedding of the lining produces menses.

Fertilization

Fertilization can interrupt the last series of events in the luteal phase. A fertilized egg begins to produce a hormone called human chorionic gonadotropin (HCG). This hormone moves into the blood stream and supports continued functioning of the corpus luteum, keeping estrogen and progesterone levels high enough to prevent the uterine lining from shedding until the placenta is able to provide these hormones. The corpus luteum must continue to function for 7–9 weeks after conception for a pregnancy to continue (Hatcher et al., 1994).

Fertilization of the egg occurs in the fallopian tube and involves a complex series of biochemical events that occur in the interaction of sperm and egg. Many separate events have to be accomplished for fertilization to be successful and the genetic contribution of the man and the woman to be combined. Early cell division occurs in the fallopian tube for the first 2 days, supported by cells that have accompanied the egg and fluid from the tube itself. The ball of cells then travels to the uterus where it continues to develop for several days before beginning the implantation process. Implantation is another complex biochemical process in which cells from the embryo literally grow into the uterine lining. Approximately 50% of embryos do not survive this complex process of fertilization and implantation. The chances of survival increase to 85% if the embryo survives the first 2 weeks of pregnancy (Hatcher et al., 1994).

Other Effects of Menstrual Cycle Hormones

The hormones involved in the menstrual cycle affect several other body structures and functions.

Cervix

Changes in the cervical mucus caused by stimulation of the mucus-secreting glands in the cervix by hormones has already been described. The cervical os (opening to cervix) widens during the first half of the cycle and then closes during the second half of the cycle (Lichtman & Papera, 1990). It is at its widest point during ovulation.

Breast Tissue

Breast tissue responds to stimulation by hormones. Size, sensitivity, and nodularity are highest in the second half of the cycle (Lichtman & Papera, 1990).

Vagina

The cells lining the vaginal walls undergo characteristic changes under the influence of first estrogen and then progesterone.

Basal Body Temperature

Shifts in hormone levels affect the temperature-regulating center in the hypothalamus. A small rise in temperature occurs around ovulation and is sustained throughout the second half of the cycle because of the presence of progesterone (Hatcher et al., 1994).

Senses

The five senses reach a peak in sensitivity at ovulation. In addition, the appetite center is affected, usually increasing appetite in the second half of the cycle. Brain waves change during the cycle. Study results have shown that an increased alertness, a sense of well-being, and sexual arousal occur during the first half of the cycle, and a decrease in short-term memory and attention occurs during the second half of the cycle (Lichtman & Papera, 1990).

Fluid Balance

The complex systems involved in salt and water balance in the body are influenced by hormone fluctuations associated with the menstrual cycle. These fluctuations can result in an increase in fluid retention during the second half of the cycle (Lichtman & Papera, 1990).

Other Factors Affecting the Menstrual Cycle

Because the hypothalamus is primarily responsible for initiating and orchestrating menstrual cycle events, other influences can have a profound effect on the menstrual cycle. Not only must the hypothalamus release specific hormones, but the quantity and timing of release must follow a specific pattern to result in proper stimulation of the pituitary gland and thus a normal cycle. This can be easily thrown off by external influences on the brain. Stress, diet, and excessive exercise all influence brain chemistry (Northrup, 1994). Irregular periods and amenorrhea (lack of period) can both occur as a result of stress. Medications and social drugs that affect neurotransmitter function can profoundly affect the menstrual cycle (Lichtman & Papera, 1990).

New Developments

In the continuing investigation of the menstrual cycle, new hormones are being discovered that may hold future promise for birth control. These include hormones found in the ovary that the ovary uses to control events in the maturation of its follicles. They include inhibin, which suppresses FSH release, and activin, which promotes FSH release. These hormones may prove useful in developing new birth control substances that alter the menstrual cycle to regulate fertility (Hatcher et al., 1994).

A word of caution is in order. One needs to be aware that a delicately balanced and finely tuned "whole system" is being tampered with. Altering one part may have wide-reaching effects that may take years to uncover. Caution is a wise choice as technology often suffers from lack of a broad vision.

CONCLUSION

The monthly menstrual cycle is the primary bodily event that occurs uniquely in women from menarche to menopause. Hormones have powerful as well as subtle influences on the body's physiologic responses, as well as on the way human beings think, feel, and sense. Even at the conclusion of such a rigorous scientific overview, one can appreciate why the ancients held this process in awe. Educating patients about the menstrual cycle by using age-, education level, and culturally appropriate materials can help them understand the normal functioning of their bodies and dispel myths and fears, as well as empower them to make informed choices.

EXAM QUESTIONS

CHAPTER 2
Questions 4–14

4. The hypothalamus sends messages directly to the

   a. ovary.

   b. uterus.

   c. adrenal glands.

   d. pituitary gland.

5. Ovulation is triggered by a surge of which hormone?

   a. Estrogen

   b. Progesterone

   c. Luteinizing hormone

   d. Follicle-stimulating hormone

6. The egg follicle is stimulated to grow and develop primarily by which hormone?

   a. Progesterone

   b. Gonadotropin hormone

   c. Follicle-stimulating hormone

   d. Testosterone

7. Estrogen is produced by the

   a. pituitary gland.

   b. hypothalamus.

   c. uterus.

   d. ovaries.

8. The primary hormone produced in the luteal phase of the menstrual cycle is

   a. estrogen.

   b. luteinizing hormone.

   c. progesterone.

   d. follicle-stimulating hormone.

9. Fertilization usually takes place in

   a. the uterus.

   b. the fallopian tube.

   c. either the uterus or the fallopian tube.

   d. the internal os of the cervix.

10. Approximately _____% of embryos do not survive the process of fertilization and implantation.

    a. 10

    b. 35

    c. 50

    d. 75

11. Progesterone is made in the

    a. hypothalamus.

    b. pituitary gland.

    c. ovary.

    d. uterus.

12. During the menstrual cycle, the presence of progesterone causes the basal body temperature to

   a. increase.

   b. decrease.

   c. remain unchanged.

   d. peak and then decrease.

13. Fertile cervical mucus has a consistency that is described as

   a. tacky.

   b. thick and opaque.

   c. clear and stretchy.

   d. creamy white.

14. Stress, or extremes of exercise or diet, can alter the menstrual cycle by its effects on the

   a. pituitary gland.

   b. adrenal glands.

   c. hypothalamus.

   d. ovary.

CHAPTER 3

SEXUALITY

CHAPTER OBJECTIVE

After completing this chapter, the reader will be able to recognize the diversity of human sexual expression, describe normal sexual function, identify common problems that occur related to sexuality and describe the role of health care providers in counseling women experiencing sexual difficulty.

LEARNING OBJECTIVES

After studying this chapter, the reader will be able to

1. discuss some of the influences that can affect sexual response.

2. describe the normal sexual response cycle for men and women.

3. identify problems with sexual function and possible causes.

4. describe the diversity of sexual preference and alternative sexual lifestyles.

Key Words

* Dyspareunia
* Refractory period
* Vaginismus

INTRODUCTION

In the animal kingdom, sexual practices are so wildly diverse and at times humorous that the sexual practices of human beings seem a bore by comparison. Take the sheepshead fish, for example: It can turn off its female genes and turn on its male genes to take over when the dominant male dies.

Understanding the complex tapestry of sexuality is an important part of the knowledge base of the health care provider in counseling clients about birth control and family planning, as well as in assisting clients to enter into and sustain healthy relationships. In addition to biologic functions, sexuality involves identity roles, relationships, perceptions, and expectations. Sexuality is tied integrally to self-esteem (Kozier, Erb, Blais & Wilkinson, 1995). In addition, cultural groups have their own practices and values centered around sexuality with regard to homosexuality, husband-wife roles, nudity, and sexual expression. All are influenced by religious values as well (Hatcher et al., 1994).

When problems with sexual function arise in a relationship, health care providers are often the first source of feedback and information and the first nonjudgmental ear. The more health care providers expand their knowledge base and comfort zone around sexual issues, the better prepared they are to put clients at ease.

Sexuality is tied integrally to issues of pregnancy prevention and transmission of infection

(Hatcher et al., 1994). The rise of infection with HIV has changed sexuality forever and increased awareness about transmission of all sexually transmitted infections (Finer & Zabin, 1998). The challenging task for health care providers and clients is to maintain a high motivation for finding ways to keep sex pleasurable and infection free (Hatcher et al., 1994).

HUMAN SEXUAL PHYSIOLOGY

Sexual arousal and sexual expression differ for every individual, as well as for the same individual from one time to another or with different partners. A wide range of intimate expression can be enjoyed. The common denominator is consensual touching; that is, both partners agreeing to and enjoying the experience of sexual intimacy. Sexual intercourse, as it is usually described, is only one of many ways to enjoy this intimacy (Hatcher et al., 1994).

Women tend to be whole-body oriented for sexual touching and vary greatly in what kind of stimulation produces orgasm. The highest areas of sensitivity for women are the clitoris, the inner surfaces of the labia minora, and the first inch and a half of the vagina (Hatcher et al., 1994). Some women's breasts are very sensitive; some are not. Anal sex is very stimulating for some women, but not for others. It is common to find women who achieve orgasm but not during penile-vaginal contact. Some women have an area of sensitivity called the G spot, about half way between the back of the pubic bone and the cervix along the vaginal wall. This is a normal variation. Orgasm from this area may result in the rhythmic expulsion of fluid from the urethra. The fluid is not urine but is similar to prostatic fluid in men (Hatcher et al., 1994). This variation of orgasm has not been well studied, nor is it well understood (Boston Women's Health Book Collective, 1992).

There is a wide range of normal sexual response in women. Often women learn that vaginal intercourse should be the route to orgasm. As the body of research has grown on female sexual response, this view has fallen by the wayside (Boston Women's Health Book Collective, 1992).

Sexual Response Cycle

The sexual response cycle consists of four parts:

Excitement Phase

In the excitement phase pelvic engorgement, involving erection in men and vaginal lubrication and vasocongestion of the vagina and labia in women, takes place. The vagina lengthens and swells. Both men and women experience an increase in muscle tension, heart and respiratory rates, and blood pressure. The focus of attention becomes more and more centered on sexual matters (Stenchever, 1996).

Plateau Phase

In the plateau phase engorgement is sustained, as is the increased muscle tension and respiratory rate. The labia minora and vagina appear red and puffy with vasocongestion. The breasts may swell, and the nipples become erect. The clitoris may become sensitive and retract under the clitoral hood. This period may vary from minutes to hours (Stenchever, 1996).

Orgasm

During orgasm, rhythmic contractions of pelvic voluntary and involuntary muscles occur in both sexes. In men, ejaculation of semen results; in women, a type of ejaculatory fluid may be emitted from the urethra. Women typically require longer to reach orgasm than men. Women have a shorter refractory period than men, that period during which another erection or orgasm could not occur. In women the refractory period is short, and women are physiologically capable of moving from plateau to orgasm, back to plateau, and then to orgasm one time or several times. For men, the refractory period varies from 5–15 minutes in young men to 18–24 hours in men by the age of 60 years. There is a wide range of individual variation in men and women (Hatcher et al., 1994).

Resolution

Resolution is the final stage of the sexual response cycle. The body returns to the preexcitation phase, muscles relax, and heart and respiratory rates and blood pressure return to normal levels. This can occur with or without orgasm (Lichtman & Papera, 1990).

Sexual Dysfunction

Because sexual function is interconnected with psychologic and emotional concerns, the health care provider's attempts to find the source of sexual dysfunction for a client must take into account a broad range of issues, including the following (Hatcher et al., 1994):

- Fear of
  - pregnancy
  - infertility
  - contracting an infection
  - pain
- Type of birth control method used
- Discrepancies in sexual desire
- Religious and cultural taboos
- Medications that cause a
  - decrease in libido
  - failure to achieve or sustain an erection in men
- Issues in the relationship around trust, control
- Self-esteem and body-image issues
- Poor communication between partners

Common Sexual Problems for Women

Low Libido

There are many reasons for a lack of sexual interest, including those listed earlier. Some birth control pills can decrease libido. Changes in hormone levels associated with increasing age and medications, such as antihypertensives and antidepressants, can also have an impact on sexual interest and function (Hatcher et al., 1994).

Dyspareunia

Dyspareunia is the term used for pain with intercourse. Dyspareunia can have several causes, including a physiologic cause such as an infection or a gynecologic disorder such as endometriosis. It also can be due simply to insufficient lubrication. A history of sexual trauma or abuse or other predominantly psychologic factors may be at the root of the problem. Health care providers should first consider this primarily a physical problem until proven otherwise. A thorough history, physical examination, and appropriate tests should be obtained.

Vaginismus

Defined as spasms of the perineal muscles surrounding the vagina, vaginismus occurs in response to attempted penetration of the vagina. These contractions may be so intense as to preclude insertion of the penis or even a tampon. Rarely, this condition may be due to a structural problem detected on examination. More often, however, it is related to a fear response, either to a first pelvic examination or to attempted intercourse and the potential loss of control involved. In some women vaginismus develops as a result of sexual trauma. Women can be taught to dilate their own vaginas as part of the treatment, by using their own finger or other devices, and can be taught relaxation techniques as well (Hatcher et al., 1994).

Lack of Orgasm

Lack of orgasm is the most common sexual problem encountered in women. It varies widely, occurring in women who have never experienced orgasm or women who have had orgasms but are currently unable to have them to women who have orgasms only in certain situations. Sex therapists in general do not believe that women physiologically lack the capacity to learn to be orgasmic (Hatcher et al., 1994). Learning to have a first orgasm can be relatively easy for a woman and may involve masturbation, use of a vibrator, or involvement of the partner. Learning to have an orgasm in every desired situation or with high frequency may be less easy for many women, and it often involves practice and experimentation and working through emotional and psychologic issues and inhibitions.

It is beyond the scope of this course to describe fully the causes and treatment options for sexual problems. Many good sources of information and training in this area are available.

SEXUAL PREFERENCE— LESBIANISM

In the past 15 years in the United States the lesbian community has grown and flourished. Lesbians are numerous in every ethnic group, socioeconomic class, and political persuasion. Although most historical records do not discuss lesbian influence, research is uncovering a lesbian culture dating back to ancient times (Boston Women's Health Book Collective, 1992). As with all minority groups, discrimination is a very powerful and predominant force in American society. American culture assumes heterosexuality. This assumption has far-reaching implications for the willingness of individuals and society as a whole to accept and welcome differences. A strong lesbian culture has developed that supports and nurtures women who are making the choice to love women as their primary relationships.

Lesbians, as do all men and women in American society, face the developmental task of finding their identity. The development of a sexual self-concept is a complex process. There are a number of components described by psychologists, including the following (Kozier et al., 1995):

- Biologic sex
- Gender identity—sense of being male or female, masculine or feminine
- Gender role—how a person expresses his or her sexuality as male or female
- Sexual identity—sexual orientation, preference for a person of the same or opposite sex

Some of the myriad influences involved in developing identity are described in relation to adolescence in chapter 4. This process is made more difficult for women who choose to be lesbians through the widespread discrimination and intolerance for nonheterosexual sexual preference.

Health Issues

Perhaps the most serious health issue for lesbians is avoidance of needed medical care because of fear of discrimination. Health care providers frequently assume heterosexuality, often forcing a woman to discuss her sexual preferences whether she would chose to do so or not to avoid an inevitable discussion about birth control. Health care providers as a group are often not very well informed about lesbian health issues. Women in general have been neglected in health research for many years, and research on the special needs of the lesbian population is limited (Boston Women's Health Book Collective, 1992).

The following five topics are pertinent to a health care provider understanding the health and sexual issues for lesbians:

1. **Sexually transmitted infections:** All sexually active lesbians need to be concerned about sexually transmitted infections, although woman-to-woman transmission of this type of infection is much lower than in heterosexual relationships. Because the organisms causing some

sexually transmitted infections are present in blood and vaginal secretions, sexual activities other than traditional intercourse can result in transmission of organisms from one individual to another, as can intravenous drug use. Viruses such as herpes and the genital wart virus are transmitted by skin-to-skin contact, and they can be transmitted from woman to woman. Safe(r) sex is important for lesbians as well as heterosexual or bisexual women (Boston Women's Health Book Collective, 1992).

2. **Alcoholism, substance abuse:** Traditionally, bars have been the places where lesbians have been able to feel comfortable in a public social setting, so alcohol has played a large role in the lives of many lesbians. The effects of discrimination add to the stresses of life for lesbians of every ethnic and socioeconomic group, compounding the stresses already known for heterosexual populations. During the past decade there has been a growth of self-help and treatment opportunities specifically for lesbians (Boston Women's Health Book Collective, 1992).

3. **Bisexuality:** Some women find themselves drawn to both women and men, or they may find during different periods of their lives that their sexual preference changes.

4. **Celibacy and abstinence:** The choice not to be sexually active for life (celibacy) or for a certain time (abstinence), is a personal one that is based on many factors. These include upbringing, religious beliefs, and goals. The choice may be one of avoidance on the basis of previous trauma. The health care provider may be in a position to help clients explore this decision.

5. **Self-stimulation:** Masturbation is a natural part of childhood experimentation, and it can be a healthy way for adult women to learn more about their own sexual response. It can be a form of erotic play between partners of either sex, or a form of sexual pleasure for women who do not have partners (Boston Women's Health Book Collective, 1992).

CONCLUSION

Sexuality is an enlivening and pleasurable part of life. Problems centering around sexuality are common and can be devastating to clients and their relationships. A sensitive, well-informed, open, and relaxed health care provider can be a lifesaving influence for women experiencing sexual difficulties. There is wide sexual diversity among the population of women that is seen in the health care setting, and health care providers should not assume heterosexuality. Health care providers need to be informed about the special requirements and needs of the populations they serve and be sensitive to women's rights to privacy regarding their sexual preference.

EXAM QUESTIONS

CHAPTER 3
Questions 15–23

15. The most serious issue in medical care for Lesbians is

    a. failure to seek medical care in a timely manner.

    b. sexually transmitted infections.

    c. sexual dysfunction.

    d. abnormal Pap smear findings.

16. The refractory period refers to

    a. initial excitement before orgasm occurs.

    b. the period after orgasm when heart and respiratory rates return to resting level.

    c. the period after orgasm in which another orgasm cannot occur.

    d. another term for the plateau period.

17. The resolution phase occurs

    a. only after orgasm.

    b. with or without orgasm.

    c. just before orgasm.

    d. only occasionally.

18. Women who have difficulty having an orgasm are considered to be physiologically

    a. incapable of orgasm.

    b. capable of orgasm.

    c. deficient in the hormone estrogen.

    d. deficient in the hormone progesterone.

19. Which Lesbians need to be concerned about sexually transmitted infection?

    a. Lesbians who have previously had sex with men

    b. All sexually active Lesbians

    c. Lesbians who are former intravenous drug users

    d. Lesbians who have had sex only with women

20. The female sexual response cycle includes what four phases?

    a. Arousal, plateau, resolution, excitement

    b. Plateau, orgasm, relaxation, excitement

    c. Vasocongestion, arousal, intercourse, resolution

    d. Excitement, plateau, orgasm, resolution

21. Pain during intercourse is called

    a. cervicitis.

    b. endometriosis.

    c. dyspareunia.

    d. vaginismus.

22. The most common sexual concern for women is

    a. failure to reach resolution.

    b. inability to achieve excitement.

    c. difficulty having an orgasm.

    d. inability to accept penetration.

23. The common denominator of healthy sexual intimacy is

    a. mutual orgasm.

    b. adequate foreplay.

    c. consensual touching.

    d. frequent sexual contact.

CHAPTER 4

SPECIAL ISSUES IN HEALTH CARE FOR YOUNG WOMEN

CHAPTER OBJECTIVE

After completing this chapter, the reader will be able to discuss the events that occur during the process of sexual maturation and identify issues that are pertinent to the patient population undergoing sexual maturation (i.e., adolescents), including physiologic and anatomic changes, emotional and social development, self-esteem, and sexuality. The reader will also be able to describe health challenges faced by adolescents and identify ways to ease adolescents' experience with the first pelvic examination, as well as ways to counsel and educate adolescents on health issues pertinent to this group.

LEARNING OBJECTIVES

After studying this chapter, the reader will be able to

1. describe the changes that occur during puberty.

2. differentiate between normal and abnormal changes associated with puberty.

3. discuss psychosocial issues in adolescent development.

4. describe health issues pertinent to the teen-age population.

5. describe health risks for teen-agers.

6. describe the components of self-esteem and clues to observing low self-esteem.

Key Words

- Menarche
- Piaget
- STI

INTRODUCTION

Adolescence is a time of enormous change and tremendous vulnerability. Young people are experimenting, taking risks, and moving farther and faster, perhaps, than at any other time in their lives. At the same time, teen-agers lack experience and often good judgement. Because of this, the teen-age population is especially vulnerable to health risks. Traffic accidents and suicide are primary causes of death in this age group (Lichtman & Papera, 1990). Sexually transmitted infections (STIs) have reached epidemic proportions (Centers for Disease Control and Prevention, Division of STD Prevention, 1997). Unwanted pregnancy rates are higher in the United States than for any other developed country. Health care providers have a challenging task: to provide nonjudgmental, non-patronizing care for young people while calling them to higher degrees of self-responsibility. Promoting self-esteem is key to the success of health education efforts.

PUBERTY

Puberty is a developmental process, not a single event, that occurs over time. It causes profound changes in every aspect of the developing young woman.

The onset of puberty is variable, and results of studies have shown that it is influenced by heredity, socioeconomic status, nutrition, endocrine function, body weight, percentage of body fat, physical activity, altitude, illness, stress, and abuse or neglect (Lichtman & Papera, 1990). The maturation of the central nervous system, including the hypothalamus, is a crucial yet poorly understood part of this process. The hypothalamus seems to reach a level of maturity that results in an increased responsiveness to hormones produced in the ovaries. The hypothalamus also starts to increase its own hormonal secretion. It is the activation of the feedback loops between the brain and the ovaries that will ultimately result in the initiation of the menstrual cycle. Increasing levels of sex hormones produced by the ovaries influence the whole body, resulting in the development of secondary sex characteristics (Lichtman & Papera, 1990).

The sexual maturation process (or puberty) occurs over a 3- to 5- year period beginning around age 9 years, with a growth spurt, followed by growth of internal and external genitalia, breast tissue, and axillary and pubic hair (see *Figure 4-1).* The first menstrual flow, termed menarche, usually occurs around 13 years of age, although the normal range is by 10–16 years of age (Lichtman & Papera, 1990). Even after initiation of menses, it may take an average of 12–18 months for the cycles to stabilize as the feedback loops and receptors in the nervous system complete the maturation process. It is common for young women to have cycles in which ovulation does not occur (Lichtman & Papera, 1990).

Trends in the Age of Menarche

The average age of menarche in the United States is 12.2 years. One hundred years ago it was at age 17 years. In China, the average age is 15–17 years (Kradjian, 1994). Daughters and granddaughters of Asian women who are raised in America have the same early menarche as American women. Researchers at Duke University have found that about half the girls in America begin breast development or pubic hair development (or both) by age 9 years (Kradjian, 1994). The most plausible explanation for this has to do with the increase in dietary fat consumed by Americans. Other cross-cultural studies show similar findings: Native people who eat their traditional low-fat diets tend to have late menarche. After emigrating to America and adopting a high-fat, high-protein diet, young women from these same cultures tend toward earlier menarche (Kradjian, 1994). Young women that have early menarche also have greater body weight. This trend could partly be due to healthy increases in fat, but an important cause is thought to be unhealthy increases in consumption of animal products, especially animal fat (Kradjian, 1994).

A potential factor in menarche that has not been well researched is the role of hormones in animal products. It is known that hormones are stored in fat cells. When animal fat is consumed, any hormonal residues will get passed on in the food. This could be a large source of hormone stimulation. Further research needs to be done (DeMarco, 1996).

PERIOD OF ADOLESCENCE

In contrast to many traditional cultures, in Westernized cultures a prolonged period of development is considered to be a normal and even critical period to prepare young people to meet the demands of a complex society. The basic psycho-

FIGURE 4-1

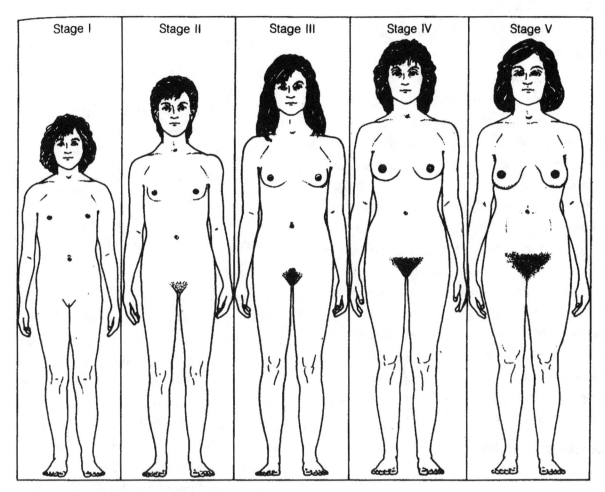

Stages of female breast and pubic hair development.

Stage I   Preadolescent. Juvenile breast with elevated papilla and small flat areola. No pubic hair, fine hairs cover genital area.

Stage II   Breast bud forms with hormonal stimulation, papilla and areola elevate to small mound, areola increases diameter. Sparse distribution of long slightly pigmented straight hair appearing bilaterally along medial border of labia majora.

Stage III Continued enlargement of breast bud further elevates papilla, areolar continues to enlarge, no separation of breast contours noted. Pubic hair pigmentation increases, hair curls and spreads sparsely over mons pubis.

Stage IV   Areola and papilla separate from the contour of breast to form secondary mound. Pubic hairs continue to curl and become coarse, number of hairs increases.

Stage V   Mature. Areolar mound recedes into general contour, papilla continues to project. Pubic hair attains adult feminine triangular pattern, spreads to medial thigh.

Source: Griffith-Kenney, J. *Contemporary Women's Health,* 2725 Sand Hill Road, Menlo Park, CA 94025: Addison-Wesley, Health Sciences Division.

logic task is to formulate and consolidate an adult identity (Lichtman & Papera, 1990). Complex forces from within the individual and the outside world combine to make this process one of great depth and magnitude.

Identity, or self-concept, has a number of different elements, including cultural, social, gender, sexual, personal, and spiritual influences. Developing autonomy with one's family; developing an active sexual life; peer relationships; social responsibility; value systems; an orientation toward the future; and issues of body image, self-esteem, and competence are all part of identity formation. This search for identity and self-expression can include a wide range of experimentation, including choice of clothing, use of make-up, and use of drugs and alcohol and other kinds of risk-taking behavior. In the area of sexuality, experimentation may include masturbation, sexual fantasy, and a wide range of sexual play, including homosexual experiences, and may or may not include having sexual intercourse (Kozier et al., 1995).

Changes in Cognition

Piaget, a well-known psychologist who developed theories about how mental functioning matures, characterizes the cognitive shift that occurs in adolescence as a movement from concrete to abstract reasoning (Lichtman & Papera, 1990). Until this developmental milestone is achieved, the young person may have difficulty planning for the future or seeing that behavior may have predictable consequences. In addition, egocentrism tends to characterize adolescence, which creates a myth of invulnerability. For example, this way of thinking often leads young women to think they can be sexually active and will not get pregnant (Lichtman & Papera, 1990).

It is often difficult for caregivers to realize that young women who look fully physically mature may have a totally different way of viewing the world and thinking through issues in their lives

than might be expected of mature-looking individuals. Caregivers have to make a cognitive shift to understand and reach them.

Self-Esteem

Each person's self-concept is like a collage. At the center are the beliefs and images most vital to the person's identity. They constitute the core self-concept—for example, male/female, attractive/unattractive, competent/incompetent. Individuals behave as they perceive themselves, so a person's self-perception becomes a self-fulfilling prophecy.

There are a number of components to what is termed a self-concept, including the following:

Body Image

Body image is how a person perceives the size, appearance, and functioning of the body and its parts. It includes an intellectual component (body image) and a body sensation component (how one feels and experiences oneself as a physical being, including sensory perceptions such as pain and pleasure). Body image is developed throughout childhood but particularly during adolescence from others' attitudes and responses, the individual's own exploration, and cultural and societal values (Kozier et al., 1995).

Role Performance and Role Mastery

Role performance and role mastery is how to act appropriately. People need to know who they are in relation to others and what society expects (Kozier et al., 1995).

Personal Identity

Personal identity is a person's sense of his or her individuality and uniqueness, beliefs, values, talents, and interests (Kozier et al., 1995).

Low Self-Esteem

Health care providers who work with adolescents need to be sensitive to communications of low self-esteem. Kozier and colleagues (1995) list the following cues to low self-esteem, which can assist the health care team in their assessment and counseling of young clients:

- Avoidance of eye contact

- Stooped posture

- Hesitant speech

- Overly critical attitude regarding self or others

- Frequently apologetic

- Unable to accept positive feedback

- An "I don't care" attitude

- Indecisiveness

- Failure to complete or follow through on tasks

- Expression of feelings of worthlessness or isolation— "Nobody cares"

- Not seeking help when needed

- Lack of effective problem-solving skills

- Unrealistic, vague goals

- Exhibiting of inappropriate attention-seeking behaviors (or the opposite)

- Lack of energy or enthusiasm

- Poor grooming

In addition, people with low self-esteem generally exhibit illogical and distorted thinking, which then perpetuates the existing low self-esteem. Common types of illogical thinking include the following (Kozier et al., 1995):

- Catastrophizing (tending to think the worst)

- Minimizing or maximizing (minimize positives and maximize negatives), black and white thinking

- Overgeneralizing (thinking that something that happened in one situation will happen in all situations)

- Self-referencing (believing that others are very concerned with one's own thoughts and actions, shortcomings, and mistakes)

- Filtering (selectively pulling details out of context, usually negative content)

These signs need to be taken seriously. It is important for caregivers to know the limits of their role in a given setting, as well as to familiarize themselves with community services available to teen-agers in the area of counseling, peer support, and school services. For health education to be successful, teen-agers need to have the personal skills to commit to consistent, positive health behaviors. A young client may need long-term counseling and should be referred for such. A caregiver's ability to provide compassionate and sensitive care will perhaps set the stage for a young client to trust enough to stay involved.

Positive Self-Esteem

The following are possible strategies caregivers can use to promote a positive self-esteem for clients (Kozier et al., 1995):

- Assist in identifying the client's areas of strength.

- Help the client define clear, realistic goals, as well as plan for their accomplishment.

- Encourage a change in language patterns from passive to more active to help the client assume greater responsibility for her own power. For example, encourage a change from "I can't" to "I choose not to."

- Guide the client in developing more positive thoughts and images about self by

 — modeling positive self-statement.

 — providing honest positive feedback and praise.

 — using visualization to envision a goal and its accomplishment.

 — eliciting accomplishment the client feels good about. Have clients make a list of accomplishments, behaviors, and characteristics about themselves that are positive.

- Show physical affection as appropriate.

- Take time to interact with the client. Depending on the limits of the health care setting, plan for several visits.

- Help the client establish a sense of purpose and belonging.

Clearly, these strategies cannot be used in isolation by one health care provider. They must be applied in a coordinated effort with others who play an important role in the client's life if this is desired by the client. Educating the family about how to promote self-esteem in the child may be a crucial part for a health care provider in developing a successful plan of care.

HEALTH ISSUES IN ADOLESCENCE

There are several health issues that are particularly pertinent to adolescence.

Traffic Accidents, Homicides, and Suicides

According to Lichtman and Papera (1990), the leading causes of death in adolescents are traffic accidents, homicides, and suicides. They note that a suicide attempt that results in death is often preceded by 50–200 unsuccessful attempts. In addition, women in this age group are two to three times more likely to commit suicide than young men.

Nutritional Deficits/Eating Disorders

Because adolescence is a time when body image and self-esteem are being developed so intensely, young women are particularly vulnerable to inadequate nutritional intake, as well as to disorders that have more extreme psychologic and emotional components and can be life threatening. Influence of peers and the media is so powerful that this can be a difficult area in which to provide positive guidance for young women. By supporting individuality and positive creative expression, the

health care provider can help teen-agers find themselves amongst the jungle of impressions and influences and give them the self-esteem to want to care for themselves.

The following information on three key health issues can assist health care providers in addressing the needs of adolescents:

Nutritional Deficits

Bone density reaches its peak in adolescent women after approximately 2 years of normal menstrual periods (*Depo-Provera and Bone Density,* 1998). Regular menses depends on adequate body adipose tissue (Lichtman & Papera, 1990). Young women need adequate protein, vitamins, and minerals to support their development and maintain adequate immune responses. In addition, popular birth control methods, such as the pill and the injection, can interfere with the body's utilization and assimilation of some vital nutrients. A multivitamin–mineral supplement is a good general recommendation for all teen-agers.

Anorexia Nervosa and Bulimia Nervosa

Anorexia nervosa is a form of severe and deliberate self-starvation and distortion of body image, which, if left untreated can be fatal (Kozier et al., 1995). Bulimia nervosa is another syndrome in which binging and then purging, with laxatives or vomiting, occur. This can result in severe tooth decay from regurgitation of stomach acids, damage to the esophagus, and electrolyte imbalances, which can also be life threatening (Kozier et al., 1995). These two illness patterns, involving severe emotional, psychological, and physical distress, are reaching epidemic proportions in our society and are prevalent especially among white women, both teenage and adult. Discussion of factors affecting self-esteem and body image can be found in other portions of this text. During assessment and counseling of women, health practitioners need to be attentive to indicators of low self-esteem and poor body image, as described in other chapters, for possible indications of eating disorders. Please see the Resource Guide for in-depth literature on this topic.

Sexually Transmitted Infections (STIs)

Many factors have influenced the rising epidemic of STIs among the teen-age population. The statistics are sobering. Infection with HIV is on the rise as a leading cause of death in women age 15–25 years (Hatcher et al., 1994). The incidence of cervical cancer is rising among young women. Some of the factors involved in these increases include

- the asymptomatic nature of many STIs.

- multiple sexual partners, which includes serial monogamy (series of partners with which the client has a monogamous relationship).

- inconsistent use of barrier methods of birth control.

- lack of understanding about STIs.

These issues will be discussed in greater detail in chapter 7.

Birth Control

Why do so many adolescent women fail to use contraception? Results of one large survey of never married, sexually active women showed that a large proportion did not think they were going to have intercourse (Abma, Driscoll & Moore, 1998). This is especially true of those just beginning to be sexually active. Half of all initial adolescent pregnancies occur within the first 6 months after initiation of intercourse, and 20% occur within the first month alone (Hatcher et al., 1994). Study findings have revealed an average of 23 months' delay between initiation of sexual relations and the first family planning visit (Finer & Zabin, 1998). Results of more recent studies have shown a promising trend: Adolescents are increasing their use of birth control methods, especially condom use, at first intercourse whether or not they have seen a health care provider for contraception (Finer

& Zabin, 1998). This indicates that health education efforts are having an important impact.

Some of the special concerns of this age group include

- possible confidentiality issues with parents.

- compliance issues.

- age-related health issues.

See chapter 5 for more discussion of birth control methods.

Tobacco/Social Drug Use

Teen-agers are using a wider range of substances at younger ages than ever before. Use of these substances has a profound impact on the short- and long-term health of adolescents.

Tobacco use increases the risk of a number of diseases, including cervical cancer, breast cancer, chronic lung disease, chronic cardiovascular disease, and asthma (Boston Women's Health Book Collective, 1992).

Substance abuse is associated with an increase in risky behaviors, including sexual activity among adolescents. It is beyond the scope of this course to discuss this area in detail.

Undesired Sexual Activity/Rape

Adolescent women are particularly vulnerable to various forms of sexual harassment, coercion, and rape. Peer pressure, feelings of invulnerability, risk-taking behavior, unpredictable situations, dating with unfamiliar men, substance abuse, and lack of experience contribute to this vulnerability.

Rape is generally underreported and underprosecuted. The person committing the rape is often someone known to the individual. Date rape often occurs in which the young woman participates in voluntary sexual play but does not consent to sexual intercourse. Findings from the 1995 National Survey of Family Growth show that an important percentage (9%) of young women age 15–24 years report that their first sexual experience was nonvoluntary (Abma et al., 1998). Further, of the women who described their experience as voluntary one fourth indicated that although they had consented, they had not wanted intercourse to happen (Abma et al., 1998). The greater the age difference between male and female, the greater the incidence of unwanted sex. In addition, the partner's condom use accounted for most of the reported contraceptive use at first intercourse for both groups of women, although the use of condoms was significantly less for those reporting unwanted sexual intercourse. This indicates that a large number of young women feel a lack of control over their sexuality in these circumstances (Abma et al., 1998).

Sex education needs to include information about sexual harassment, sexual coercion, and rape. Young women need to be given the tools to recognize and avoid potentially dangerous situations. Self-defense courses are widely available. The health care provider needs to become familiar with community resources as well as the specific requirements in the state for reporting sexual abuse and violence. Licensed health care providers are often required by law to report any mention of abuse by the client whether or not she wishes to report it herself. The health care system is often the first contact for a young person who has been raped or coerced into sexual activity.

Rape represents an often life-threatening attack and has a profound psychologic and emotional impact. Physical evidence needs to be gathered according to a very time-specific protocol, especially if the evidence is to be of use in court. Young women especially tend to delay reports of rape or sexual coercion because of confusion and embarrassment and fear. This is a very difficult and delicate situation, and it needs to be handled by trained healthcare providers (Stenchever, 1996).

Incest and Family Violence

Stenchever (1996) has noted that incest and violence are widespread in the United States across all socioeconomic, education level, and ethnic groups. Stenchever also noted that estimates indicate approximately 10% of all childhood abuse cases involve sexual abuse, and perhaps 350,000 or more children in the United States each year are victims of sexual abuse. The actual figures are probably higher due to underreporting. In addition, 15%–25% of adult women and 12% of adult men experience incest in their childhood. As many as 80% of childhood sexual assaults are perpetrated by a parent, guardian, family member, or maternal significant other. Abma and associates (1998) comment that tragically enough, young women who were raised in families with abusive patterns often tend to find themselves in situations that resemble those of their upbringing. Results of studies have shown that women who lived apart from their parents before age 16 years and women whose parents abused alcohol or illegal drugs were more likely to have unwanted intercourse at a younger age (Abma et al., 1998).

Young women with a history of sexual abuse may have great difficulty forming a positive sexual identity, as well as have emotional and functional sexual problems that need to be addressed by providers with special training. It is the task of nurses and other primary health care providers to be attentive to cues from clients that underlying abuse issues may play a role in current problems. These signs include expressions of shame, guilt, and anger; unexplained physical complaints; sleep disturbances; school problems; and problems developing relationships (Stenchever, 1996).

Unintended Pregnancy

One in eight women age 15–19 years in the United States becomes pregnant each year. This proportion has changed little since the 1970s (Hatcher et al., 1994). The United States leads almost all other developed countries in the world in rates of teen-age pregnancy, abortion, and child-bearing, even though the rates of sexual activity are similar (Hatcher et al., 1994). Findings from the recent National Survey of Family Growth (completed in 1995) showed that the highest rate of unintended pregnancy occurred among teen-agers age 18 years and younger, and approximately 83% of these pregnancies were unintended (Henshaw, 1998). The rates were highest for unmarried, poor, and Black and Hispanic women. The proportion of pregnancies that ended in abortion increased among women age 20 years and older, but decreased in younger women who are now more likely than older women to continue their unplanned pregnancies (Henshaw, 1998).

Health care providers need to consider seriously what is missing from not only their health care system, but also the whole approach to young people in American culture (Hatcher et al., 1994). Unwanted pregnancy rates are clearly linked to socioeconomic status, which is further associated with deficits in health care access, education, and opportunity. Large societal efforts involving every aspect of social inequality need to be directed toward turning these statistics around. Results of international studies show that countries in which pregnancy rates are lowest have contraceptive supplies widely available and free or at low cost. In addition, sex education is widespread and emphasized in the mass media, and schools are closely linked with adolescent birth control clinics (Hatcher et al., 1994). Although almost everyone would seem to agree that teen-age pregnancy is a problem in the United States, there is such a wide range of opinion and belief about these issues that there is no agreement on a way to approach the problem (Hatcher et al., 1994).

THE FIRST PELVIC EXAMINATION

The first pelvic examination has been described as a rite of passage into American womanhood. This first experience can set the stage for the entire future of a woman's relationship with the health care system. The first examination and often subsequent examinations can be anxiety producing. Sources include fear of pain, embarrassment about undressing, feelings of vulnerability about having the body viewed and touched by a stranger, and fear of an abnormality. In addition, cultural differences and language barriers may need to be addressed.

Health care providers can do much to minimize these concerns and create a positive first experience (Lichtman & Papera, 1990):

- Take time to establish a comfortable rapport.

- Remember that 90% of communication is non-verbal.

- Pay attention to your own as well as the client's nonverbal cues.

- Reassure the client of confidentiality.

- Take a thorough history.

- Explain in advance exactly what is to occur (in the order of occurrence), and make sure that everything is understood.

- Be sure that all the client's questions and concerns are answered before the examination is begun.

- Use illustrations and models; show the speculum.

- Teach relaxation breathing techniques in advance.

- If desired, welcome a friend or family member.

- Let the client know before her body is touched.

- When beginning a pelvic examination, touch the client's thigh before touching her genitalia.

- Offer a mirror to view the cervix if desired.

- Maintain the client's privacy.

- Let the client know what you are seeing; reassure her of normalcy.

- Teaching and counseling should be done in the native language with sensitivity to cultural issues.

COUNSELING AND EDUCATION OF ADOLESCENTS

The following tips can assist health care providers in working with adolescents and their special issues in health care:

- Be aware that learning about how one's body functions can be fun, an ordeal, or even frightening for some women. It is important for health care providers involved in education to be sensitive to their audience. This includes finding out what information they already bring to the session, how accurate it is, who they heard it from, and how much emotional content is mixed with the actual information.

- Find out what *they* want to learn about. It is an art to draw out people's interests, pique their curiosity, and help them discover themselves. Health care providers have so much information that they believe needs to be communicated that they may get so involved in their teaching that they fail to ignite the spark that will result in communications being received and retained.

- Avoid overwhelming clients with too much information at once.

- Use visual aids. Many people learn primarily visually; others, by listening or writing. Help clients get a visual picture of what is being described.

- Make the session interactive as much as possible. Ask questions; ask clients to describe their own experience.

- Create hypothetic situations. This makes the discussion more true to life.

- Be relaxed, create a comfortable environment, and be humorous. Set the audience at ease as much as possible.

- When talking to a group, create a format for anonymous questions. Bring 3 × 5 cards and pencils. This allows more open discussion by creating the privacy to ask "secret" questions.

- Provide simple reading materials for clients to take home.

- If possible, have a follow-up session or find out if there is any interest in peer education. Young people listen to their peers. Give them resources for their further exploration.

CONCLUSION

Adolescence is a critical time. Events occurring, choices made, and habits acquired during this period can have serious and permanent consequences. It is the role of health care providers to find effective ways of working with young clients, helping them to establish and practice consistent behavior that will enhance their health.

Health care organizations can do much to enhance their relationship with the teen-age population by

- offering flexible hours.

- having close geographic accessibility.

- providing transportation schedules.

- letting clients know about free or government-supported services available to them.

- informing young clients of their rights to confidentiality. Findings from recent studies have confirmed that practitioners who assure their young clients of confidentiality find that these young people, many of whom are at high risk for sensitive health problems, are more likely to reveal sensitive information and return for repeat visits (*When Physicians Assure Confidentiality*, 1998).

EXAM QUESTIONS

CHAPTER 4
Questions 24–31

24. The first menstrual period is called

    a. amenorrhea.

    b. menarche.

    c. dysmenorrhea.

    d. menopause.

25. The first evidence of puberty (or sexual maturation) is

    a. the first menstrual period.

    b. growth of pubic hair.

    c. a growth spurt.

    d. budding of the breasts.

26. After the first menstrual period it may take, on average, _____ for cycles to become regular and stable.

    a. 2 years

    b. 3 months

    c. 6 months to 1 year

    d. 12–18 months

27. The developmental milestone that occurs in adolescence is a shift in the way of thinking from

    a. primary reasoning to future orientation.

    b. identification with the mother to separate self sense.

    c. concrete to abstract reasoning.

    d. concentration on self to focus on others.

28. Bone density reaches its peak in adolescent women

    a. after about 2 years of normal menstrual periods.

    b. when the breasts are fully grown.

    c. when the growth spurt is complete.

    d. when menarche occurs.

29. One leading cause of death in women age 15–25 years is

    a. suicide.

    b. anorexia nervosa.

    c. HIV.

    d. ovarian cancer.

30. Sexually transmitted infections

    a. are often asymptomatic.

    b. usually produce some symptoms in women.

    c. always produce symptoms.

    d. usually result in vaginal discharge.

31. _____ of all adolescent first pregnancies occur in the _____ of initiation of intercourse.

    a. Twenty percent / first year

    b. Thirty percent / first month

    c. Fifty percent / first 6 months

    d. Seventy-five percent / first 3 months

CHAPTER 5

BIRTH CONTROL METHODS AND REPRODUCTIVE CHOICES

CHAPTER OBJECTIVE

After completing this chapter, the reader will be able to identify current methods of birth control, as well as ways to counsel women in choosing a method of contraception that best suits their needs. The reader will also be able to recognize current choices available to women for pregnancy termination, including emergency contraception (the morning after pill) as well as identify trends and statistics on birth control in the United States.

LEARNING OBJECTIVES

After studying this chapter, the reader will be able to

1. identify the methods of birth control currently available in the United States.

2. describe the pros and cons of each method.

3. identify the components of counseling for unintended or unwanted pregnancy.

4. describe the options for procedures for pregnancy termination.

5. discuss current trends in use of birth control methods in the United States.

Key Words

- Depo-Provera
- ECP, MAP
- Medical abortion
- National Survey of Family Growth
- Thromboembolic disease
- Vasectomy

INTRODUCTION

Although they are vitally important areas of women's health, birth control methods and reproductive choices are fraught with controversy. Women's religious values, constitutional rights, concept of family, and hopes for their children—as well as young people's rights for autonomy, privacy, and respect—are all on the line. Technology has not yet created a perfect birth control method. There is a wide range of opinion in the adult community about when sexual activity should begin. Abstinence is still the only perfect method for preventing unwanted pregnancy, but efforts to promote abstinence in the young population have not been successful (Hatcher et al., 1994). All groups on either side of the controversy have to ask themselves if this is realistic in today's society. As nurses who work in health care settings are confronted by these issues, they are challenged to find their own personal values, as well as to provide nonjudgmental care for their patients. A crucial aspect of health care is to promote self-esteem in clients, so that the choices they make for themselves are positive and practiced consistently.

One of the crucial issues in decision making for contraception is preventing the transmission of sexually transmitted infections (STIs). Unfortunately, the most convenient, longer acting birth control methods currently available offer minimal, if any, protection for STIs. In addition, many clients choose these methods because they are so "hassle free", and it may be difficult for them to accept adding a barrier method (Hatcher et al., 1994).

Note: The terminology in common use for "sexually transmitted disease" (STD), has been replaced by "sexually transmitted infection" (STI). STI will be used throughout the course.

UNINTENDED PREGNANCY

According to the 1995 National Survey of Family Growth (as reported by Henshaw, 1998), the unintended pregnancy rate in the United States declined by 16% between 1987 and 1994, from 54 to 45 pregnancies per 1,000 women of reproductive age (15–44 years old). This is probably due to the increased use of contraception and use of more effective contraceptive methods. Even with a decline in percentages, it is estimated that in 1994 approximately 1.22 million births were from unplanned pregnancies, and adding abortion there were 2.65 million unintended pregnancies. This represents almost half (49%) of all pregnancies for that year. The survey reveals further that among women who experienced an unintended pregnancy, 54% had an abortion and 46% carried the pregnancy to term. 58% of women who had abortions were using a birth control method during the month they became pregnant. What may seem surprising is that 48% of women who had an unplanned birth had been using a contraceptive method during the month they became pregnant. So for all unintended pregnancies combined, more than half the women got pregnant while using a contraceptive method. This finding reveals that a large segment of women are taking some action to prevent pregnancy, but they may need more education and encouragement for consistent and correct use of their chosen methods. In addition, there is still a large population of women who have yet to choose and use a contraceptive method.

EFFECTIVENESS OF BIRTH CONTROL METHODS

How effective are birth control methods? This is a commonly asked question, and unfortunately there is no simple answer. Hatcher and associates (1994) discuss many factors that make an accurate determination of failure rates very difficult, as outlined in the following discussion.

Statistically, failure rates are influenced by many factors, including age, socioeconomic status, educational level, cultural and lifestyle factors. Consistency and correctness of use and duration of use of a particular method also affect failure rates. Failure rates as they are often reported include women who are infertile and would not get pregnant without the method. Failure rates for a particular method would then be artificially low. In addition, no reliable method has been found to adjust for frequency of intercourse. Failure rates are often defined as failure with "perfect" use and "typical" use. "Perfect" use of a method is correct use of the method every time intercourse takes place. Failure rates for "typical" use are higher, reflecting occasions of incorrect use or failure to use the method (Hatcher et al., 1994). All of these factors interact to make birth control statistics ballpark figures rather than an exact science.

Therefore Hatcher and associates (1994) emphasize that when counseling clients who are considering which birth control method would be most appropriate, effectiveness statistics are secondary to finding a method which will be used properly and consistently. This requires a careful evaluation of the individual's lifestyle and personal preferences, including safety, cost and convenience.

REVIEW OF BIRTH CONTROL METHODS

It is beyond the scope of this course to provide all details needed to counsel women adequately on each method of birth control. The health risks of some methods can be more serious than those of other methods. Therefore, careful evaluation of the client's personal and family health history as well as sexual history needs to be completed by a nurse practitioner, physician's assistant, or physician before any method, however appropriate to the client's other needs, is prescribed. Fitting all the pieces together can be challenging for the health care provider, and members of a health care team have different roles to play in this process of evaluation, counseling, and teaching. This section is designed to introduce the basics of each method. Please refer to the bibliography and resource guide at the end of the course for more in-depth information.

Hatcher and colleagues (1994) note that a perfect birth control method does not yet exist. Contraceptives are imperfect and can fail even the most diligent user. Methods such as the birth control pill, IUD and the injection offer superior protection against pregnancy in comparison to barrier methods, but have more potential for health risks and side effects. Barrier methods, especially male and female condoms, are superior in their protection against sexually transmitted infections, with minimal risks and side effects, but are not as effective in preventing pregnancy. Using a condom along with an appropriate method which provides superior pregnancy protection is the best option currently available.

Natural Family Planning/Fertility Awareness

There are several variations within the natural family planning/fertility awareness form of birth control. All are based on daily recording and charting of physiologic changes that occur normally during the menstrual cycle; that is, changes in basal body temperature and cervical mucus (Kass-Annese & Danzer, 1992). This method permits identification of fertile and nonfertile days.

There are a number of specific rules that must be applied to determine when unprotected intercourse could safely happen (Kass-Annese & Danzer, 1992):

- **Basal body temperature (BBT):** The BBT cannot be used to predict ovulation. However, it can indicate when ovulation has occurred. (See the glossary for a more complete description.)

- **Cervical mucus changes:** The texture and the consistency of cervical mucus change in response to the influence of first estrogen and then progesterone. Mucus on a typical fertile day is of egg-white consistency, clear, and stretchy.

Health care providers need special training to counsel clients on fertility awareness methods, and in some states certification is needed as well. Several sessions are usually required in which the client learns to be sensitive to her fertility signs as she charts them for several months. Individual patterns are determined. The rules are learned, and decisions are made about abstinence vs. other forms of contraception during fertile days. A strong level of commitment is required, as are comfort with body processes and good communication between partners (Kass-Annese & Danzer, 1992).

Oral Contraceptive Pills (OCPs, OCs, or Combination Pills)

Oral contraceptive pills contain a synthetic estrogen and progestin. Neither is chemically identical to the hormones that the body produces naturally, but each is close enough to exert similar effects. Since approval of OCPs by the Food and Drug Administration (FDA) in 1960, most research has been directed at reducing the effective dose and thereby reducing the risk of serious side effects. Most pills used today are considered low-dose pills.

Method Of Action and Formulation

According to Hatcher and colleagues (1994), the estrogen component of OCPs primarily affects the pituitary gland to inhibit ovulation. Other effects of the estrogen component are to accelerate transport of the egg, inhibit implantation, and promote premature degeneration of the corpus luteum. The progestin component changes the cervical mucus, making it more hostile to sperm transport.

Hatcher and colleagues (1994) further note that pills are formulated in two ways: with a fixed estrogen-to-progesterone ratio or with three different ratios during the cycle, attempting to approximate more closely cyclic hormonal changes in the natural cycle. In all formulations the first 21 pills contain hormones, and the final 7 pills have no hormone component.

Risk Factors

Hatcher and colleagues (1994) note the following with regard to risks with OCP use. In general, oral contraceptives pose few serious health risks to most users, and these risks certainly are not as great as pregnancy-related complications. The most serious risk of all, death, is extraordinarily low for most women. Other major health risks are uncommon, and they are most likely to occur in women with underlying medical conditions that may be influenced by hormonal contraceptive methods.

Four specific risks warrant consideration:

1. **Cardiovascular risk:** According to Hatcher and associates (1994), the most serious and well-documented risks of OCPs are those affecting the circulatory system. They further note that an increased risk of death in users of OCPs caused by cardiovascular disease is concentrated in women older than 35 years of age, especially smokers. In addition, venous thromboembolic disease is the leading cause of death attributed to OCs because estrogens promote blood clotting. Hatcher and colleagues advise that clients in their midthirties should be evaluated for cardiovascular risk before OCPs are prescribed. Smokers age 35 years or older should not use an estrogen-containing contraceptive. They also note that age increases the risk of having other unhealthy conditions, such as high blood pressure and diabetes, which put women at an increased risk of complications from OC use.

2. **Cancer:** Hatcher and colleagues (1994) have also addressed the risk of cancer with OCP use. Oral contraceptives offer protective effects against endometrial and ovarian cancer. The subject of breast cancer is more controversial. The jury is still out in determining an association between breast cancer and use of the pill. Certain subpopulations may be at increased risk. Women with long-term pill use, particularly before the first full-term pregnancy, are the subgroup most consistently identified as being at increased risk. More research is needed to clarify the matter. Combined with other risk factors such as smoking, OC use may be part of a more complex risk picture.

3. **HIV:** Recent study findings (*Does the Pill Help Spread HIV?*, 1998) have shown that women already infected with HIV who used OCPs were more likely than nonusers infected with HIV to have infected cells detected in cer-

vical secretions, resulting in an increase in risk of transmission during sexual activity or birth. This was also true for the injectable contraceptive. Why this occurred was not clear.

4. **Chlamydial infection:** Study results (Stenchever, 1996) have revealed an increased risk of acquiring chlamydial infection among pill users. This is probably due to changes in the cervix, which expose more of the inner, more delicate cervical cells to possible infection. A combination of OCPs and condom use may be a good solution to the risk:benefit picture.

Contraindications

The contraindications to use of OCPs include the following (Hatcher et al., 1994):

- Thromboembolic disorder (or history of)
- Stroke
- Cardiovascular disease
- Reproductive cancer
- Benign or malignant liver tumor or impaired liver function
- Pregnancy
- Gallbladder disease
- Undiagnosed abnormal vaginal bleeding
- Age 35 years and older with a history of smoking
- Hypertension
- Severe headaches

Benefits

Study findings have shown that the birth control pill decreases the risk of ovarian cyst formation, as well as of ovarian and uterine cancer (Hatcher et al., 1994). The risk of ectopic pregnancy is almost eliminated because ovulation is inhibited. There is a decreased incidence of iron deficiency anemia and less dysmenorrhea.

Effectiveness

Failure rates with use of the birth control pill are in the range of 0.1%–3% in the first year of use (Hatcher et al., 1994).

Side Effects

Manufacturers have aimed at reducing hormone levels in the birth control pill to reduce both dangerous and annoying side effects. The risk of dangerous side effects is minimal, but it increases with age, smoking, and the presence of other diseases.

Danger signs with use of the pill include the following (Hatcher et al., 1994): jaundice (indicating liver toxicity); abdominal pain (possible gallbladder disease); and severe headache, vision changes, eye problems, numbness in an extremity, chest pain, calf pain, and shortness of breath (all indicating the possibility of a blood clot). Any of these symptoms require immediate evaluation. Other side effects, which can be annoying but certainly not life threatening, include mood changes, hair loss, nausea, breast tenderness, weight gain, darkening of the skin, and an increase in headaches (Hatcher et al., 1994). These side effects are the most common reason why women stop taking their birth control pills.

Minipill

The minipill is a variation of oral contraception which is composed of only a synthetic form of progesterone, or progestin with no estrogen component. It is a more appropriate pill for certain groups of women. It is often prescribed for nursing mothers because estrogen inhibits lactation while progestins do not. Both hormones have been detected in breast milk. It is also prescribed for women who have medical conditions that would prohibit the use of estrogen, such as women with cardiovascular disease (see OCP's) (Stenchever, 1996).

Because it is a progestin-only pill, the minipill has fewer side effects than the combination pill, but it is also less effective. In contrast to the combined pill, each minipill contains hormones and must be taken at the same time each day to maximize effectiveness. Use of the minipill carries an increased risk of ectopic pregnancy because the progestin slows the movement of the small hairs in the fallopian tube which help the fertilized egg travel toward the uterus, thus slowing its movement and increasing the risk of implantation in the tube (Stenchever, 1996).

Depo-Provera Contraceptive Injection

In the United States, the only approved injectable form of birth control is medroxyprogesterone acetate (Depo-Provera), a type of progestin or synthetic progesterone that is given by intramuscular injection and formulated for release over a 3-month period. Since its approval in 1992 by the FDA, it has been an increasingly popular birth control method, especially for teen-agers. Depo-Provera has been in use worldwide for a number of years. Other injectable contraceptives with a shorter duration of action are also available in other countries.

Method Of Action and Administration

Depo-Provera prevents pregnancy in three ways (Hatcher et al., 1994). It

1. stops eggs from ripening and inhibits ovulation.

2. changes the cervical mucus, making it difficult for sperm to get to the uterus.

3. changes the lining of the uterus, making it inhospitable to implantation.

Stenchever (1996) provides the following on administration of Depo-Provera. Ideally, Depo-Provera therapy is begun during the first 5 days of a normal menstrual cycle to minimize the risks of prior pregnancy. An injection is given every 10–12 weeks because the chances of pregnancy increase after 12 weeks. The preferred injection site is in the muscles of the hip. The deltoid muscle may be used if it is of adequate size, and it should be used for obese women to ensure that the medication is injected into muscle tissue. The injection site should not be massaged.

Risk Factors

Two specific risks warrant consideration:

1. **Cardiovascular risk:** This is an area of ongoing research. Although the use of Depo-Provera carries none of the estrogen related cardiovascular risks. Use of Depo-Provera does not elevate blood pressure, the progestin has the potential for adversely affecting blood lipids and glucose metabolism (Hatcher et al., 1994). Studies thus far have been inconclusive and further research is needed to clarify this issue. This will be particularly important as this method becomes more popular for women over 35 years of age.

2. **Cancer:** Stenchever (1996) reports that the studies that have been done on breast cancer risk and use of Depo-Provera have revealed inconclusive evidence, and more research needs to be done. He notes further that although results of studies with animals have shown an increased risk of breast cancer with Depo-Provera use, this drug acts differently in animals than in humans beings. Thus these study findings cannot be used to predict effects in women.

Contraindications

The contraindications to use of Depo-Provera include the following (Hatcher et al., 1994):

• Pregnancy

• Acute liver disease or liver tumor

• Undiagnosed vaginal bleeding

• Active thromboembolic disease

• Breast cancer

Other Possible Contraindications

Depending on the protocol of the facility, other possible contraindications could include the following (Hatcher et al., 1994):

- History of depression
- Seizure disorder (with treatment with phenytoin [Dilantin])
- Diabetes
- Hypertension
- Active gallbladder disease
- History of heart attack or stroke

Effectiveness

According to Hatcher and colleagues (1994), Depo-Provera is an extremely effective method of birth control, with failure rates of less than 1%. One of every 300–400 women receiving Depo-Provera will become pregnant.

Side Effects

One of the disadvantages of Depo-Provera use is that any side effects that do occur have to be endured for the duration of the drug's activity in the body. There is no antidote to Depo-Provera. In addition to depression, headaches, nervousness and fatigue, two common side effects are menstrual irregularities and weight gain:

1. **Disruption of the menstrual cycle:** This is the most common side effect of Depo-Provera therapy. With continued use of Depo-Provera, most women cease to have periods altogether or have occasional spotting. Some women have excessive or irregular bleeding that needs to be managed with hormone therapy or nonsteroidal antiinflammatory drugs such as ibuprofen (Hatcher et al., 1994).

2. **Weight gain:** Depo-Provera seems to cause an increase in appetite. Most women do gain some weight, which is not fluid retention. This is usually about 5 pounds the first year, increasing to 8 pounds after 2 years and 14 pounds after 4 years (Hatcher et al., 1994).

3. **Mood alterations:** Depo-Provera has been found to exacerbate depression in some women and should not be given to women with a history of depression.

Other less common side effects include insomnia, breast tenderness, hair loss, bloating, nausea, acne, and hot flashes (Hatcher et al., 1994).

Reproductive Effects

It can take between 9 and 14 months for a woman to conceive after stopping Depo-Provera therapy. Her menstrual cycles may take 6 months or longer to return to a normal pattern (Hatcher et al., 1994). At 2 years after discontinuation, pregnancy rates are the same as those for non–Depo-Provera users (Stenchever, 1996).

Lactation Effects

Depo-Provera does not inhibit lactation, so it is considered a good birth control method for lactating women. It is, however, detectable in breast milk (Stenchever, 1996).

Bone Density Effects

The following discussion on the bone density effects of Depo-Provera is gleaned from an article published in the January 1998 issue of *Contraceptive Technology Update:* "Depo-Provera and Bone Density."

Because Depo-Provera does not contain estrogen and it suppresses normal estrogen production by the body, bone density loss can occur during use. This is of concern especially for young women, whose bone density is increasing during the teenage years (*Depo-Provera and Bone Density,* 1998).

There are many questions to be answered in the area of bone density effects. It is known that bone density decreases during use of Depo-Provera. However, what occurs when Depo-Provera is discontinued? Does bone density return to pre-drug initiation levels for all populations? Are their differences associated with long-term vs. short-term use? How does Depo-Provera affect the teen-age population or the population over age 35 year?

Presently, clinicians are keeping a cautious eye on the subject. In light of this concern, some practitioners are delaying giving Depo-Provera to teen-agers who have not completed at least 2 years of regular menstrual cycles. Calcium supplements are recommended for women, especially teen-agers who are receiving Depo-Provera. Regular exercise, which promotes and maintains bone density, is also advised. Some health care practitioners are considering adding some form of estrogen (oral or transdermal patch) for those women receiving Depo-Provera who are at an especially high risk for bone loss because of family history or other risk factors. More research is needed to clarify this issue.

> *Notes to the reader:* One cannot help but have some concern that the normal menstrual cycle is being profoundly disrupted in women who use Depo-Provera as a contraceptive method. What does this mean for the long-term health of women? As has been discussed previously, hormones have profound effects on many organs and tissues in the body, including various centers in the brain. The hormonal methods of birth control are an experiment women are participating in worldwide. It is not known as yet what price is being paid in terms of long-term health, nor what the long-term benefits might be, for use of this effective and convenient birth control method.

Norplant System

Levonorgestrel (Norplant System) is a set of 6 matchstick-sized hormone-containing capsules made of flexible tubing. It is implanted just beneath the skin of the upper inner aspect of the arm, with use of a local anesthetic. The implant uses a synthetic progestin, which becomes effective 24 hours after the capsules are placed. The implants contain no estrogen and continue to release progestin and provide protection for 5 years, at which time they need to be removed. The Norplant System was approved by the FDA in 1990, and it has been used worldwide since the early 1980s (Hatcher et al., 1994).

Advantages

Norplant is a very effective birth control method. It can be reversed by removal of the implanted rods. It holds the advantage of requiring no "daily maintenance," and may be a good method for women who have a difficult time remembering to take a pill or have poor compliance when using a barrier method (Stenchever, 1996).

Contraindications

The contraindications to the use of the Norplant System include the following (Stenchever, 1996):

- Active thrombophlebitis or thromboembolic disease
- Undiagnosed vaginal bleeding
- Acute liver disease
- Benign or undiagnosed liver tumors
- Suspected pregnancy
- Known or suspected breast cancer

Effectiveness

Hatcher and associates (1994) note that during the first year after insertion, statistics show only one pregnancy in 500 users. The Norplant System loses effectiveness as the 5-year mark approaches.

Side Effects

As with Depo-Provera, the menstrual bleeding pattern is disrupted and irregular bleeding is common with the Norplant System (Hatcher et al., 1994). Other side effects include headache, infection at the site of insertion, weight gain, breast tenderness, acne, and mood changes. There can be difficulty in removal because fibrous tissue tends to develop around the capsules (Stenchever, 1996).

Study findings have shown that women who do continue to have a normal menstrual cycle with the implant have a higher risk of pregnancy because they may continue to ovulate regularly (Stenchever, 1996). In those women who continue to ovulate, growth of extra follicles may occur. These growths are similar to ovarian cysts and may twist or rupture, requiring surgery. However, most disappear on their own without intervention.

Reproductive Effects

After removal of the system, regular menstruation usually returns within 30 days. The hormone is no longer detectable within 2 days after removal, and pregnancy rates are comparable to those in nonusers (Stenchever, 1996).

Emergency Contraceptive Pill (ECP)

Also called the morning after pill (MAP) or postcoital contraception, the ECP is a form of emergency contraception. It is not considered to be a method of birth control, but is to be used after a contraceptive accident or an incident of unprotected intercourse.

For best effectiveness, the ECP should be initiated within 72 hours after intercourse, although some practitioners are extending this time a bit in individual cases. After ruling out an existing pregnancy, certain formulations of birth control pills are prescribed according to a specific protocol, given in two doses spaced 12 hours apart. The ECP may delay menses slightly. If no menses occurs within 3 weeks, the client needs to return for a pregnancy test (Hatcher et al., 1994).

Method Of Action

The ECP works by changing the chemical balance of the reproductive system, preventing either fertilization or implantation.

Risks

The ECPs are safe for most women. Women with common reasons for avoiding combined pills as an ongoing contraceptive can safely take pills as an emergency contraceptive. This applies to the following women (Hatcher, 1998):

- Women who are
  - older than 35 years of age who smoke
  - diabetic and have vascular disease
- Women with a history of
  - severe migraines
  - thromboembolism
- Women with benign or malignant liver tumors

Contraindications

The use of the ECP is contraindicated in the presence of severe migraines with neurologic impairment.

Effectiveness

The ECP is about 97% effective (Stenchever, 1996).

Side Effects

Minimal side effects occasionally occur, including breast tenderness, headaches, nausea, or vomiting.

Intrauterine Devices (IUDs)

Intrauterine devices are small plastic devices that are inserted into the uterus. Depending on the type, they also contain copper or a type of progestin. A string is tied to the device, and this string extends through the cervix and into the vagina just an inch or so.

History

The first forms of IUDs, centuries ago, were pebbles inserted into the uteruses of camels, so they would not get pregnant during long journeys (Boston Women's Health Book Collective, 1992). No one understands exactly how the IUD works. It is thought that the uterus has a foreign-body response. It sends white blood cells and a variety of chemicals to the site, which interferes with sperm transport and survival and thus changes the uterine environment. The presence of the IUD may affect the egg itself by slowing down the activity of the fallopian tubes. The hormone-containing IUDs prevent buildup of the uterine lining. Study findings have revealed an absence of fertilized eggs in women who use IUDs, which indicates that the method seems to exert its effects before fertilization rather than by preventing implantation (Stenchever, 1996).

The IUD has had an unfortunate history in the United States. Introduced in the 1960's they rapidly gained popularity because they provided women with a highly effective and "carefree" and cost effective method of birth control. However, the safety of the IUD has always been a controversial issue. The FDA withdrew several IUD's from the market because of a high incidence of serious side effects. The Dalkon Shield, the most well-known of the IUD's taken off the market, resulted in ten maternal deaths due to midtrimester septic abortion. Several others were removed from production as well because of the serious side effects of increased incidence of uterine perforation, strangulated bowels, and tendency to embed within the uterine wall. Another IUD, the Lippes Loop was taken off the market by its manufacturer after two national studies published in 1985 reported an increased incidence of pelvic inflammatory disease and subsequent tubal infertility compared with other IUD's. Another factor which contributed to complications among IUD users was the widespread practice in the 1960's of having multiple sexual partners, thus increasing the risk of sexually transmitted infections which often lead to pelvic inflammatory disease. The popularity of the IUD of course plummeted as a result of these serious complications, and most of the remaining IUD's were taken off the market due to falling profits (Lichtman and Papera, 1990).

A second generation of IUD's have been reintroduced, constructed so as to minimize the chances of infection. These devices are considered an excellent contraceptive choice for women who are not at risk for contracting a sexually transmitted infection. The Copper T-380A or Paraguard is a T-shaped device containing copper, which creates an inhospitable environment for egg and sperm. It is effective for 10 years. The Progestasert is also T shaped, and contains a progestin which thickens cervical mucous and may also reduce cramping and bleeding during menses (which may increase with IUD use). The Progestasert needs to be replaced each year (Lichtman and Papera, 1990).

Risk Factors and Contraindications

Practitioners are advised to screen clients carefully for risk factors and contraindications. Contraindications include active pelvic infection, as well as known or suspected gonorrhea or chlamydial infection or pregnancy.

Protocols vary from one agency to another. Other conditions in which the IUD is often contraindicated include the following (Hawkins, Roberto & Stanley-Haney, 1993):

- Multiple sexual partners
- Recent or recurrent pelvic infection
- Abnormal uterine bleeding
- Impaired immune response (related to diabetes, steroid therapy, HIV infection)
- Allergy to copper
- Abnormal Pap smear findings
- Valvular heart disease
- Cervical or uterine malignancy
- Fibroids or other uterine abnormality
- History of ectopic pregnancy

Effectiveness

According to Hatcher and colleagues (1994), perfect use and typical use failure rates with the IUD are almost identical. They note that the rate of accidental pregnancy in the first year of use for women who use the Progestasert IUD is 2.0% with typical use and 1.5% with perfect use. For women who use the Copper T-380A, the first year failure rate for typical use is 0.8%, with that for perfect use being 0.6%.

Side Effects

Some women have heavier periods or more cramps while using this method. Clients should be taught to watch for signs of infection, as well as to check the length of the string after each menstrual period (Stenchever, 1996). The string length is the means to determine that the IUD has remained in its proper placement and has not receded up into the uterus nor has become partially expelled. Any changes in string length should be reported immediately to the healthcare provider.

Infection

The highest risk of infection with an IUD is during the first 3 months of use, because of bacteria entering the uterine cavity at the time of insertion (Stenchever, 1996). Serious pelvic infection (PID) can cause infertility.

The infection rate is low. Study findings show 1.38 per 1,000 women per year contract PID (Hatcher et al., 1994).

Pregnancy

If a woman does get pregnant with an IUD in place, the risk of ectopic pregnancy (tubal pregnancy) is great (Stenchever, 1996). Lack of menstrual period in a woman who uses this method of contraception should be evaluated immediately. In rare cases the IUD punctures through the uterine wall during insertion (perforation). It is also rare for an IUD to become embedded in the wall of the uterus (Hatcher et al., 1994). Spontaneous expulsion occurs in 2%–10% of IUD users and is most likely to occur during the first few months after insertion (Hatcher et al., 1994). Women need to be taught to check their string regularly.

BARRIER METHODS

As Hatcher and colleagues (1994) note, in contrast to hormonal birth control methods barrier methods do not alter the physiology of the menstrual cycle. In addition, barrier methods, some more than others, offer protection against not only unwanted pregnancy but also STIs. Proper and consistent use of these methods is the key to contraceptive effectiveness. As will be evident from the effectiveness rates, there is a big difference in effectiveness between typical use and perfect use. Therefore, a crucial role for nurses is education of clients on the correct use of these methods appropriate to age, prior experience, culture, and educational level, with adequate time for demonstration and practice.

Condoms

As noted by Stenchever (1996), surprisingly widespread approval of condom use in the United States is a relatively new occurrence. In fact, their sale was outlawed by Congress in 1873. In some states it was a criminal offense for one person to inform another that use of a condom might prevent pregnancy. Similar laws remained in effect in some states until 1975.

Male Condoms

There are three types of male condoms currently on the market: latex, lambskin, and polyurethane. The polyurethane condom has been approved by the FDA for use only by people who are allergic to latex (Hatcher et al., 1994). Both the latex and the polyurethane condoms prevent transmission of viruses; the lambskin condom does not (Stenchever, 1996). The market is currently exploding with creative condom variations, including lubricated and nonlubricated (usually with a spermicide), contoured, ribbed, colored, and flavored ones.

The polyurethane condom (Avanti) has recently been reformulated in response to the high breakage rates associated with its use (four times those of latex condoms). It is thicker and stronger, but it is still approved for use only by clients who are allergic to latex. This condom may gain wider approval when more studies have been done to determine its effectiveness. One advantage of this condom is that it can be used with oil-based lubricants, whereas latex condoms will deteriorate quickly with oil-based products and must be used only with water-based lubricants.

Effectiveness: Typical use of latex condoms shows a failure rate of 12% in the first year; with perfect use, 3% in the first year (Hatcher et al., 1994).

Proper Use: Hatcher and colleagues (1994) provide the following tips for proper use of the male condom:

- Never use oil-based lubricants (e.g., household oils or massage oils) because they quickly break down the latex.

- Remove air from the reservoir tip before application.

- After ejaculation, withdraw the penis before an erection is lost, by holding the base of the condom to prevent leakage.

- If breakage occurs, call a clinic for emergency contraception.

- Never reuse a condom.

Female condom ("Reality")

Approved by the FDA in 1993, Reality is a prelubricated sheath made of polyurethane. It is inserted vaginally up to 8 hours before intercourse.

The female condom provides a physical barrier that completely lines the vagina and partially shields the perineum. The soft, loose-fitting sheath contains two flexible polyurethane rings. One ring is placed inside, at the closed end of the sheath. The other ring remains outside the vagina, providing protection to the woman's labia and base of the man's penis during intercourse (Hatcher et al., 1994).

The sheath is prelubricated on the inside. The lubricant is dimethicone, which is not a spermicide but is commonly used in the medical field as a skin protectant.

Advantages: The main advantages of the female condom barrier method are that it offers the protection from pregnancy and STIs of the male condom, but it is controlled by the woman (Stenchever, 1996). The female condom also offers more protection for both men and women because more of the female external genitalia are covered. This may offer added protection against transmission of herpes or genital warts (*The Female Condom*, 1997).

Reality can be used if one of the partners has a latex allergy. There have been no reported alterations in vaginal flora, nor irritation to the urinary tract, associated with its use (*The Female Condom*, 1997). Both are common in diaphragm users.

Effectiveness: In preventing pregnancy, the effectiveness of Reality has been shown to be comparable to other barrier methods with consistent and correct use. In addition, results of laboratory studies have shown that it is an effective barrier to viral transmission of known STIs (*The Female Condom*, 1997). In these studies the hepatitis B virus, actually one-fourth the size of the HIV virus, was blocked by the female condom.

Results of one study (*The Female Condom*, 1997) that tested leakage after use showed that the female condom had a 0.6% leakage rate, whereas the male condom had a 3.5% rate. The female condom showed superiority over the male condom in terms of tears and breaks. The female condom also proved superior in a study (*The Female Condom*, 1997) comparing spillage of semen for both types of condoms. An estimated 97% reduction in risk of HIV infection with correct and consistent use was reported in another study (*The Female Condom*, 1997). The female condom rates favorably overall as an acceptable and effective barrier method.

FIGURE 5-1

REALITY
Female Condom Insertion & Positioning

1. Inner ring is squeezed for insertion

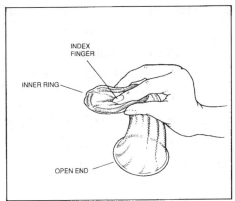

INDEX FINGER

INNER RING

OPEN END

3. Inner ring is pushed up as far as it can go with index finger

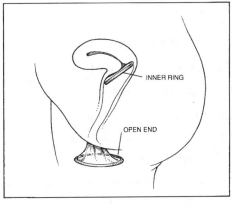

INNER RING

OPEN END

2. Sheath is inserted, similarly to a tampon

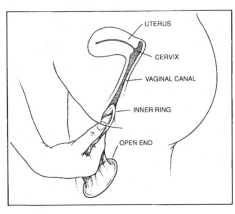

UTERUS

CERVIX

VAGINAL CANAL

INNER RING

OPEN END

4. REALITY in place

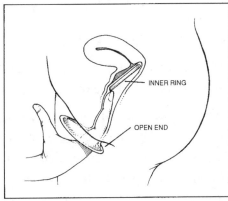

INNER RING

OPEN END

Source: REALITY® female condom, The Female Health Company, 875 N. Michigan Ave., Suite 3660, Chicago, IL 60611; http://www.femalehealth.com.

Three studies have been completed to date that measure the contraceptive efficacy of the female condom (Leeper & Stein, 1998). The most recent study was completed in Japan, and results show a probability of becoming pregnant within 6 months of less than 1% during perfect use and approximately 3% during typical (inconsistent and sometimes incorrect) use. The study that was done in the United States to support the application for approval by the FDA revealed a somewhat higher accidental pregnancy rate in the first 6 months of perfect use of 2.6%, with 12.4% for typical use. A third study completed in England revealed a somewhat higher pregnancy rate of 15% for typical use.

Proper Use: The female condom may take some practice to insert (see *Figure 5-1*) and use correctly. Clients should practice insertion before using it for sexual intercourse. One problem is that the outer ring can be pushed inside the vagina during sex. Use of more lubricant usually solves this problem. The penis can slip to the side of the device during insertion and may have to be guided into the vagina.

With some practice, the female condom is hardly noticeable, and its loose-fitting construction allows more comfort and sensitivity for the male partner.

The following tips on use of the female

condom can be helpful for clients (*REALITY® Female Condom,* 1997):

- Use the female condom every time sex occurs.

- Use a new condom with each sex act.

- Do not use a male and female condom at the same time.

- Use more lubricant as needed.

- Use care in handling; be careful of jagged fingernails or rings that could tear the condom.

Cost: The female condom is more expensive than the male condom, on average $2 per condom. Many state-funded programs that pay for male condoms also cover the female condom, making this an affordable option for many clients of low income.

Spermicidal Preparations

Hatcher and colleagues (1994) provide the following review on spermicides.

Unfortunately, spermicidal preparations are often used without the addition of another barrier method, resulting in a higher failure rate. Ideal use is as an adjunct to other barrier methods. These preparations consist of a spermicide (usually nonoxynol-9) in a base of foam, cream, or jelly. Contact allergy to these products is the main side effect. New on the market is a contraceptive film that is folded and placed against the cervix at least 5 minutes before intercourse. It melts and adheres to the surface of the cervix.

Hatcher and colleagues (1994) note further that spermicidal preparations have been shown to alter normal vaginal flora and can make a woman more prone to vaginal infections. Recent study findings have also indicated that some women have a reaction to spermicides, resulting in irritation of the vaginal mucosa. This can compromise the integrity of the lining of the vagina and make it easier for viral infections, allowing viruses such as HIV to enter the blood stream.

Diaphragm

A soft, dome-shaped device with a firm rim, the diaphragm is inserted up to 6 hours before intercourse and holds spermicidal jelly up against the cervix. It must be left in for 8 hours after the last intercourse. If intercourse occurs more than once, the diaphragm is not to be removed, and another dose of spermicide is to be inserted into the vagina with each intercourse (Hatcher et al., 1994).

There are several types of diaphragms available. Some are made with latex, and some are made with silicon. Diaphragms can be cared for easily by washing them in warm soapy water and drying them before storage. The client needs to inspect the diaphragm before each use by checking for holes. The diaphragm should be refitted after a weight gain or loss of 10 pounds or after pregnancy and birth. The diaphragm does confer some protection against STIs, and results of studies have shown that cervical cancer rates are decreased in users of this method (Hatcher et al., 1994).

Effectiveness

With perfect use, there is a 6% failure rate. With typical use, 18% of users will get pregnant in a year (Hatcher et al., 1994).

Side Effects

Diaphragms can cause irritation to the lower urinary tract, increasing the client's susceptibility to bladder infection. They have been shown to alter the normal vaginal flora, which can make a woman more prone to vaginal infections.

Cervical Cap

Stenchever (1996) has provided an informative review on the cervical cap. He notes that it makes sense to cover the cervix to prevent pregnancy; women have done so since ancient times. In the Mediterranean, half a lemon filled with honey was placed over the cervix as birth control. In modern days, a cup-shaped latex device that fits directly over the cervix has been developed. This device

FIGURE 5-2 *1 of 2*
Insertion of the Cervical Cap

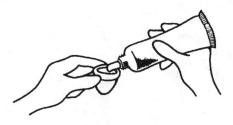

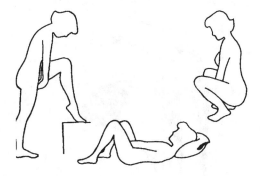

FIG. I
Fill cap 1/3 full with spermicidal cream/jelly

FIG. II
Prepare to insert the cap by squatting, lying down or standing with one leg up on a stool. In addition, bear down as though having a bowel movement.

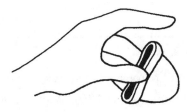

FIG. III
Fold cap and hold between fingers of one hand. Gently part lips of the vagina and insert cap into the vagina.

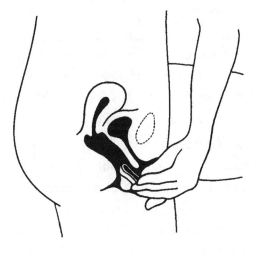

FIG. IV
Hold cap pinching the sides together. Reach back to place cap on the cervix.

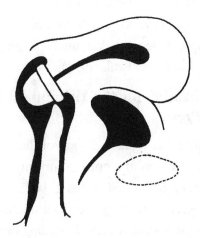

FIG. V
Check placement of the cap with index and middle finger. The cervix should be completely covered by the cap. The dome should feel soft with some dimpling.

Source: Gallagher, D. M. & Richwald, G. A. (1989). *Fitting the cervical cap: A handbook for clinicians.* Los Gatos, CA: Cervical Cap Ltd.

FIGURE 5-2 *2 of 2*
Insertion of the Cervical Cap

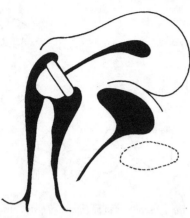

FIG. VI
Feel the cervix underneath the dome. Press gently on the dome to dimple it and apply suction/ seal. Next spin the cap one quarter turn to increase the seal.

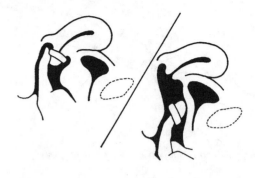

FIG. VII
To remove the cap, tip the side with the index finger to break the seal, then gently pull cap down and out.

has been used successfully in Europe for many years, and it was finally approved for use in the United States by the FDA in 1988, after much lobbying by women's health organizations.

Stenchever (1996) notes that the cervical cap is more difficult to fit than a diaphragm because proper fit depends on the angle of the cervix and uterus (see *Figure 5-2),* and the device is only available in four sizes in the United States. It offers the advantage of minimal spermicide use (a small amount is placed in the cup), and it can be left in place for 48–72 hours (convenient if the client is going camping, for example), although this can cause some cervical irritation. The cap must be left in a minimum of 8 hours after the last intercourse. With multiple intercourse, there is no need to insert more spermicidal jelly as with the diaphragm.

Contraindications

Contraindications to use of the cervical cap include history of toxic shock syndrome, abnormal Pap smear findings, or allergy to latex.

Effectiveness

For nulliparous women, with 1 year of typical use the failure rate is 18%. With 1 year of perfect use the failure rate is 9% (Hatcher et al., 1994).

Side Effects

The cap has the potential to irritate the cervix, especially if it is left in frequently for the maximum time limit. Because of this, a part of the protocol for cervical cap fit is normal Pap smear findings. A second Pap smear 3 months later is advised (Hatcher et al., 1994).

Sterilization for the Woman (Tubal Ligation)

The tubal ligation is one of the most popular methods of contraception currently favored by women in the United States as well as worldwide. Considered permanent, reversal of this procedure has varying success rates depending on the method used, the age of the woman, and the length of the remaining tubes. Overall, sterilization is one of the safest, most economic, and effective birth control methods available to women who have completed child bearing (Hatcher et al., 1994).

The decision to become sterile is often not made easily. There are often strong feelings involved. Clients need correct information, a chance to air their feelings, and a complete discussion of the pros and cons of this procedure and other birth control methods.

According to Lichtman and Papera (1990), federal sterilization regulations were passed in 1979 to stop sterilization abuse. This was spearheaded by feminist and health activists in response to abusive practices such as performing sterilization without the woman's knowledge of its permanence. Other abuse situations included threatening to stop welfare benefits or obtaining consent under duress of labor or birth. The federal guidelines apply only to federally funded programs, however. These include that

- consent must be obtained by someone other than the physician performing the procedure.

- the client must be informed of the irreversible nature of the procedure.

- other birth control options must be explained.

- there is a 30-day waiting period required after signing of the consent for the performance of the procedure.

Counseling Tips for Couples Considering Sterilization

Lichtman and Papera (1990) have provided the following suggestions to help couples gain clarity about their decision to choose sterilization:

- Look for women who are at risk of regretting the decision; that is, women

  — who have given very little thought to their decision.

  — who have made the decision alone.

  — who show indications of being under pressure from others.

  — who are currently under a great deal of personal stress.

- Consider patterns of previous decision making. Does the client usually stick to decisions made or regret and reverse them?

- Propose situations for client consideration that might help clarify the choice. Examples include

  — death of children.

  — change of spouse.

  — death of spouse.

Techniques

There are a number of techniques used, all involving blocking the fallopian tube so the ovum and sperm cannot meet (Hatcher et al., 1994). These techniques include electrocautery, clips, rings, and removal of a part of the tube. Usually female sterilization is done under local anesthesia as a laparoscopy. It usually is an outpatient procedure and takes less than an hour. Most women resume normal activity in 2–4 days. Less frequently, sterilization is performed under general anesthesia as a minilaparotomy. Surgeons are experimenting with performing this surgery through the cervix (Hatcher et al., 1994). Tubal ligation can be performed during a cesarean section, after vaginal delivery, after abortion, or at a time unrelated to pregnancy or its termination (Hatcher et al., 1994).

Complications

Recovery is most often uneventful, with mild discomfort at the incision site or mild abdominal and shoulder pain due to the gas used in the surgery to inflate the abdomen. More serious complications are rare and include infection, hemorrhage, and anesthesia-related complications. Death is extremely rare. Long-term complications include the failure of sterilization, resulting in pregnancy (with a high rate of ectopic pregnancy)—as well as scarring and adhesions, which can result in pelvic pain (Stenchever, 1996). Some women report changes in their menstrual cycles or painful periods. No explanation has been found as yet for these problems.

Effectiveness

A failure to prevent pregnancy occurs in only 0.4% of women in the first year (Hatcher et al., 1994).

Sterilization for the Man

Male sterilization or vasectomy is more effective, less expensive, and safer than female sterilization. It is technically easier to perform with local anesthesia, generally as an outpatient procedure.

The vas deferens is blocked by tying, cutting, cautery, or mechanical plugs to prevent sperm passage. Reversal has functional success rates in the range of 16%–79%, depending on type of procedure, time interval between original surgery and reversal, and presence of sperm antibodies (Hatcher et al., 1994).

FUTURE BIRTH CONTROL METHODS

Hatcher and colleagues (1994) provide a thorough discussion on the wave of the future for birth control methods. The following information, with the exception of the section on injectables, is gleaned from their discussion. The comments on injectables are based on an article published in the January 1998 issue of *Contraceptive Technology Update*. The reader is referred to both sources for more in-depth information.

New methods of birth control are being researched in both public and private sectors with several goals in mind:

- Creating female-controlled methods that protect against both pregnancy and STIs

- Improving hormone-delivery systems to lessen bleeding disruption, which occurs frequently with progestin-only methods

- Reducing costs of hormonal birth control methods

- Continuing research on birth control vaccines for both men and women

- Creating birth control methods that are easier to use and have reduced side effects

Mechanical Barrier Methods

Four mechanical barrier methods are either on the market or soon to be released:

1. Lea's Shield, a one-size-fits-all diaphragm-like device

2. Femcap, a cervical cap-like barrier method, which is available in several sizes

3. Disposable diaphragm, a throwaway version of the diaphragm that releases the spermicide nonoxynol-9

4. Polyurethane condoms, which are already on the market and being improved to reduce breakage and slippage rates

Chemical Barrier Methods

Research in the area of chemical barrier methods is focusing on development of new spermicidal-delivery systems, which would improve spreadability and cohesiveness for better protection against STIs and pregnancy. Alternatives to nonoxynol-9 are being researched, which might lessen the irritation to vaginal tissue associated with nonoxynol-9.

Hormonal Methods

Research on hormonal methods is focusing on the development of (1) new forms of synthetic progesterone, which are longer acting, and (2) new delivery systems, including implants, vaginal rings, creams, suppositories, and injectables.

Implants

The following three implants are in development:

1. Implanon, a single progestin implant effective for 2–3 years

2. Norplant II, an improved version of the Norplant System that contains two rods instead of six

3. Biodegradable implants, in which the carrier of the hormone degrades in the body and does not need to be removed

Vaginal Rings

Vaginal rings are another form of hormone-delivery system being tested. Some contain a progestin only; some are a combination of estrogen and a progestin.

Injectables

The World Health Organization is testing a number of injectables, including longer acting progestins and combinations of estrogen and progestins. One such injectable is Cyclo-Provera. It contains both a synthetic estrogen and progesterone, and it looks promising that it will be approved by the FDA.

Male Hormonal Methods

Also under investigation are hormone-delivery systems for men with the use of synthetic forms of testosterone. Forms include injectables and implants.

IUDs

New IUDs are being studied, some of which contain a progestin. Devices, called "frameless" IUDs, are being researched that have structures that eliminate pressure on the uterine wall. One such device is a biodegradable cone.

Vaccines

In development are vaccines for both men and women. These vaccines act by either preventing implantation or inhibiting fertilization in women or by preventing sperm production in men.

SUGGESTIONS FOR CONTRACEPTIVE EDUCATION AND COUNSELING

The health care provider can apply the following strategies in educating and counseling clients on contraceptive use:

- Begin a counseling session by assessing clients' current knowledge of, level of prior experience with, and misconceptions about birth control methods. Peers are most young clients' primary source of knowledge about sex and contraception.

- Ask questions; find out what clients want to know.

- Explore with clients their individual needs, prior experiences, lifestyle factors, frequency of intercourse, situations in which intercourse usually occurs, confidentiality issues, number of partners, cultural and religious beliefs, and motivating factors.

- Present the pros and cons of each method.

- Present questions and situations for clients to consider. Help clients think through how they might react to various situations. Role play. For example, have clients consider that if their parents do not know they are using the pill, where are they going to keep it so they will be sure to take it every day? Or, if they only have intercourse once or twice a month, do they think they will remember to take the pill every day?

- Work with clients to problem solve creatively. For example, consider that if they think they might have sex on a date, why don't they insert the diaphragm or female condom before they go? Advise clients to take a condom with them, not to depend on their partners to remember theirs. Or, if they only have sex at their boyfriend's house, will they remember to have the diaphragm with them? Why not keep one diaphragm at the partner's house and carry one or keep one at home?

- Follow up with clients to evaluate effectiveness and use of the method. Be sure to have the client contact you if she is experiencing any side effects and is considering not using her method, or if she is finding that she is not being consistent.

- Promote self-responsibility; encourage decision-making skills.

- Encourage clients' partners to be involved.

- Be nonjudgmental in working with young clients. Health care providers who have attitudes and judgments about what is right and wrong for their clients will not be able to be open enough to tune into their needs. If health care providers believe that sex is wrong before a certain age or before marriage, they really cannot be effective in providing services for this age group. Health care providers need constantly to examine their biases and beliefs.

PREGNANCY TERMINATION

Pregnancy termination can be spontaneous (miscarriage) or induced (abortion). Termination of an unwanted pregnancy has been legal in the United States since 1973. Procedures performed after the first trimester are subject to individual state law.

The issue of abortion provokes strong feelings in most people, either pro or con. The issues involved are deeply personal ones and need to be accorded due respect. Health care providers need to consider the issues involved and come to their own conclusions, present accurate information, and provide nonjudgmental counseling and supportive care for clients having abortion procedures.

An Historical Perspective

Lichtman and Papera (1990) describe several events that have led to the modern state of pregnancy termination.

Throughout history women in all cultures have used abortion as a solution to unwanted pregnancy. Before the late 1800s abortion was not addressed in U. S. law, but by 1880 every state had passed some kind of abortion law. During the 100 or so years during which pregnancy termination was not legislated, abortion remained an option mostly for economically privileged women, deemed necessary by the medical establishment for the woman's physical or psychologic health. It was socially acceptable because the decision to terminate the pregnancy was made by the physician, not the woman. Abortion law reform came gradually state by state until 1973 when the Supreme Court ruled on the test case, *Roe v. Wade.* The ruling states that during the first 3 months of pregnancy the decision to abort could be made by the woman and her physician without interference of the state. After the first trimester, states could impose their own regulations. This resulted in an immediate decrease in mortality from illegal abortion from approximately 39.3 during the 5-year period 1972–1976 to 0 in 1979. Abortion-related morbidity also greatly decreased.

Preabortion Counseling

There are a number of areas that need to be addressed when a woman finds out she has an unintended pregnancy. Crucial to the process is a nonjudgmental person with whom to explore feelings. Each woman has different needs (Lichtman & Papera, 1990):

- The woman must be helped to deal with her feelings. Accidental pregnancy often triggers a reassessment of a woman's entire life-goals. Most often there are feelings of being overwhelmed. Women may need time to process their feelings before they are ready to receive more information. More than one visit may be necessary.

- There should be a thorough discussion of options, including adoption and the different kinds of abortion procedures appropriate for the woman's situation.

- Pregnancy confirmation paper work should be completed to obtain state aid for the woman as needed for the procedure.

- The woman should be prepared for the abortion, including being told what to expect during the abortion procedure itself, discomforts, medication options, safety, risks and complications, and information on self-care after the procedure.

- The woman needs to know that ultimately the decision must be hers and for her own reasons.

- Some women delay seeking pregnancy confirmation because of irregular menses, denial, lack of knowledge about normal cycles, lack of access to abortion services, lack of knowledge about options, and cost.

Abortion Procedures

Study findings have revealed that abortion procedures performed in a physician's office with the use of local anesthesia have a lower complication rate and are more cost effective than procedures performed in a hospital for first and early second trimester abortions (Stenchever, 1996). Initial screening is important to rule out problems, such as bleeding disorders or cardiac problems, that might warrant an inhospital procedure. A urine human chorionic gonadotropin level, hematocrit, and Rh typing are done before the procedure. Counseling is followed by the client's giving informed consent. The type of procedure depends on the length of the pregnancy.

Vacuum Aspiration With or Without Curettage

Vacuum aspiration with or without curettage is the most common method used for first trimester and early second trimester abortion procedures. Common practice for women at 10 weeks or more, is to use a sterile piece of seaweed called *Laminaria japonica* or in some cases a synthetic dilator, which is inserted into the cervix the day before the abortion procedure (Lichtman & Papera, 1990). It absorbs moisture from the body fluids and expands, slowly dilating the cervix and softening it, so the procedure is easier and accomplished more safely (Lichtman & Papera, 1990). Some providers offer prophylactic antibiotic therapy. The procedure generally lasts 2–3 minutes, after which clients are escorted to an after-care room where vital signs and bleeding are monitored for 15–30 minutes, self-care instructions are given, and a 2-week follow-up visit is scheduled. Clients who are Rh negative receive an injection of immune anti-D globulin (RhoGAM) to prevent blood incompatibility problems in future pregnancies.

Dilation and Evacuation

According to Lichtman and Papera (1990) for the second trimester (i.e., 13 weeks and longer) dilation and evacuation (D&E) is the safest abortion method. This method combines dilation, suction and curettage, and possibly use of forceps. Dilation and evacuation is also the safest up to 20 weeks and has major advantages over the older techniques. Use of *Laminaria japonica* is essential to prepare the cervix adequately, greatly decreasing the risk of uterine perforation.

Labor Induction

Lichtman and Papera (1990) note that another method for pregnancies that are in late second trimester or longer (after 16 weeks) is labor induction. This method involves an injection of saline or prostaglandin into the amniotic fluid surrounding the fetus. This provokes uterine contractions and expels the fetus and placenta from the uterus. This procedure is usually done in the hospital with medications to ease the discomfort of labor and delivery. A short hospital stay may be recommended.

Medical/Chemical Abortion

Methotrexate/Misoprostol

Schaff, Eisinger, Franks & Kim (1996) describe the use of methotrexate and misoprostol in early abortion. Administration of these drugs as an abortion method is appropriate for women whose pregnancies are at 4–8 weeks. After a vaginal sonogram is performed to confirm pregnancy and date of conception, an injection of methotrexate is given. This drug is approved by the FDA, but not specifically for this use. According to FDA regulations, drugs can be used for a purpose other than that for which they received original approval. Methotrexate is a drug that stops rapidly growing cells, and it is used in chemotherapy and the treatment of other conditions. The woman is advised not to eat specific foods high in the B vitamin folate, which interferes with the action of the drug.

Schaff and colleagues (1996) note that 1 week later, the woman returns to the clinic. Tablets of a prostaglandin, misoprostol, are inserted into her vagina, placed near the cervix, and held in place with a tampon. The prostaglandin tablets induce contractions of the uterus to expel the contents of the uterus. She remains supine for 30 minutes, at which time she can return home and is asked to recline. She is given prescriptions for acetaminophen with codeine and prochlorperazine (Compazine) to use as needed for cramping and nausea. Usually within 1–3 hours, she proceeds to have a miscarriage, often accompanied by a large degree of cramping, bleeding, and possibly nausea and vomiting. She returns the next day for a sonogram to confirm that her pregnancy has been terminated. If not, the cycle of tablet insertion is repeated, and she returns a week later for another sonogram. If unsuccessful, she can wait up to 3 weeks for the pregnancy to pass on it's own, or have a surgical procedure—protocols depend on the health care setting.

RU486

RU486 is an antiprogestational pill that blocks the action of progesterone on the uterine lining, thus creating an environment in the uterus that is not conducive to implantation (*Medical Abortion,* 1992). Without this hormonal support, implantation and pregnancy are unlikely. With the RU486 procedure, the woman is required to remain at the health care setting for observation and monitoring during the miscarriage. This is a disadvantage logistically, financially, and emotionally. RU486 has been used successfully in other countries but has not yet been approved for use in the United States. Clinical trials are currently in progress (Silvestre et al., 1990).

After-Care for Abortion

Immediate after-care for the client who has undergone an abortion procedure consists of monitoring vital signs and assessing for evidence of bleeding, as well as administering Rho(D) immune globulin to women who are Rh negative. A lower dose of Rho(D) immune globulin is available as MICRhoGAM or MiniDose for abortions at less than 13 weeks (Lichtman & Papera, 1990).

Abortion Complications

Complications can occur with any type of pregnancy termination, including miscarriage. Recovery for first and early second trimester abortion procedures is most often uneventful.

Complications can include the following (Hatcher et al., 1994):

- Missed procedure. This is more common in early pregnancy termination when the embryo is very small and may be missed.

- Retained tissue

- Infection

- Excessive bleeding

- Perforation of the cervix or uterus at the time of the procedure

- Tearing of the cervix

- Allergic reactions to drugs or the anesthetic agent

Offices or clinics in which abortion procedures are performed are required to have an emergency cart on hand and a registered nurse on staff who is familiar with emergency procedures.

Self-Care After an Abortion Procedure

It is normal to experience some bleeding and cramping during the 2 weeks after an abortion procedure. Pregnancy symptoms should subside gradually, although some symptoms such as nausea generally disappear shortly after the procedure. It is also normal to experience emotional ups and downs during this period.

The client should receive instructions on self-care after the procedure. These include the following (Lichtman & Papera, 1990):

- Watch for signs of infection, including fever, chills, smelly discharge, continuous severe abdominal pain, and heavy bleeding.

- Take your temperature daily (call the physician if higher than 38°C [100°F]).

- Do not use tampons until the follow-up visit in 2 weeks.

- Do not put anything in the vagina until after the next check-up—no douching, no baths, no intercourse.

- Avoid lifting or heavy exercise.

- Drink lots of fluids, and eat well to aid the body in recovery.

- Take the full course of any medications prescribed, even if no symptoms are experienced.

Long-Term Effects of Abortion

Misconceptions about the safety of abortion and its long-term effects on fertility are common. Abortion is safer than term delivery. Study findings have shown that fertility is not altered by the abortion procedure itself (Stenchever, 1996). Complications such as infection can result in infertility if not treated in a timely manner.

Study results have shown that the most important factor affecting a woman's reaction to her abortion is the level of support provided by those who are important to her (Lichtman & Papera, 1990). Findings from research over the past 20 years have revealed few long-term psychiatric sequelae to abortion (Lichtman & Papera, 1990). This is not to say that it cannot be an extremely difficult and stressful process for many women.

CONCLUSION

Choosing an appropriate birth control method can be challenging for both client and health care provider. It requires careful consideration of each woman's individual needs and should always include a consideration of preventing STIs. Women who experience an unwanted pregnancy need to be informed fully about their options. If they choose to have an abortion, they need to be informed about the procedures available to them and guided through the process with respect and sensitivity.

EXAM QUESTIONS

CHAPTER 5
Questions 32–44

32. The most common reason why women stop taking their birth control pills is

    a. misunderstanding instructions.

    b. fear of sexually transmitted infections.

    c. side effects.

    d. confidentiality issues with parents.

33. Depo-Provera has no effect on

    a. blood pressure.

    b. mood.

    c. the menstrual cycle.

    d. bone density.

34. Depo-Provera should not be given to women who have a history of

    a. problems with oral contraceptives.

    b. menstrual irregularities.

    c. depression.

    d. sexually transmitted infection.

35. The most common side effect of the Norplant System is

    a. headache.

    b. irregular bleeding.

    c. anxiety.

    d. infection at the implantation site.

36. For the highest level of effectiveness, the emergency contraceptive pill should be taken by the client

    a. between 2 and 36 hours after intercourse.

    b. within 72 hours after intercourse.

    c. 72 hours after intercourse.

    d. any time after intercourse.

37. The greatest danger of infection with the intrauterine device occurs during the

    a. first 3 months after insertion.

    b. first 6 months after insertion.

    c. first year after insertion.

    d. menstrual period.

38. One of the main advantages of the female condom is that it

    a. is less expensive than birth control pills.

    b. does not interfere with the spontaneity of sex.

    c. is controlled by the woman.

    d. can be reused.

39. The only method of birth control that is 100% effective is

    a. the intrauterine device.

    b. abstinence.

    c. sterilization.

    d. Depo-Provera.

40. First trimester and early second trimester surgical abortions can be performed more safely by using

    a. general anesthesia.

    b. local anesthesia.

    c. an intravenous sedative.

    d. no anesthesia.

41. The National Survey of Family Growth (Henshaw, 1998) has found that more than half of women who seek abortion

    a. were not using any birth control method.

    b. were using a birth control method.

    c. never used a birth control method.

    d. used condoms as their birth control method.

42. For surgical abortion procedures, *Laminaria japonica* is used to

    a. dilate the cervix at the time of the procedure.

    b. prevent excessive bleeding.

    c. dilate the cervix before the procedure.

    d. empty the contents of the uterus.

43. During a chemical abortion, the insertion of prostaglandin tablets into the vagina is for the purpose of

    a. inducing contractions of the uterus.

    b. stopping the growth of rapidly dividing cells.

    c. preventing bleeding.

    d. preventing the embryo from attaching to the uterine wall.

44. A woman comes to your facility for counseling to choose a birth control method. You would begin to work with her by first

    a. describing all the different methods on the market.

    b. asking her if she had unprotected sex.

    c. listing the pros and cons of each method.

    d. finding out what she already knows about birth control methods.

CHAPTER 6

INFERTILITY

CHAPTER OBJECTIVE

After completing this chapter, the reader will be able to recognize that the evaluation and treatment of infertility has seen more change in the past two decades than perhaps any other area of women's health. The reader will also be able to identify trends in fertility among women and men, and the process involved in fertility evaluation as well as recognize currently available tests, procedures and new technologies for infertility.

LEARNING OBJECTIVES

After studying this chapter, the reader will be able to

1. define infertility.

2. describe current trends in the incidence of infertility and the probable reasons for these trends.

3. describe the process a couple typically goes through in being evaluated for infertility.

4. explain the definitions of the new technologic procedures.

5. describe the different procedures now available for assisted reproduction.

6. identify psychosocial issues that have an impact on infertile couples.

7. identify resources for women and couples seeking infertility information.

Key Words

- Agglutination
- ARTs
- Assisted hatching
- BBT charting
- DES
- Endometrial biopsy
- GIFT
- HCG (Human Chorionic Gonadotropin)
- ICSI
- Laparoscopy
- Micromanipulation
- PID
- Pituitary desensitization
- Postcoital test
- Semen evaluation
- SPA
- TET
- ZIFT

INTRODUCTION

The proportion of women in the United States between the ages of 15 and 44 years who reported some form of impairment in their fertility rose from 8% in 1988 to 10% in 1995 (Chandra & Stephen, 1998). This represents an increase from

4.6 million to 6.2 million women (Chandra & Stephen, 1998). Interestingly enough, the *proportion* of women who sought help for infertility (44%) did not increase in this period, but the *numbers* of such women grew by 30% (Chandra & Stephen, 1998). These women tended to be older, had a higher income, and were more likely to be married than women in the general population not reporting fertility impairment. Study findings indicate that this dramatic increase occurred because the large baby-boomer group, many of whom delayed childbearing, had reached their later and less fertile reproductive years (Chandra & Stephen, 1998). This represents a broad social change, new in the history of the United States, which is having an impact in every social arena.

According to Chandra and Stephen (1998), baby-boomers tend to marry late and delay childbearing within marriage. Not only are there more women in older age groups, but more of these women are attempting to have first and subsequent births at older and less fertile ages.

Hatcher and colleagues (1994) note that pelvic inflammatory disease (PID) caused by sexually transmitted infections (STIs) is another important factor in infertility. They comment further that if the trend in STIs continues, this will account for an ever-increasing percentage of the infertility statistics in the future as more young women, who have the highest rates of STIs, attempt childbearing.

DEFINITIONS

Hatcher and colleagues (1994) have summarized the following terms on the basis of the World Health Organization's definitions of infertility:

- **Primary infertility:** The couple has never conceived despite unprotected intercourse for at least 12 months. It is further defined for each member of the couple as never having con-

ceived or initiated a pregnancy in this or another relationship.

- **Secondary infertility:** The couple has previously conceived (or both members of the couple have previously conceived or initiated a pregnancy) but is subsequently unable to conceive despite exposure to unprotected intercourse within the last 12 months.

- **Pregnancy wastage:** The woman is able to conceive but unable to carry the fetus to a viable age.

- **Subfertility:** The couple has difficulty in conceiving jointly because both partners may have reduced fertility.

PROBABILITY OF CONCEPTION

In addressing the probability of conception, Hatcher and colleagues (1994) note that among the fertile population each cycle represents about a 20% chance of pregnancy. With the use of this figure, 95% of couples conceive by the 13th cycle. Only a minority of *infertile* couples will never conceive without technologic intervention. The majority may just take longer to conceive.

REQUIREMENTS FOR FERTILITY

The following requirements have been set forth for fertility in men and women (Hatcher et al., 1994):

For the Male Partner:

- Normal reproductive structures for the manufacture and maturation of sperm

- Normal count, motility, and morphologic characteristics of sperm

- Adequate sexual drive

- Ability to maintain an erection and achieve normal ejaculation

For the Female Partner:

- Adequate sexual drive
- Normal reproductive anatomy
- Cervical mucus conducive to sperm survival and transport
- Ovulatory cycles
- Functional fallopian tubes
- Uterus that develops an environment favorable to implantation
- Normal hormone balance
- Normal immunologic response to sperm
- Adequate nutritional status to maintain a pregnancy

RISK FACTORS FOR INFERTILITY

Infertility can be attributed to problem sources in either partner, reduced fertility in both partners, or factors as yet unknown. Prevalent factors include the following:

- Female pelvic factors: 30%–40%
- Male factor infertility: 30%–40%
- Combined male and female factors: 10%–15%
- Unknown factors: 5%–10%

Health care workers consider eight risk factors in particular with infertility, and each is highlighted next.

Age

One of the eight risk factors in infertility is age, and age comes into play for both women and men. Hatcher and colleagues (1994) provide a good overview, as well as report findings from several studies, in this section on age and infertility.

Age does not have a great effect on fertility in most women until they are in their late 30s. A woman older than 35 years of age is twice as likely to be infertile as a 25-year-old. Older women may not be infertile, but they take longer to conceive than the standard definition and thus may be considered infertile.

Hatcher and colleagues (1994) note that the number of miscarriages increases with age, as do problems with the embryo, implantation site, or hormone balance. Study results indicate that the aging egg is a major factor in infertility for older women. Results of studies that have been done with women by using assisted fertilization technology have shown that the main determining factor in the success of a donated egg is the age of the donor, regardless of the age of the recipient.

To date, age has been less studied in men than in women (Hatcher et al., 1994). In men, there is an increased risk of sperm chromosomal abnormalities with age. Men are three times more likely to initiate a pregnancy at 25 years of age than at 40 years. More important than fertility itself, with increasing age in men there are issues of frequency of intercourse and problems with sexual function possibly related to medications or surgery.

Sexually Transmitted Infections

Hatcher and colleagues (1994) have addressed another factor in infertility: STIs. In doing so, they have also noted several statistics and study findings related to PID specifically.

Sexually transmitted infections are one of the most important risk factors in infertility for both men and women. The incidence of PID has risen over the past 20 years to 1 million reported cases per year. Pelvic inflammatory disease can cause permanent damage to the ovaries and fallopian tubes. In addition, because a large percentage of common STIs are asymptomatic, the damage occurs perhaps without the woman ever knowing it until she tries to conceive. Study findings have shown that half the women diagnosed with tubal infertility have no history suggesting PID. This type of infertility represents about 10% of infertile women. Exposure to STIs also increases the risk of cervical dysplasia and cervical cancer, both of which may require surgical intervention. This intervention could have an impact on fertility or the ability of a woman to carry a fetus to term.

Lifestyle

In the following section Stenchever (1996) has described several lifestyle factors related to infertility, again reporting findings from research into these areas.

Studies to determine the effects of lifestyle on fertility are difficult to do because lifestyle factors are usually not isolated. All the following have been found to have a negative effect on fertility: alcohol, social drugs, caffeine, and cigarettes. Results of studies in men who smoke have revealed nicotine in seminal fluid, decreased sperm count and motility, and alterations in the structure of sperm. In women, smoking is associated with decreased fertility and an increased rate of spontaneous abortion and ectopic pregnancy. Smoking is an important risk factor for cervical cancer. Menopause has been found to occur earlier in smokers, indicating that smoking has effects on hormone balance and possibly the health of the ovaries.

Activities that cause an increase in the scrotal temperature of men, such as the use of hot tubs and tight clothing, can decrease fertility as well.

Environmental Pollution

As reported by Stenchever (1996), toxic trace metals (e.g., mercury and cadmium), textile dyes, dry cleaning fluid, and many chemicals commonly found in the workplace and home can have an impact on fertility. Often, exposure occurred years before infertility was diagnosed.

Raloff (1994) reports that environmental pollution is an area of increasing concern with the advent of chemicals that are estrogen "mimics." He further reports that findings from animal studies show a profound and frightening array of short- and long-term alterations in fertility, as well as reproductive anomalies in the offspring.

Medications

Stenchever (1996) comments that a number of medications can cause impotence or affect sperm count (or both). These include narcotics, tranquilizers, antidepressants, and antihypertensives. Ovulation can be inhibited by barbiturates and narcotics. Other drugs are associated with miscarriage and birth defects. Chemotherapy may permanently impair fertility.

Surgery

Removal of or damage to reproductive structures, nerve damage in the genital area, and adhesions from pelvic surgery can directly or indirectly cause infertility (Stenchever, 1996).

Radiation

Depending on the site, dose, and duration of exposure, radiation can lead to structural damage and cause an increase in chromosomal aberrations (Stenchever, 1996).

Exposure to Diethylstilbestrol (DES)

Prenatal exposure to DES can impair fertility in both men and women (Stenchever, 1996).

THE FIRST STEP—INITIAL ASSESSMENT OF THE INFERTILE COUPLE

Consider the circumstances that prompt a woman or a couple to seek infertility evaluation. They have tried for months or perhaps years to conceive, and they are finally admitting "failure." The emotional impact of the entire process has already had profound implications for the self-esteem of each member of the couple, their sexual interaction with one another, and their relationship altogether. What they are faced with is possible solutions and no guarantees, which range anywhere from simply reeducation and changes in lifestyle and timing of intercourse to complex hormone manipulation or surgery. The process of evaluation and treatment can be lengthy and costly, taxing the personal, financial, and coping resources of the couple. They also look forward to an intense scrutiny into what is usually the most private and intimate part of their relationship.

Nurses play a special role in the field of infertility evaluation and treatment. They are educators, ensuring that couples are provided with culturally sensitive, readable, and understandable information and sources for further information. They are also caregivers as they provide couples with emotional support, ensure as much privacy as possible, answer questions and concerns, and allow the couple time to express their feelings and find an attentive and compassionate ear.

Stenchever (1996) notes that most of the initial routine evaluation can be conducted at a family planning clinic or by a general practitioner or gynecologist, and it begins with a complete history and physical examination for each partner. A number of tests will be recommended, which range from charting of cyclic temperature fluctuations, semen analysis, and hormone testing to more invasive diagnostic procedures for both partners. Findings from this level of testing will diagnose the infertility problem in approximately 60% of infertile couples. Stenchever comments that referral to a specialty center should be done if pregnancy has not been achieved within 1 year of developing a plan or within 6 months if the woman is older than 35 years of age.

Stenchever (1996) also reports that the history and physical examination are crucial in the search for a diagnosis. They should include the following:

- For women:
  — Menstrual history
  — Pregnancy history
  — Evidence of any weight gain, hirsutism, or acne
  — Diet
  — Exercise practices
  — Environmental exposures
  — Exposure to DES
  — Substance use or abuse
  — Medical conditions (e.g., infections, exposure to tuberculosis, chronic illness)
  — Sexual history (e.g., birth control methods, number of partners, STI exposure and treatment)
  — Surgeries, especially those involving the reproductive system
  — Psychosocial and cultural histories
- For men:
  — Evidence of exposure to environmental toxins
  — Current or history of infection (e.g., mumps, urinary tract infection)
  — History of trauma to the scrotal area
  — Lifestyle and cultural issues
  — Surgeries
  — History of undescended testes, hernia, or other abnormalities of the reproductive system

Education is a primary focus in infertility evaluation. The couple needs to comprehend the changes that occur during the menstrual cycle, so that they can understand how to optimize their fertility. They also need to understand the procedures and tests that will be done to evaluate fertility. They should be informed why and when specific tests will be performed, as well as of the necessary preparation, possible discomfort, and anticipated recovery time.

Tests and Procedures

According to Stenchever (1996), a complete workup should be done even if abnormalities are found on a particular test. Crucial tests should be repeated after corrective suggestions have been initiated, with enough time in between for these corrections to have an effect. For example, because sperm takes about 10 weeks to mature, any changes would not be apparent for several months.

Evaluation of the Man

For the infertile couple, evaluation of the man can include the following: semen analysis, postcoital test, sperm penetration assay (SPA), hormone tests, and surgical diagnostic interventions. The following discussion on these five areas, along with cited statistics and research study findings, are gleaned from the information provided by Stenchever (1996) in his book, *Office Gynecology*.

Semen Analysis

Normal sperm production is a continuous process, not cyclic. An immature sperm takes about 2.5–3 months to reach maturity. The first test performed for men during an evaluation for infertility is a semen evaluation. Variations in the sperm count of healthy men are so great that any abnormal result should be checked again.

The level of sophistication in testing different factors involved in male fertility has increased dramatically in recent years with the advent of computer-assisted analysis. The World Health Organization has established standards for semen analysis. Most variations will be accounted for by two to three separate analyses over a 3 month period. Semen analysis includes evaluation of factors, such as volume; pH; sperm count; consistency of seminal fluid; morphologic characteristics and motility of sperm; and signs of infection, inflammation, or agglutination.

Postcoital Test

The ability of sperm to function properly has been the subject of new advances. The standard test done for this purpose up until the past decade was the postcoital test. This test is used to assess the number of sperm present in cervical mucus 8–12 hours after intercourse, as well as their level of forward movement. So it is a measure of the ability of sperm to stay alive and travel through cervical mucus. (See the glossary for a description of the steps involved in doing a postcoital test.)

Sperm Penetration Assay

Successful fertilization involves a complex series of biochemical steps that occur when the sperm interacts with the egg. The latest testing methods are being developed to assess different aspects of this process. The new group of tests, called SPA, include analysis of the ability of sperm both to shed its protein coating and to release the enzymes needed to penetrate the egg.

Hormone Tests

Hormone imbalance in men can be another cause of abnormal sperm production, and hormone testing might be included in the male workup.

Surgical Intervention

Surgical intervention may be indicated to evaluate for possible tubal obstructions. In addition, radiographic studies, with the use of contrast dye injected into the vas deferens or ejaculatory duct, might be performed. A testicular biopsy may be done to confirm evidence of the development of structures needed to support normal sperm maturation.

Evaluation of the Woman

For the infertile couple, evaluation of the woman must include documenting ovulation, determining patency of the fallopian tubes, and diagnosing cervical or uterine factors.

Current technology lacks the ability to assess the complex functioning of the fallopian tube and its role in fertilization. The fallopian tube has chemical as well as muscular and ciliary activities that contribute to fertilization and development of the embryo and its transport into the uterus. New technology is being developed to evaluate this aspect of fertility more directly.

Charting of Fertility Signs

Stenchever (1996) notes that the most basic and least expensive tests involve charting of events (i.e., changes in basal body temperature and cervical mucus) that occur during the menstrual cycle. He comments further that approximately 15%–20% of infertility can be attributed to failure to ovulate.

1. **Basal body temperature (BBT) charting:** Stenchever (1996) has provided the following overview of BBT charting.

    The charting of the BBT consists of documenting the changes that occur in the BBT with ovulation. The temperature-regulating centers in the hypothalamus are controlled in part by progesterone levels. After ovulation, when the progesterone levels increase dramatically, there is a rise in temperature of approximately 0.28°C (0.5°F). This rise in temperature indicates that ovulation has already occurred and thus it *cannot* be used to predict ovulation. The temperature normally stays elevated for a minimum of 11 days. Large deviations from this may indicate other cycle abnormalities. Several months of charting are usually requested.

2. **Cervical mucus charting:** DeMarco (1996) has provided helpful information on cervical mucus charting, including the availability of over-the-counter (OTC) testing devices.

    The documentation of changes in the consistency of cervical mucus is another time-tested way of indicating ovulation. The increase in estrogen levels that occurs around midcycle causes changes in the cervical mucus

from tacky, opaque mucus to a clear, stretchy, slippery, and thinner consistency. This type of mucus resembles egg white and is termed *spinnbarkeit*. It does not break when stretched between thumb and forefinger. If observed under the microscope, this mucus has an organized fernlike pattern. This is because of glycoproteins (molecules made of sugars and protein) in the mucus that line up to create a pathway for sperm to travel up the cervical canal. These glycoproteins also provide nutrients for the sperm. It is amazing how nature has provided the perfect environment. Some women never manufacture this kind of mucus because of infection or injury to the endocervical glands, which produce mucus. Or they may have congenital or hormone abnormalities. This test should be repeated if it yields abnormal results.

Several OTC devices are available for identifying fertile-type mucus. These kits test for an electrical change, which occurs in cervical mucus and in saliva as a result of hormone-induced chemical changes. Cervical mucus is also *not* an accurate predictor of ovulation.

Predicting Ovulation

DeMarco (1996) has also discussed ways to predict ovulation. She reports that in the past 10 years more accurate tests have been developed.

An OTC kit is on the market that measures the levels of luteinizing hormone (LH) in urine. The LH surge precedes ovulation by 24–28 hours. This test both predicts and verifies ovulation and can be used to time intercourse.

Hormone Tests

Stenchever (1996) has discussed how hormone tests can be used to evaluate fertility in a woman. Specific blood tests can be done to evaluate the functioning of the thyroid gland and adrenal glands, as well as to assess the levels of hypothalamic, pituitary, and ovarian hormones:

1. **Serum progesterone levels:** Progesterone is measured in the middle of the second half of the cycle (luteal phase). Adequate levels of this hormone are an indication that ovulation has occurred, and that the corpus luteum has formed fully and is functioning adequately to produce the progesterone needed to provide a receptive environment for implantation (Stenchever, 1996). If ovulation does not occur, serum progesterone levels will be below normal range.

2. **Serum estrogen levels:** The test of serum estrogen levels measures levels of estrogen produced by the granulosa cells of the ovary in the first half of the cycle. This estrogen is needed for adequate maturation of the ovarian follicle before ovulation can occur (Stenchever, 1996).

Procedures

Five procedures can be used to evaluate fertility in a woman:

1. **Endometrial biopsy:** Hatcher and colleagues (1994) report that the thickness and glandular structure of the endometrial lining of the uterus undergo dramatic changes in response to first estrogen and then progesterone. They note that results from a sampling of the lining can be correlated with serum progesterone levels to determine whether the uterine environment is conducive to implantation.

2. **Ultrasound techniques:** According to Stenchever (1996), ultrasound techniques can be used to pinpoint pelvic abnormalities, as well as to evaluate the growth and development of the ovarian follicle and the corpus luteum.

3. **Hysterosalpingogram:** Stenchever (1996) notes that the hysterosalpingogram is used to evaluate tubal patency and gather information about the internal anatomy of the uterus and fallopian tubes. A contrast dye is injected into the uterine cavity, allowing these structures to be visualized. He comments further that in some cases this test can be used to open a blockage in the fallopian tube. It is performed in the first half of the menstrual cycle.

4. **Falloscope:** The falloscope is currently being developed to allow direct access to the fallopian tube, with the eventual development of instruments to sample tubal secretions and reestablish tubal patency (Stenchever, 1996).

5. **Laparoscopy:** With a laparoscopy, a scope is inserted through a small incision in the woman's umbilicus, allowing direct visualization of pelvic structures and surgical removal of adhesions and lesions of endometriosis (Stenchever, 1996).

COUNSELING, REFERRALS, AND TREATMENT

The health care provider can assist couples with infertility through several strategies and interventions.

Timing of Intercourse

According to Hatcher and colleagues (1994), the simplest intervention, which for some couples might be the missing link in achieving pregnancy, is counseling the couple about the events of the menstrual cycle and how to maximize their chances of conceiving on the basis of timing and interval of sexual intercourse (SIC). They note that infrequent SIC is a common cause of infertility, and the recommendation is to have SIC every other day around the time of ovulation. Less frequent SIC may miss ovulation; more frequent intercourse decreases sperm count.

DeMarco (1996) notes that the timing of intercourse before ovulation is crucial. Sperm can survive for more than 72 hours in the female genital tract. The ovum has a shorter life span of only 12 hours if unfertilized. The actual time an egg is able to be fertilized is thought to be only a few hours. Thus sperm need to be present before or shortly after ovulation.

The timing of intercourse needs to be determined in relation to the woman's menstrual cycle. For example, a woman with short cycles and a long menses may need to have SIC during her menses to conceive. Cultural and social taboos that center around SIC during menses may prove to be a barrier to fertility. Education of the couple may help solve the problem.

Lifestyle Changes

Other simple interventions for infertility involve general changes in lifestyle. For women, these include

- changing
  - the diet.
  - exercise patterns to prevent exercise-induced amenorrhea (lack of menses).
- establishing adequate weight for a regular menstrual cycle to occur.
- avoiding the use of cigarettes, alcohol, social drugs, and caffeine.
- reducing exposure to chemicals.

For men, "keeping cool"—that is, avoiding hot tubs and tight-fitting clothes, which increase scrotal temperature—may help.

Techniques of SIC

According to Hatcher and colleagues (1994), positions that maximize the exposure of sperm to the cervix will enhance the chances of success. For example, a woman with a uterus tilted forward would do best by lying on her back with hips elevated. By having the woman stay in this position for 20 minutes after SIC, the sperm will have time to pool around the cervix.

Use of Lubricants

Some lubricants contain spermicide and should not be used. In addition, some may set up an allergic, inflammatory reaction.

Douching

Douching counteracts efforts to achieve pregnancy (Hatcher et al., 1994).

Antibiotics

Antibiotics may be indicated for signs of infection in either partner.

Structural Abnormalities

Any existing structural abnormalities should be corrected if possible.

Hormonal Interventions

Intervention with hormones may be indicated for either partner.

Surgical Intervention

Stenchever (1996) reports that the presence of fibroids can result in implantation failure by creating a chronic inflammatory response in the uterus. A myomectomy can be performed.

Fertility Drugs

Certain drugs can be used in varying combinations to stimulate ovulation and, depending on the extent of intervention involved, the development of multiple ovarian follicles. During treatment with these drugs, SIC is timed carefully around ovulation as determined by techniques already discussed, including BBT and cervical mucus charting. Infertility drugs increase the likelihood of multiple gestation.

Four fertility drugs are of particular interest to health care providers working with couples with infertility problems: clomiphene citrate (Clomid®, Serophene®), menotropins (Pergonal®), follitropin beta (Follistim®), and follitropin alpha (Gonal-F®).

Each drug is described briefly in the discussion that follows. The information—including any cited statistics—was gleaned from several online articles available through the Internet from the Reproductive Science Center of the Bay Area Fertility & Gynecology Medical Group, Inc., and each article has been cited at the end of the respective discussion on these drugs. Please refer to the bibliography for more information on retrieving these sources for further study.

1. **Clomid or Serophene:** Clomid or Serophene was first introduced in the late 1950s. This drug is used to induce ovulation by acting directly on the hypothalamus. It is useful for women who fail to ovulate because of a problem at the hypothalamic or pituitary level.

   When given early in the menstrual cycle, clomiphene citrate suppresses the amount of natural estrogen and "tricks" the pituitary gland into producing more follicle-stimulating hormone (FSH) and LH, which cause maturation of a follicle and ovulation. About 70% of women will ovulate, and about 40% of those will become pregnant without any further assistance.

   The woman should be monitored with daily urine LH tests and examined with ultrasound when the LH surge occurs to signal impending ovulation. Clomiphene citrate may cause blurred vision, ovarian cysts, pelvic discomfort, hot flashes, insomnia, and irritability. Multiple pregnancy may occur; about 6% of women who receive this drug develop twins ("Clomiphine Citrate [Clomid] [Serophene]," 1995).

2. **Pergonal:** Pergonal is a naturally occurring hormone (FSH and LH) extracted from the urine of postmenopausal women. When given as an injection to premenopausal women according to a specific timing protocol, this hormone stimulates the maturation of ovarian

follicles containing the eggs ("Pergonal and Metrodin," 1998).

3. **Follistim and Gonal-F:** Follistim and Gonal-F are both new and purer forms of FSH with a more predictable bioeffect. These drugs are not obtained from the urine of menopausal women but from genetic technology. Advantages include that there is less local reaction at the injection site, and the injection can be given subcutaneously with a small needle. Thus it is easier for the client to give herself injections ("Gonal F/Follistim Gonadotropins," 1998).

As with most drugs, complications and side effects can occur with fertility drugs. These sequelae are related to hyperstimulation of the ovary, leading to the possibility of increased ovulation and multiple gestations and premature delivery. Hyperstimulation results in temporary enlargement and swelling of the ovary with lower abdominal pain and pressure, weight gain, and swelling. These signs will usually resolve spontaneously with rest and no intercourse, but occasionally hospitalization is needed for observation of the woman and fluid hydration ("Overview of Assisted Reproductive Technologies," 1995).

The incidence of multiple gestation is approximately 15%–20%, with 75% of these being twins and 25% being triplets. Eighty percent of successful pregnancies produce one fetus. Results of some studies have revealed a slight increase in ovarian cancer in women who have taken fertility medications ("Pergonal and Metrodin," 1998).

Non–Drug-Related Therapies

Sperm Donation

According to Hatcher and colleagues (1994), sperm donation is the simplest and least expensive way to treat male factor infertility. Particular attention must be paid to assuring that the sperm does not carry any disease. They note that criteria for preparation, storage, and screening are set by the American Fertility Society. Its current recommendation is to use sperm that has been frozen and quarantined for 6 months to ensure that it is disease free.

Artificial Insemination

Artificial Insemination bypasses problems with cervical mucus by instillation of a small amount of specially prepared sperm into the uterus (Stenchever, 1996).

Stress and Fertility

Findings from a number of recent studies suggest that stress may hinder female fertility ("New Hope for Infertility," 1997). A new study, funded by the National Institute of Mental Health, is underway to evaluate the relationship among stress, depression, and infertility. This is a 5-year study of 120 infertile couples conducted by the Behavioral Medicine Infertility Program. Women have been assigned to one of three groups: a mind-body program, a support group, or a group to receive routine care only. Results are not due out until next year, but preliminary reports reveal that infertile women were anxious and depressed on a scale comparable to that in women with cancer, heart disease, or AIDS. The purpose of the study is to help women learn skills for stress reduction and to rediscover the joy of their lives and relationships. An unexpected side effect is occurring, as reported in preliminary findings: 44% of participants have gotten pregnant within 6 months, compared with an 18% pregnancy rate due to chance alone ("New Hope for Infertility," 1997). (See the for more information about this study.)

ASSISTED REPRODUCTIVE TECHNOLOGIES (ARTs)

On July 25, 1978, an event occurred that changed the course of human society forever: the birth of the first baby conceived through in vitro fertilization (IVF)—the first "test tube baby," Louise Brown (Stenchever, 1996). The technology has been proliferating at a rapid rate ever since, and with it there has been increasing success in achieving pregnancy. With the advent of this capability has come the need to consider the whole depth and array of ethical issues that this realm of "possibility" has opened up. Nurses and clients alike are challenged to come to grips with these ethical dilemmas, so that nurses can provide, and clients can receive, nonjudgmental care.

Approximately one third of infertile couples are appropriate candidates for ARTs. Which procedures are selected depends on the circumstances of the couple; that is, the causes of infertility, age of the woman, financial considerations, and individual beliefs and values.

Once again, information in the following sections has been gleaned from several online articles available through the Internet from the Reproductive Science Center of the Bay Area Fertility & Gynecology Medical Group, Inc., and included in the bibliography. For more in-depth information on the typical cycle in ARTs, cryopreservation, and specific ART procedures—that is, in vitro fertilization/embryo transfer (IVF/ET), gamete intrafallopian transfer (GIFT), and zygote intrafallopian transfer/tubal embryo transfer (ZIFT/TET)—please refer to "Overview of Assisted Reproductive Technologies" (1995). For information on intra-cytoplasmic sperm injection (ICSI) and testes/epididymis sperm aspiration (TESA) procedures, refer to "IVF with ICSI" (1996); for the assisted hatching procedure, "Assisted Hatching," (1995/1996); and for oocyte donation, Weckstein (1996).

Typical Cycle

All ARTs involve a number of steps that are initially similar ("Overview of Assisted Reproductive Technologies," 1995). The first step is to stimulate the ovaries to produce multiple eggs, which will be retrieved from the ovary to be used in one of the ART procedures. Beginning about 1 week after ovulation, the woman undergoes a vaginal ultrasound for evaluation of her ovaries. Then she begins receiving the medication teuprolide acetate (Lupron). This drug prevents an early LH surge, which would stimulate the ovaries to release eggs prematurely. It does this by acting on the hypothalamus. This is called pituitary desensitization. Side effects of the drug include hot flashes, headaches, and vaginal dryness.

The woman gives herself Lupron daily as a subcutaneous injection in the thigh. Menses usually begins as usual about 1 week later. Another vaginal ultrasound is done on about day 2 of the period. If the ovaries are normal, the woman is given a date to start one of the drugs that will stimulate multiple follicles to develop. The ovary-stimulating drugs are given by injection daily for 5–6 days. Blood estrogen levels are monitored, and a vaginal ultrasound is performed every few days, with adjustment of medication dosages being made each time on the basis of findings. When the eggs are at the right maturation level, the next part of the procedure is begun ("Overview of Assisted Reproductive Technologies," 1995).

To give the eggs a final growth spurt, the client gives herself an injection of the hormone human chorionic gonadotropin (HCG). The egg retrieval procedure is scheduled for the next day.

Egg retrievals are performed almost exclusively with the aid of ultrasound guidance without laparoscopy. A needle is advanced through the back of the woman's vagina into the ovaries, and the eggs are suctioned from the ovaries. The procedure takes about 20–30 minutes. Risks include infection, bleeding, and, rarely, injury to bowel or bladder. The woman is kept at the office where the procedure was performed for 2 hours and then returns home, possibly with slight lower abdominal discomfort and light vaginal bleeding. Injections of progesterone are begun to prepare the uterine lining

for implantation. Once the eggs have been retrieved, the husband provides a sperm specimen after 3–5 days of abstinence from sexual intercourse. The next step is determined by which type of ART procedure is appropriate for the client, based on the reasons for infertility—both male and female ("Overview of Assisted Reproductive Technologies," 1995).

Oocyte Donation and Cryopreservation

Two techniques—oocyte donation and cryopreservation—may come into play in the typical ART cycle, depending on the individual woman or couple.

According to Weckstein (1996), oocyte donation provides an alternative for women who have had their ovaries removed or whose infertility is due to failure to mature an egg. It is often used with women who are older than 38 years of age when the chances of pregnancy from their own eggs seem to be low. Donor ova are used, and they are retrieved from a young woman—who has a surplus of oocytes—while she is undergoing IVF. Each facility who offers this ART has its own guidelines regarding knowledge of who the donor is. Some facilities discourage or prohibit "known donor" oocytes or "known donor" sperm (or both) (Weckstein, 1996).

With cryopreservation ("Overview of Assisted Reproductive Technologies," 1995), embryos not used in a particular ART cycle are frozen and stored for future use. They can remain viable for long periods. This allows the attempts to achieve pregnancy to be repeated without the need for another round of chemical stimulation of the ovaries or having to repeat the procedures for egg retrieval. About half the frozen embryos survive the thawing process. Approximately 18% of frozen embryos result in pregnancy. Several ethical issues need to be considered ("Overview of Assisted Reproductive Technologies," 1995), including answers to questions, such as; Which of the

---

FIGURE 6-1
Steps of In Vitro Fertilization

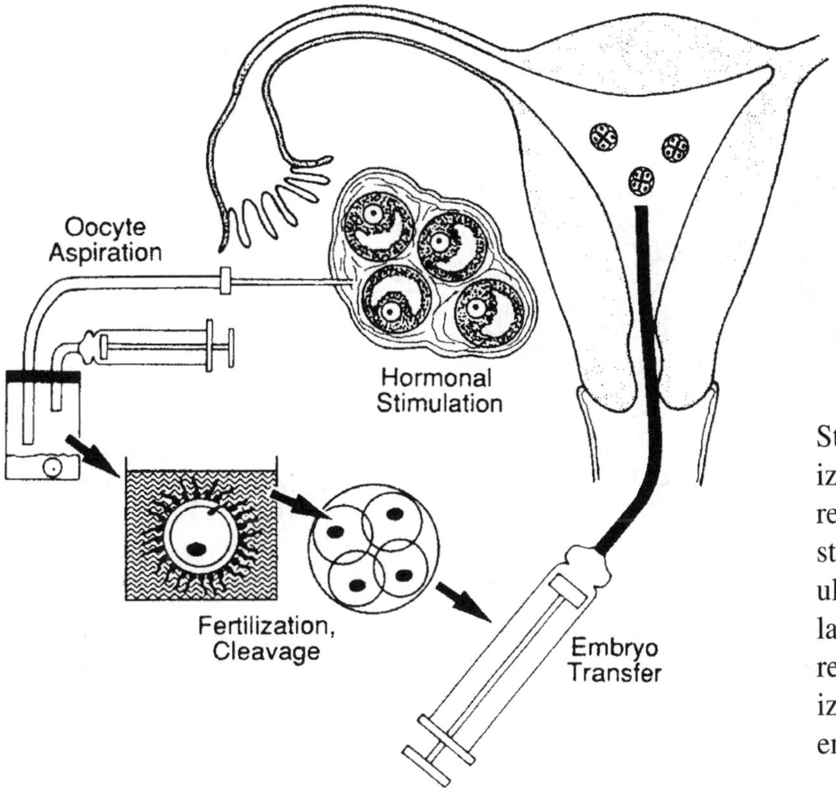

Oocyte
Aspiration

Hormonal
Stimulation

Fertilization,
Cleavage

Embryo
Transfer

Steps of in vitro fertilization and embryo replacement are ovarian stimulation, monitoring, ultrasound or laparoscopy, oocyte retrieval, in vitro fertilization, and uterine pre-embryo replacement.

Source: Scott, J. R., Disaia, P. J., Hammond, C. B. & Spellacy, W. N. (Eds). (1994). *Danforth's obstetrics and gynecology* (7th ed.). Philadelphia: J. B. Lippincott.

---

embryos does one choose to use and what is to be done with a client's unused embryos?

Available Procedures

IVF/ET

In vitro means "in glass," referring to a natural process that is performed outside the body. It is from this literal translation that the term test tube baby arises ("Overview of Assisted Reproductive Technologies," 1995).

With IVF/ET ("Overview of Assisted Reproductive Technologies," 1995), an egg (oocyte) is taken from the female (partner or donor) and placed in a culture dish with sperm from the male (partner or donor). Conditions are carefully controlled. After fertilization, the embryo is allowed to grow 1–3 days. The single egg cell, con-

taining genetic contribution from male and female, begins to divide. Transfer of the growing embryo into the uterus is usually done at the 2- to 12-cell stage. This is one IVF/ET cycle. (See *Figure 6-1.*) Because IVF bypasses the fallopian tubes, clients with blocked or absent fallopian tubes, pelvic adhesions, or history of multiple tubal pregnancies are the appropriate candidates for IVF. Because eggs are retrieved from the ovary by using new methods that gain access to the ovary through the vagina, no laparoscopy is needed.

GIFT

The GIFT procedure uses unfertilized oocytes which have been aspirated from the woman's ovary during a laparoscopy. These are combined with prepared sperm and placed in the fallopian tube (see *Figure 2-2*). this technique most closely

FIGURE 6-2
Steps of Gamete Intrafallopian Transfer

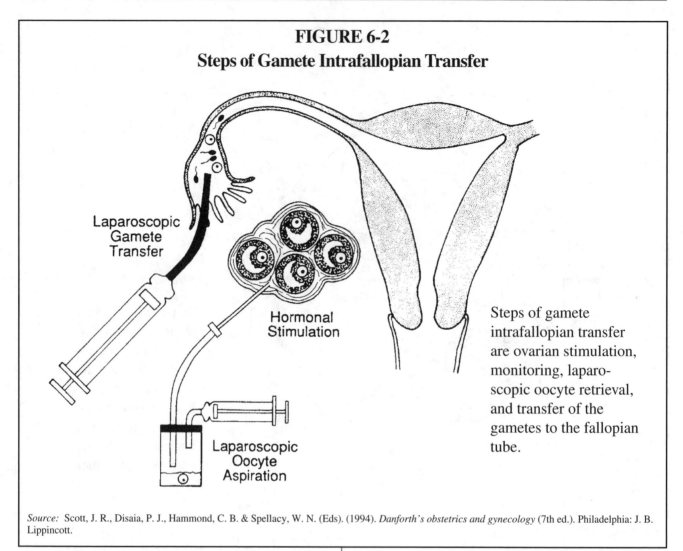

Laparoscopic
Gamete
Transfer

Hormonal
Stimulation

Laparoscopic
Oocyte
Aspiration

Steps of gamete
intrafallopian transfer
are ovarian stimulation,
monitoring, laparo-
scopic oocyte retrieval,
and transfer of the
gametes to the fallopian
tube.

Source: Scott, J. R., Disaia, P. J., Hammond, C. B. & Spellacy, W. N. (Eds). (1994). *Danforth's obstetrics and gynecology* (7th ed.). Philadelphia: J. B. Lippincott.

resembles the natural fertilization process in which fertilization occurs in the fallopian tube where oocyte and sperm meet. If the egg is fertilized it arrives naturally into the uterus without any interference. The disadvantage of this procedure is taking the risk that none of the oocytes placed in the fallopian tube will get fertilized by the sperm, since unfertilized oocytes are used. Patency of the tube below the placement site can also be a problem which could result in a tubal (ectopic) pregnancy. Pregnancy rates are higher with GIFT than with IVF by 5–10% ("Overview of Assisted Reproductive Technologies," 1995).

ZIFT/TET

The ZIFT/TET ("Overview of Assisted Reproductive Technologies," 1995), are modifications of the GIFT and IVF procedures in which fer-

tilization is determined before the egg is transferred to the fallopian tube. This procedure is helpful when the male factor predominates and the woman's fallopian tubes are functioning normally. The disadvantage of this group of procedures is that two surgical procedures are required—one to aspirate eggs from the ovary and one to transfer fertilized eggs into the fallopian tube. The cost of this procedure is accordingly higher.

ICSI

The ICSI ("IVF with ICSI," 1996) is a micromanipulation procedure in which a single sperm is injected directly into the egg, bypassing the outer coverings of the egg. If the egg is fertilized, the embryo is inserted into the uterus. This is a breakthrough in technology that has occurred during the past 3 years. It is used for men with very low sperm numbers or sperm motility.

TESA

In a TESA ("IVF with ICSI," 1996), sperm are aspirated directly from the testes or epididymis and used in conjunction with the ICSI procedure. The TESA can be used in men with vasectomy or who had a failed vasectomy reversal.

Assisted Hatching

Assisted hatching ("In Vitro Fertilization [IVF] - Including [Assisted Hatching]," 1995/1996) is a form of micromanipulation of the egg itself. A hole is made in the egg's outer covering, presumably assisting in fertilization. This procedure is used to improve chances of successful pregnancy with women who have a history of implantation failures or whose eggs have a thick covering. It is also used in women age 39 years or older.

Advances

Stenchever (1996) reports that progress is being made continually in success rates with ARTs. This is due to the discovery of ways to enhance the quality of sperm and egg with new protocols that combine various hormone and drug regimens and refine the timing of intrauterine insemination. Advances are also being made in establishing an optimal culture environment that more closely resembles tubal secretions. Embryo biopsy techniques that are used in the diagnosis of genetic disorders before implantation are in development. This would open up pregnancy options to couples who are avoiding conception because of the risk of transmitting a known genetic disorder to their newborn (Stenchever, 1996).

Complications

There are two complications associated with ARTs:

1. **Spontaneous abortion:** The rates for spontaneous abortion in ARTs are slightly higher than

for naturally occurring pregnancies ("Overview of Assisted Reproductive Technologies," 1995).

2. **Multiple pregnancy:** There is a higher incidence of twins and multiple pregnancies after the transfer of multiple eggs (Lichtman & Papera, 1990).

Adjunct Support

Genetic counseling and amniocentesis (Stenchever, 1996) may be indicated with ARTs, as well as in naturally occurring pregnancies. Indications for these interventions will depend on family history and age of the couple.

Success Rates

The success rate for ART has improved steadily since these procedures were introduced in the late 1970s. In most cases, success may require more than one attempt before conception occurs. However, this is true even of normally fertile couples who have only an 18%–25% chance of achieving pregnancy within any given month (Stenchever, 1996). Couples who use ART procedures have a chance of pregnancy that compares favorably with that of a fertile couple (Stenchever, 1996). The Center for Disease Control keeps detailed yearly statistics on all aspects of ART, including success rates for the different techniques. These reports can be accessed via the Internet. You will find their web site listed in the bibliography.

Standards and guidelines for ART procedures are set by the American Society for Reproductive Medicine. Stenchever (1996) notes that in choosing an ART center, clients need to become knowledgeable about differences in protocols and criteria for accepting clients, as well as how the center reports its success rates. He comments that often the "take home baby" rate is very different from the overall pregnancy rate.

Costs

The ARTs are very expensive. Couples can spend up to $30,000, depending on the procedures and the number of cycles required to achieve a successful pregnancy ("New Hope for Infertility," 1997). Most health insurance providers pay for only a limited portion of fertility evaluation and treatment. Government funding for couples of low income is limited and varies from state to state. Income level is tied to access perhaps more than in any other area of women's health.

ADOPTION

According to Hatcher and associates (1994), many infertile couples will choose adoption. This process can also be lengthy and frustrating, although the number of possibilities for adoption has expanded in recent years. Open adoption, which involves cooperation between adoptive and birth parents, is one option. In addition to licensed adoption agencies, sources for possible adoption connections include clergy, attorneys, independent adoption agencies, and friends. Children from other countries or with special needs can often be adopted with a shorter waiting period.

PSYCHOLOGIC AND EMOTIONAL ASPECTS

It is evident that infertility is an extremely complex, deep, and multifaceted area of health care. Some of the factors that add to the stress of the situation include the following:

- Age of the couple and time pressure to achieve pregnancy

- Previous pregnancies in this or other relationships in one or both spouses
- Differences in desire to achieve a pregnancy between members of the couple
- Pressures from extended family
- Religious beliefs
- Financial resources
- Career choices

Stenchever (1996) reports that normal reactions to the diagnosis of infertility include those that have been identified for other grieving processes: surprise, denial, isolation, anger, guilt, sorrow, and, finally, resolution. Depression and prolonged stress are common, and they may have a profound impact on the life of the individual and the health of the relationship. Stress itself has unknown but possibly profound effects on fertility (Stenchever, 1996).

CONCLUSION

The health care team is challenged to accomplish the infertility evaluation and treatment in a thorough, timely, and sensitive fashion. Members of the health care team may need to set the stage and tone of intimate discussions involving details of sexuality and other private aspects of the couple's life together. Difficult ethical decisions also need to be discussed in an honest, forthright, and nonjudgmental manner. It is important that members of the health care team know themselves and understand their own beliefs and biases, so that they can truly assist couples in making their own informed choices.

EXAM QUESTIONS

CHAPTER 6
Questions 45–50

45. Primary infertility in a couple is defined as a couple who has never conceived despite unprotected intercourse for at least

    a. 6 months.

    b. 1 year.

    c. 18 months.

    d. 2 years.

46. Female pelvic factors account for approximately what percentage of infertility?

    a. 10%–15%

    b. 75%

    c. 30%–40%

    d. Less than 10%

47. Women are asked to chart their basal body temperature and cervical mucus characteristics for evidence of

    a. ovulation.

    b. sexually transmitted infection that could interfere with fertility.

    c. blockage of the fallopian tubes.

    d. changes in the lining of the uterus.

48. A hysterosalpingogram is a diagnostic test used to determine

    a. hormone insufficiencies.

    b. abnormalities of ovulation.

    c. patency of the fallopian tubes.

    d. presence of cysts on the ovaries.

49. In vitro fertilization (IVF) is most appropriate for

    a. all infertile women.

    b. women who do not ovulate regularly.

    c. women who have a blockage of the fallopian tubes.

    d. women who want to know the sex of their child.

50. Gamete intrafallopian transfer (GIFT) involves placing

    a. an unfertilized egg into the uterus.

    b. an unfertilized egg into the fallopian tube.

    c. a fertilized egg into the uterus.

    d. a fertilized egg into the fallopian tube.

CHAPTER 7

SEXUALLY TRANSMITTED INFECTIONS

CHAPTER OBJECTIVE

After completing this chapter, the reader will be able to recognize the most common sexually transmitted infections (STIs), as well as modes of transmission, treatment options, prevention, self-care, and practicing of safer sex in relation to these infections.

LEARNING OBJECTIVES

After studying this chapter, the reader will be able to

1. identify the common sexually transmitted infections.

2. describe the symptoms and modes of transmission for the most common sexually transmitted infections.

3. discuss treatment options.

4. describe safer sex practices.

5. discuss health education, prevention, and self-care for sexually active clients.

Key Words

- PID
- Safer sex

INTRODUCTION

In recent years, there has been a spread of a number of STIs. Some are more life threatening than others, but each takes its toll—both physically and emotionally. Individuals younger than age 25 years account for the majority of people affected (Hatcher et al., 1994). It is urgent that young people be helped to understand the seriousness of sexual activity and the consequences of risky behaviors.

Serious long-term effects of STIs can include blockage of the fallopian tubes leading to infertility, high risk of ectopic pregnancy, chronic pelvic pain, increased risk of liver cancer and serious liver disease, and death (Hatcher et al., 1994). For most STIs, women suffer more long-term reproductive consequences than men, and women are more likely than men to acquire an infection from any single sexual encounter (Hatcher et al., 1994). Because of the asymptomatic nature of many STIs, especially in women, treatment is often delayed. This factor increases the likelihood of more serious long-term consequences (Lichtman & Papera, 1990).

It is beyond the scope of this course to provide complete treatment protocols for each disease, because protocols are constantly being revised. The Centers for Disease Control and Prevention (CDC) regularly publishes recommendations and updates.

CLIENT EDUCATION

There are six areas and several strategies that health care providers should focus on in educating clients about STIs:

1. Kozier and associates (1995) advise health care workers to teach sexual decision-making skills, not just facts. These skills include

    *   those needed to negotiate in a relationship.

    *   learning how to establish relationships with partners who are at low risk for STIs.

    *   operating from an internal value system, rather than under peer pressure.

2. Hatcher and colleagues (1998) describe a number of safer sex techniques (see *Table 7-1*). In addition, Hatcher and associates (1994) offer the following tips:

    *   Condoms still offer the best protection.

    *   Spermicide is less effective than condoms and may cause or exacerbate tiny abrasions on the vulva and in the vagina. Therefore, clients should check for reddened or sore areas before using such a product.

    *   Sexual contact should be avoided if the person or partner has any sore areas or lesions.

3. Health care workers should be aware that women who use non–barrier contraceptive methods usually do so for the freedom involved. It may be more difficult to influence them to practice safer sex (Hatcher et al., 1994). Therefore,

    *   inform clients that oral contraceptives cause changes in the cervix and the immune system that may make women who use them more susceptible to HIV infection ("Does the Pill Help Spread HIV?," 1998).

    *   encourage the concomitant use of barrier methods and oral contraceptives for new or

nonmonogamous relationships.

4. Partners should be involved in the discussion. Therefore,

    *   dispel any views that talking about infection and safer sex or asking about a partner's sexual history means that the client does not trust her partner. It is easy to have an STI and never know it.

    *   encourage delaying intercourse; discuss other ways to have sexual intimacy and how to make these forms of intimacy safer.

    *   confirm knowledge about proper condom use by both partners.

5. Clients should be taught

    *   to do a genital self-examination on a regular basis.

    *   not to share personal care items, such as toothbrushes or razors.

6. Health care workers should be aware of special circumstances if treatment is needed for an existing STI:

    *   Both the client and her partners need to be treated.

    *   The complete course of antibiotic therapy prescribed should be taken, even if any symptoms resolve.

    *   The couple should abstain from sexual intercourse until both partners have completed treatment to prevent reinfection.

    *   The client should be encouraged to return after treatment is completed to assess whether the infection is cured.

HIV/AIDS

Hatcher and associates (1994) have discussed HIV/AIDS in depth. Except where otherwise noted, the introduction to this topic—as well as the discussion in the subsequent sections on testing,

TABLE 7-1
Safer Sex Options for Physical Intimacy

Safe

- Sexual fantasies

- Massage

- Hugging

- Body rubbing

- Dry kissing

- Masturbation without contact with partner's semen or vaginal secretions

- Erotic conversation, books, movies, videos

- Erotic bathing, showering

- Eroticizing feet, fingers, buttocks, abdomen, ears, other body parts

- All sexual activities, when both partners are monogamous, trustworthy, and known by testing to be free of HIV

Possibly Safe

- Wet kissing with no broken skin, cracked lips, or damaged mouth tissue

- Hand-to-genital touching (hand job) or mutual masturbation

- Vaginal or anal intercourse using latex or plastic condom correctly with adequate lubrication

- Oral sex on a man using a latex or plastic condom

- Oral sex on a woman using a latex or plastic barrier such as a female condom, dental dam, or modified male condom (especially if she does not have her period or a vaginal infection with discharge)

- All sexual activities, when both partners agree to a monogamous relationship and trust each other

Unsafe in the absence of HIV testing and trust and monogamy

- Blood contact of any kind, including menstrual blood

- Any vaginal or anal intercourse without a latex or plastic condom

- Oral sex on a woman without a latex or plastic barrier such as a female condom, dental dam or modified male condom (especially if she is having her period or has a vaginal infection with discharge)

- Semen in the mouth

- Oral-anal contact

- Sharing sex toys or douching equipment

- Any sex (fisting, rough vaginal or anal intercourse, rape) that causes tissue damage or bleeding

Source: Hatcher, R. A., Trussell, J., Stewart, F. H., Cates, W., Stewart, G. K., Guest, F. & Kowal, D. (Eds.). (1998). *Contraceptive technology* (17th ed.). New York: Ardent Media.

Note to the Reader: Table 7-1 has some inaccuracies that need to be corrected. Testing for STI's including chlamydia, syphilis, gonorrhea, herpes, hepatitis B and C, as well as testing for HIV would need to be done before sexual activity which exchanges blood or semen, or involves skin to skin contact could be considered "possibly safe." In addition, other STI's, such as the human papilloma virus, may be present but undetected due to the current lack of available tests for this virus. Therefore, this kind of sexual activity, even between mutually monogamous, trustworthy partners who's tests are all negative, would still need to categorized not as safe, but as "possibly safe."

charting, special health issues for women who are seropositive for HIV, and risk to health care providers—has been gleaned from this source. Hatcher and associates cite several important statistics and results of research studies, many of which have been included here. Please refer to their book, *Contraceptive Technology.*

In reading about disease epidemics throughout history, most health care workers could never have imagined that the world's inhabitants would be experiencing some of the horrors of deadly epidemic communicable disease that are being seen today. The AIDS epidemic has touched everybody's lives, and health care providers have been affected profoundly. Many people in the United States are still somewhat immune to the fact that AIDS affects men, women, and children alike and has reached epidemic proportions. Because HIV infection can be asymptomatic for many years, many female clients are infected and do not know they carry HIV. Women who are infected with HIV have special gynecologic health issues and needs that need to be watched for and addressed.

Much progress has been made in understanding the nature of HIV and AIDS. New antiviral medications are being introduced continually. These drugs offer the hope of allowing the disease to be managed as a chronic illness for longer and longer periods. Vaccines are being researched that may eventually prevent the spread of the virus.

It is discouraging that more and more young people, especially women, are contracting HIV. In the United States, women age 15–44 years represent one of the fastest growing segments of the epidemic. Worldwide, by the year 2000 between 38 and 108 million people could be seropositive for HIV. There are 4.7 million women already infected. Women are more likely than men to acquire HIV at any one contact.

AIDS is the leading cause of death among young women in most of the world. Most of these women contracted the disease by exposure to infected men. The ratio of infected men and women worldwide is approaching 1:1. Both sexual activity and intravenous drug use play a major role in current transmission statistics.

Testing

In counseling clients about undergoing AIDS testing, it is helpful to be aware of the two types:

1. **Anonymous:** With an anonymous AIDS test, there is never a link between a name and the serum sample. A code number is given.

2. **Confidential:** With a confidential AIDS test, the name is linked to the serum sample. However, name-linked information is protected to a degree as determined by state law.

Two tests are currently being used in AIDS testing: an enzyme-linked immunosorbent assay (ELISA) and the Western immunoblot assay. Serum samples are evaluated in each.

With regard to accuracy, the ELISA and Western immunoblot confirmatory tests are very sensitive and specific, but not 100%. For a result to be reported as positive for a given serum sample, two ELISAs and one Western immunoblot are done. Results must be positive for all three. In addition, it is well known that at least 6 months must have elapsed from the time of a possible contact to the time of the test for accurate results to be obtained. This is a crucial teaching point in counseling clients about AIDS testing.

Charting

It is important for the protection of both the client and the health care practitioner that health care providers understand the regulations in their state and their facility regarding confidentiality. Some facilities keep separate charts or use a code for the HIV test. In some states removal of related information before releasing a chart is required.

Special Health Issues for Women Who Are Seropositive for HIV

In addition to having the same symptoms experienced by men, women who are seropositive for HIV often experience a constellation of gynecologic problems. They may have special psychosocial issues as well, which have an impact on their health.

1. **Gynecologic issues:**

   - **Contraception:** Intrauterine devices are contraindicated in women who are seropositive for HIV because of the immunosuppressive nature of HIV infection. Condoms should be part of any contraceptive plan.

   - **Infection:** Recurrent vaginal yeast infections are common and may require prophylactic therapy (Stenchever, 1996).

   - **Cervical disease:** For women who are seropositive for HIV, cervical disease can be much more aggressive, progressing rapidly and requiring prompt treatment and careful monitoring.

   - **Pelvic inflammatory disease:** If pelvic inflammatory disease (PID) develops, hospitalization and aggressive intravenous antibiotic treatment are necessary.

   - **Herpes:** The lesions of herpes may appear more frequently, as well as be more painful and slower to heal. Acyclovir as suppressive therapy may help control outbreaks.

   - **Pregnancy:** The risk of transmission of HIV from mother to offspring is in the range of 13%–45% but averages 20%–30%. Transmission can occur in utero, during birth, or through breastfeeding. Infants are all seropositive at birth because of maternal antibodies in the infant's blood. An accurate test can be done when the infant is 15–18 months of age.

2. **Psychosocial issues:**

   - Women who are seropositive for HIV are likely to be caregivers themselves, attending to the needs of children and spouse.

   - It may be difficult for these women to take care of themselves.

   - It may be challenging for these women to keep appointments, get adequate rest, and comply with medication regimens.

   - Oftentimes, other family members are also infected.

   - These women often have many other more immediate issues, such as housing and financial problems.

Risk to Health Care Providers

In more than 2,000 reported cases of a single needlestick or percutaneous exposure, the rate of HIV infection is about 0.3%.

CHLAMYDIAL INFECTION

Chlamydial infection is the most common STI in the United States and the leading cause of preventable infertility and ectopic pregnancy (Lichtman & Papera, 1990). In 1996 the Division of STD Prevention (1997) at the CDC reported that there were 490,000 cases of chlamydial infection, exceeding all other reportable diseases in the United States (see *Figure 7-1*). The rate for women was five times that for men. The highest rates were in adolescents, and the incidence was also related to low socioeconomic status. According to Hatcher and colleagues (1994), rates of chlamydial infection have declined in areas in which government-funded screening programs are in effect.

Symptoms

Caused by the organism *Chlamydia trachomatis*, chlamydial infection is frequently asymptomatic, especially in women (Hatcher et al., 1994). Approximately 70% of women with chlamydial

FIGURE 7-1
Chlamydia—Reported Rates: United States, 1984–1996

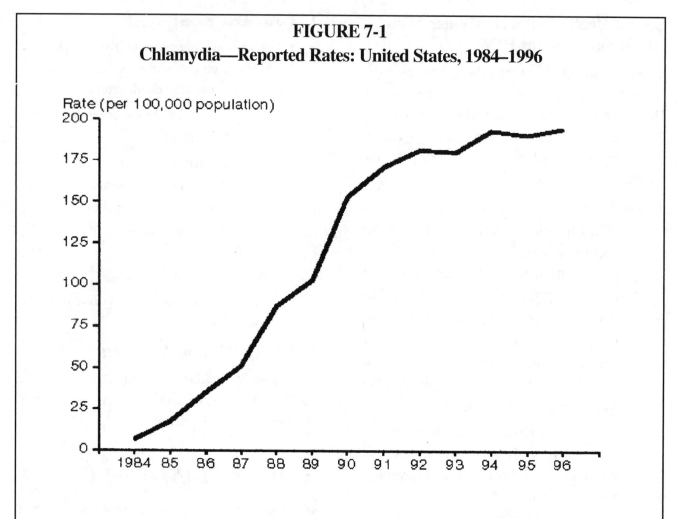

Rate (per 100,000 population)

Source: From *Sexually Transmitted Disease Surveillance, 1996* [Online], U.S. Department of Health and Human Services, Public Health Service, by Division of STD Prevention, September 1997, Atlanta: Centers for Disease Control and Prevention. Copyright September 1997 by Division of STD Prevention. In public domain. Available: http://wonder.cdc.gov/wonder/STD/STDD009/Figure_2.html

infection report no symptoms, and *Chlamydia* is the organism most often responsible for PID (Hatcher et al., 1994).

Testing

A large percentage of chlamydial infections are detected through broad-scale screening programs. A very sensitive test—the polymerase chain reaction (PCR), which detects DNA from the *Chlamydia* organism—is now available. A urine sample (obtained after a minimum of 1 hour without urinating) or a swab of the cervical tissue can be used for analysis.

Treatment

Antibiotics are the treatment of choice for chlamydial infection. (Please refer to CDC guidelines for protocols [Division of STD Prevention, 1997].)

Long-Term Complications

The Division of STD Prevention (1997) at the CDC reported that 85% of women delay getting tested and treated for chlamydial infection and gonorrhea because of vague symptoms. As the chlamydial infection spreads throughout the uterus and fallopian tubes, PID can result with its potentially permanent results. (See the section on PID.)

GONORRHEA

Gonorrhea is caused by the bacteria *Neisseria gonorrhoeae,* and it is another widespread STI (Lichtman & Papera, 1990).

According to the Division of STD Prevention (1997), gonorrhea rates have declined since the early 1970s when government screening programs began. Rates were at their lowest in 1996 since reporting first began. The rates are still higher than the national goals set by the government in Healthy People 2000.

Symptoms

Men usually have symptoms of pain with urination and penile discharge. Women may be asymptomatic. (Fifty percent of cases of gonorrhea in women are asymptomatic [Hatcher et al., 1994].) Some women report vaginal discharge, abnormal menses, or pain with urination.

Testing

Lichtman and Papera (1990) report that the primary way that gonorrhea is detected is through government screening programs. They note that the PCR used to detect chlamydial infection is also used for detection of gonorrhea. Older testing methods still in use are culture techniques requiring incubation or microscopic evaluation.

Treatment

Hatcher and colleagues (1994) report that in many areas *n. gonorrhoeae* has become resistant to the old standard of penicillin therapy. A number of different drug regimens can be used. Antibiotics that are not in the penicillin family have generally replaced the use of penicillin-related drugs, especially in locations in which resistant strains have been identified. Treatment covering possible concomitant chlamydial infection is also the standard of care.

Long-Term Complications

In up to 40% of untreated women with cervical gonorrhea PID develops, and the PID can progress to a systemic infection (Lichtman & Papera, 1990). Gonorrhea can also infect the pharynx. Clients with gonorrhea who have oral sex should be evaluated and treated for pharyngeal gonorrhea as well. Gonorrhea can be passed from mother to infant, causing infection of the infant's eyes (Hatcher et al., 1994).

TRICHOMONIASIS

Trichomoniasis is a vaginal infection that is caused by a sexually transmitted parasitic organism, *Trichomonas vaginalis* (Stenchever, 1996).

Symptoms

According to Stenchever (1996), 50% of women who have trichomoniasis are asymptomatic. "Trich" often produces a profuse, bubbly gray, green or yellow discharge with a foul odor. The discharge can be irritating and cause pain with urination.

Testing

Lichtman and Papera (1990) report that microscopic evaluation is used to confirm trichomoniasis. The parasites have a characteristic tail, which can be seen moving under the microscope. The pH of the vaginal discharge is usually higher (more basic) than normal. Other tests are less common, including vaginal culture.

Treatment

Stenchever (1996) notes that metronidazole (Flagyl) is the drug of choice for trichomoniasis, resulting in a 95% cure rate. Partners should be treated because men are often asymptomatic.

PELVIC INFLAMMATORY DISEASE

Hatcher and colleagues (1994) describe PID as an acute infection of the uterus and fallopian tubes, which can, if untreated or unresolved, result in scarring, adhesions, or blockage of the fallopian tubes. They note further that usually a number of different organisms are involved, most commonly the causative bacteria for gonorrhea or chlamydial infection as well as other bacteria. Severe infection can cause abscesses on the ovaries or fallopian tubes and inflammation of the lining of the pelvic cavity. More than 1 million cases of PID occur annually in the United States (Hatcher et al., 1994). The two greatest consequences of acute PID can be infertility and tubal pregnancy due to scarring of the fallopian tubes (Stenchever, 1996).

Risk Factors

Higher levels of PID are associated with multiple sexual partners, lower age at first intercourse, and lower economic status (Kelsey & Freeman, 1997). Douching has also been associated with an increased risk (Stenchever, 1996).

Symptoms

According to Hatcher and colleagues (1994), PID can be asymptomatic, which is very common with chlamydial infection in women, or it can cause severe pain, extreme uterine tenderness, as well as tenderness in the ovaries. The infected individual can experience extreme tenderness when the cervix is moved on examination. Fever and chills can also be present.

Treatment

Pelvic inflammatory disease can be treated on an outpatient basis, but hospitalization may be necessary, depending on the individual case (Stenchever, 1996). For patients who are being treated on an outpatient basis, reexamination within 48–72 hours is a crucial part of therapy (Kelsey & Freeman, 1997). Combination drug therapy is advised because the full spectrum of organisms involved is often not known. The CDC has specific guidelines for PID treatment, as for treatment of all STDs (Kelsey & Freeman, 1997).

HUMAN PAPILLOMAVIRUS (HPV)

According to Hatcher and colleagues (1994), HPV—also called genital warts or condyloma acuminatum—is transmitted by skin-to-skin contact. There are more than 60 viral types currently identified, several of which cause warty growths in the vagina or on the vulva, perineum, or anal area. These growths can be single or multiple, soft, and fleshy, and they are usually painless. Other strains of HPV infect the cervix and go unnoticed until findings from a routine Pap smear reveal the presence of the virus. Certain viral types are associated with the growth of abnormal cervical cells, which can lead to cancer of the cervix.

Treatment

Hatcher and colleagues (1994) note that for external warts several topical chemicals are commonly used in the office setting. The most common are "podophyllin 10%–25% in compound tincture of benzoin" (Hatcher et al., 1994, p. 91) and tricholoracetic acid. A product called podofilox is available by prescription for home application. Cryotherapy (freezing), CO_2 laser surgery, electrosurgery, or surgical removal are all treatment options, depending on severity and resistance to treatment.

A cream recently approved by the Food and Drug Administration called imiquimod (Aldara) seems to work by enhancing cell-mediated immune activity against the virus ("Warts, Frustrating But Common, Experts Say," 1997).

Please see chapter 10 for further discussion of HPV and abnormal Pap smear findings.

HERPES SIMPLEX VIRUS (HSV) TYPE 2

Herpes simplex virus type 1 is the virus that causes cold sores. Type 2 is usually found in the genital area, although the types can change location depending on sexual practices (Lichtman & Papera, 1990). Herpes is transmitted by skin-to-skin contact. An estimated 30 million Americans are infected, although most infections are asymptomatic (Hatcher et al., 1994).

Symptoms

Lichtman and Papera (1990) note that the first outbreak of herpes can cause a kind of systemic malaise, flulike symptoms, muscle aches, and headache accompanied by blisterlike lesions, which can be severe and last 4–15 days. Before an actual outbreak, there is often a period of what are called prodromal symptoms with skin sensitivity and nerve pain in the area in which the lesion will appear, followed by reddening of the skin. The lesions typically have a blisterlike appearance, are painful and sometimes itchy, and contain clear fluid. These dry up, crust over, and then heal.

Lichtman and Papera (1990) comment further that recurrent outbreaks are typically less severe, usually with minimal systemic symptoms and lesions taking up to 10 days to heal. The virus goes into a latent stage in the nerves at the base of the spine and may reactivate when the client's immune system is weakened. The lesions may occur along any skin surface supplied by that nerve distribution, including the vulva, vagina, cervix, or buttocks.

Hatcher and colleagues (1994) report that as with a number of other STIs, a client can have herpes and never have any symptoms, or she can have such mild symptoms that she would never suspect herpes unless she already knew that she had been exposed. In addition, the classic presentation of painful blister is often absent, and the virus may cause only a reddened or fissured area on the vulva, which could look like many other vulvar problems. Transmission of the virus is most likely during times when an active outbreak is occurring, and clients should abstain from contact during this time.

It is believed that transmission also occurs, although at a lower rate, between outbreaks or when there are no symptoms. Because much of the infected population is asymptomatic, it is believed that much of the transmission of HSV occurs in this group ("Herpes the Silent Epidemic," 1998).

Testing

Results of antibody testing are definitive for HSV exposure, but this test does not provide information on when exposure has occurred. Findings from a culture of the lesion are less reliable (Lichtman & Papera, 1990). A negative result does not mean there is no exposure. A positive result is definitive (Lichtman & Papera, 1990). In most people with healthy immune systems, the presence of the virus is not associated with marked illness, nor with cervical cancer as was once thought (Sifton, 1994). In women with a compromised immune system, outbreaks can be more frequent and severe.

Treatment

Acyclovir can be given for 7–10 days for the initial outbreak and for 5 days for recurrence. For clients with frequently recurring lesions, acyclovir can be taken on a daily basis for a year, at which time outbreak frequency needs to be reevaluated. It can be taken for up to 3 years (Lichtman & Papera, 1990). The medication does not eliminate the latent virus.

A newer medication, which is called valacyclovir hydrochloride (Valtrex®) and is a derivative of acyclovir, is taken only twice per day for 5 days. However, the drug is not approved for longer term suppressive therapy (*Physicians' Desk Reference,* 1998).

Some women with herpes have found that specific herbs, supplements, and dietary changes help decrease their symptoms and the frequency and severity of outbreaks. Lichtman and Papera (1990) offer the following self-help therapies for herpes prevention:

- A diet high in lysine (an amino acid that suppresses the virus) and low in arginine (an amino acid that seems to bring on outbreaks)

- Echinacea, an antiviral herb

- Vitamin C supplementation

- Zinc supplementation

Fuchs and Winograd (1985), in their book *The Nutrition Detective,* list foods to avoid (those high in arginine) and foods to include (those high in lysine) in a diet for herpes prevention:

- Foods high in arginine:
  — Nuts
  — Seeds
  — Carob
  — Whole wheat products
  — Brown rice
  — Raisins
  — Peanut butter
  — Chocolate
  — Coconut
  — Garbanzo beans
  — Oatmeal

- Foods high in lysine:
  — Fish
  — Shellfish
  — Potatoes
  — Chicken
  — Lamb
  — Beef
  — Cow's milk
  — Cheeses
  — Brewer's yeast
  — Eggs
  — Pork
  — Beans
  — Goat's milk

Lysine supplements are also available.

None of the above recommendations have been tested or approved by the Food and Drug Administration, but they are safe home remedies.

SYPHILIS

One of the oldest known STIs, syphilis is caused by *Treponema pallidum.* Unfortunately, syphilis is on the rise, reaching higher levels in the past decade than in the last 40 years (Hatcher et al., 1994). The recent syphilis outbreaks have been associated with exchange of sex for drugs, especially crack cocaine (Hatcher et al., 1994).

If left untreated, syphilis can cause severe systemic disease. Syphilis can be transmitted by means of sexual intercourse, kissing, biting, or oral-genital sex.

Symptoms

Syphilis is a complex disease, beyond the scope of this course to detail. Listed next is a basic summary of its symptoms, classified according to its three clinical stages, as well as the latent period that occurs between the first two and last.

Primary

In the primary stage a painless ulcer appears at the site of exposure, and it resolves on its own without treatment. The ulcer may go unnoticed, usually appears 1 week to 3 months after initial exposure.

Secondary

In the secondary stage a generalized malaise, skin rash, mucus patches, characteristic moist flat warts in the genital and anal areas, swollen lymph glands, and hair loss occur. If the syphilis is untreated, these symptoms resolve within 2–10 weeks.

Latent

If all the above symptoms go untreated, the disease enters a latent phase, which generally is not associated with symptoms.

Tertiary

In the tertiary stage systemic symptoms appear 1–2 years after onset of infection to as long as 30 or 40 years later. Neurologic symptoms, destruction of bone tissue, and cardiovascular disease characterize this stage (Hatcher et al., 1994).

Testing

According to Hatcher and colleagues (1994), tests for detecting syphilis depend on the stage of the disease. For primary and secondary syphilis, the material obtained from the lesion can be tested with either a darkfield microscope or a fluorescent antibody test. Blood testing is also diagnostic. Latent syphilis can be detected only by using a blood test.

Treatment

A form of penicillin is the treatment of choice for syphilis, with specific regimen and duration depending on the length of infection (Hatcher et al., 1994).

Long-Term Complications

If left untreated, syphilis can develop into systemic infection with serious neurologic and cardiac problems (Lichtman & Papera, 1990).

HEPATITIS B VIRUS (HBV)

Heterosexual intercourse is now the predominant mode of transmission of hepatitis B virus (Hatcher et al., 1994). The HBV is also transmitted by blood-to-blood contact, which can occur by sharing of razors, toothbrushes, and manicure tools, as well as through contaminated instruments for tattooing and body piercing ("Natural Help for Hepatitis," 1998). Contamination of instruments can also occur in other settings such as dental offices. This is to be distinguished from hepatitis A, which is caused by ingestion of contaminated food. Hepatitis B virus infects some 300,000 people in the United States each year ("Hepatitis A and B: Should You Be Immunized?," 1998). There has been a rising incidence among teen-agers and young adults ("Hepatitis A and B: Should You Be Immunized?," 1998).

Symptoms

Hatcher and colleagues (1994) report that most HBV infections are asymptomatic. If symptoms do occur, they can include nausea, vomiting, low energy, headache, fever, dark urine, jaundice, joint pain, and skin eruptions.

Testing

There are a number of different markers identified in a blood test, some of which indicate active infection, chronic carrier state, or past infection. About 5%–10% of adults who contract HBV become chronically infected ("Hepatitis A and B: Should You Be Immunized?," 1998).

Prevention

Vaccination is available. The CDC's current recommendations are for vaccination of adolescents; others at high risk for STIs; health care workers who have a risk of exposure; and anyone planning travel to China, Asia, or Africa. Also advised is vaccination of newborns ("Hepatitis A and B: Should You Be Immunized?," 1998).

Treatment

No effective treatments are currently available (Hatcher et al., 1994).

Long-Term Complications

Long-term complications of HBV include chronic active hepatitis, cirrhosis, cancer of the liver, liver failure, and death.

HEPATITIS C VIRUS

Largely unknown to the American public, hepatitis C has reached epidemic proportions in the United States. In an article in the July 1998 issue of *Women's Health Advocate Newsletter* ("Hepatitis C, the Silent Epidemic: Who's At Risk?"), current statistics about hepatitis C are reviewed. Approximately 4 million Americans are infected with the hepatitis C virus, with the rate of new infections estimated to be around 30,000 per year. The virus was discovered in 1989. Before that, researchers were aware that in some patients a type of hepatitis was developing that could not be traced to either hepatitis A or B. This type of infection was previously known as non-A, non-B hepatitis.

Transmission

The hepatitis C virus is spread through blood-to-blood contact. Once the virus was discovered, blood banks began testing for the virus. Blood was not tested for this virus before 1992. According to the article "Hepatitis C, the Silent Epidemic: Who's At Risk?" (1998), intravenous drug use has accounted for 60% of transmission in the past 6 years, with 20% of new cases being attributed to sexual transmission. The virus can be transmitted from mother to child, although this is rare. As with the HBV, transmission of the hepatitis C virus can potentially occur through blood contact with shared needles, razors, and toothbrushes, as well as through contaminated instruments used for tattooing or body piercing. Approximately 4% of cases have occurred in health care workers who contracted hepatitis C on the job.

Risk Factors

The following are risk factors for hepatitis C ("Hepatitis C: Testing for a 'Stealth Virus,'" 1998):

- Person who
  - had a blood transfusion before 1992
  - had a tattoo or body-piercing procedure
  - shared personal items (e.g., razor, toothbrush) with someone who is infected with the hepatitis C virus
- Transplant recipient
- Health care worker exposed to body fluids
- Intravenous drug user (current or past)
- Patient who receives hemodialysis
- Person with multiple sex partners

Symptoms

Infection with the hepatitis C virus is often asymptomatic, or initial symptoms may be mild (e.g., malaise) and easily mistaken for a cold or flu. Symptoms may be brief or intermittent, as well as go unnoticed. More prominent symptoms appear as the disease progresses and include fatigue, muscle weakness, abdominal pain, nausea, and loss of appetite. These can progress to jaundice and dark urine in the later stages of the infection.

Testing

A simple blood test can be ordered to screen for antibodies to the hepatitis C virus.

Treatment

Current treatment options are limited ("Hepatitis C, the Silent Epidemic: Who's At Risk?," 1998). Drug therapy involves two primary agents:

1. Interferon alfa-2b, recombinant (Intron A). Intron A has very specific protocols and is appropriate only for patients whose liver enzyme values (confirmed by blood test) are abnormal. Patients must be monitored closely.

2. Rebetron. Rebetron is a recently approved combination of Intron A and ribavirin (Rebetol). This drug is used for patients who do not respond to interferon or who relapse after treatment.

Both these drugs can have serious side effects.

Liver transplant is also an option, but one limited by cost, availability of organs, and eventual infection of the new liver.

Long-Term Complications

In approximately 85% of people who are infected with the hepatitis C virus a chronic infection will develop. Most of those infected are silent carriers, but in approximately 20% of chronically infected people liver disease will develop ("Natural Help for Hepatitis," 1998). The disease usually takes the form of cirrhosis—irreversible and progressive destruction of the liver. Liver cancer is another potential long-term complication of hepatitis C. Hepatitis C virus causes an estimated 8,000–10,000 deaths each year, and this number is expected to triple in the next 10–20 years ("Hepatitis C, the Silent Epidemic: Who's at Risk?," 1998).

Self-Care

No vaccine exists as yet for prevention of hepatitis C virus infection. In the April 1998 issue of *Dr. Andrew Weil's Self-Healing* newsletter, the article, "Natural Help for Hepatitis" (1998), lists the following suggestions for people with hepatitis B or C viral infection:

- Eat a low-protein, low-fat diet.
- Avoid
  — protein or amino acid supplements.
  — alcohol and tobacco.
  — exposure to toxic fumes and chemicals.
- Take
  — an antioxidant formula (including vitamins C and E, beta carotene, and selenium).

  — liver-protective herbs, such as milk thistle (*Silybum marianum*), schizandra (*Schisandra chinensis*), and maitake mushroom (*Grifola frondosa*).

- Drink plenty of water (6–8 glasses a day).
- Get
  — adequate rest.
  — vaccinated against hepatitis A. (According to the results of a study published in the *New England Journal of Medicine*, people with hepatitis C virus infection have a dramatically higher risk of dying if they eat food infected with hepatitis A virus.)

- Practice safe sex.
- Do not donate blood, tissue, organs, or semen.

LESS COMMON STIs

The 10 previously described diseases are among the most commonly seen in clients with STIs. Although they occur less commonly, the following four STIs are also of interest to health care providers who work with clients with STIs (Lichtman & Papera, 1990):

1. **Chancroid:** Chancroid is caused by the organism *Haemophilus ducreyi*. It causes painful inguinal adenopathy and is treated with antibiotics.

2. **Lymphogranuloma venereum:** Lymphogranuloma venereum is caused by *Chlamydia trachomatis*. It also produces inguinal adenopathy and is treated with antibiotics.

3. **Granuloma inguinale:** Granuloma inguinale is caused by *Calymmatobacterium granulomatis*. It is rarely seen in the United States. It causes ulcerative symptoms and is treated with antibiotics.

4. **Vulvar ulcers:** Tuberculosis can cause vulvar ulcers. A tuberculin test with injection of PPD (purified protein derivative) and chest x-ray

films are used for diagnosis. Tuberculosis should be suspected in high-risk populations.

CONCLUSION

Many of the common STIs have no symptoms. This needs to be a primary communication in health teaching. Clients need to understand that they can have an infection and not know it, they can pass an infection to their partner unawares, and their partner likewise can be infected and pass a disease innocently to them. The long-term consequences of this lack of awareness can be devastating.

One of the major obstacles in making progress in stemming the rising epidemics of STIs is that the adults do not agree on how to approach the problem of sexual activity in young people, nor on what the best solution might be. Opinion ranges from no sexual education in the schools and no condom availability to making education and barrier methods widely available. Study findings have shown that making condoms available in the schools did not increase the amount of sexual activity (Schuster, Bell, Berry, & Kanouse, 1998). Certainly no one will argue that delaying sexual activity would be a good solution, but efforts to promote abstinence have not been successful to date. Young people are having sex and at earlier and earlier ages. They are acquiring and passing on STIs. There is no time to waste.

EXAM QUESTIONS

CHAPTER 7
Questions 51–56

51. Infection with the *Chlamydia* organism is the most common cause of

    a. abnormal periods.

    b. vaginal discharge.

    c. pelvic inflammatory disease.

    d. painful periods.

52. One of the long-term consequences of untreated chlamydial infection is

    a. blockage of the fallopian tubes.

    b. increased risk of miscarriage.

    c. systemic neurologic problems.

    d. damage to the ovaries.

53. The first sign of syphilis is a sore that is

    a. painless.

    b. painful.

    c. itchy.

    d. blistery and filled with clear fluid.

54. Compared with men, what is the likelihood that women will acquire HIV at any one contact?

    a. Women are less likely than men to acquire HIV at any one contact.

    b. Women are more likely than men to acquire HIV at any one contact.

    c. Women are equally likely as men to acquire HIV at any one contact.

    d. Not enough research has been done to determine the likelihood in women vs. in men.

55. Which of the following STIs is/are often asymptomatic in women?

    a. Chlamydial infection and gonorrhea

    b. Herpes

    c. HIV

    d. All the above

56. Which of the following infections can extend into the uterus and fallopian tubes, causing pelvic inflammatory disease?

    a. Human papillomavirus infection

    b. Chlamydial infection

    c. Yeast infection

    d. Herpes infection

CHAPTER 8

PREMENSTRUAL SYNDROME

CHAPTER OBJECTIVE

After completing this chapter, the reader will be able to recognize how views about premenstrual syndrome have changed in recent years, and identify the theories that have been put forth regarding possible causes. The reader will also be able to identify the types of premenstrual syndrome, treatments and self-help approaches.

LEARNING OBJECTIVES

After studying this chapter, the reader will be able to

1. describe how views of premenstrual syndrome held by the medical community have evolved.

2. discuss possible causes of premenstrual syndrome.

3. list the different types of premenstrual syndrome and their common symptoms.

4. describe self-help and other treatment options for premenstrual syndrome.

Key Words

* Premenstrual tension (PMT)
* Prostaglandin inhibitors
* Prostaglandins

INTRODUCTION

Premenstrual syndrome (PMS) or premenstrual tension (PMT) is defined as the presence of emotional and physical symptoms and behavioral changes that occur during the second half of the menstrual cycle and cease at or within a few days after the onset of menses (Keye & Keye, 1998). The timing of the symptoms in relation to the menstrual cycle, rather than the symptoms themselves, is what is unique in this disorder. Diagnosis depends on finding that the symptoms experienced occur in this cyclic pattern, are not caused by any underlying physical or mental condition, and greatly disrupt one or more areas of the woman's life (Keye & Keye, 1998). More than 150 symptoms, ranging from mild to severe and experienced in various combinations, have been identified (Keye & Keye, 1998). These symptoms affect almost every organ system in the body (DeMarco, 1996).

Premenstrual syndrome has an interesting history. Until fairly recently, the symptoms of PMS were assumed by most of the medical profession to be part of a woman's nature, or based totally on emotion, and without any source of physiologic imbalance. Research in the field of PMS was largely ignored until the past two decades (Lichtman & Papera, 1990). As the women's movement grew in strength and awareness about women's health issues increased, views began to shift. In addition, there was an accumulating body of medical research findings that described physiologic imbalances and presented theories about what causes PMS. It came to be viewed as a complex constellation of physiologic imbalance that affects a woman's physical, emotional, and mental health (Lichtman & Papera, 1990).

PREVALENCE

Sources vary in estimates of the number of women who experience symptoms of PMS. In her book, *Take Charge of Your Body,* DeMarco (1996) estimates that up to 90% of women experience some form of PMS, however mild. Other sources report that 20%–40% of women experience some form of PMS. Recent study findings indicate that 3%–5% of women experience severe PMS (Keye & Keye, 1998).

SYMPTOMS

DeMarco (1996) has identified the most common symptoms of PMS described by women:

- Irritability
- Anxiety
- Mood swings
- Depression
- Hostility
- Headaches
- Dizziness
- Fainting
- Shakiness
- Bloating
- Weight gain
- Sugar cravings
- Constipation
- Diarrhea
- Backache

- Asthma
- Breast tenderness
- Breast swelling
- Joint pain
- Sore throat
- Cramps
- Nausea
- Insomnia
- Water retention
- Fatigue
- Increased appetite
- Cold sweats
- Hot flashes
- Lack of coordination
- Easy bruising
- Palpitations
- Hives
- Joint swelling
- Hay fever
- Migraine

These symptoms commonly occur in clusters, with women often reporting as many as 10 symptoms. Women who have severe symptoms may be prone to extremes of behavior, increasing the likelihood of accidents, alcohol abuse, and suicide attempts. For other women, symptoms may be annoying but mild.

When evaluating a woman for PMS symptoms, the health care provider must take very seriously any report of suicidal thoughts or other indication of extreme mood change. This woman will need appropriate medications, close follow-up and referrals to a qualified mental health professional. Once she is stable, lifestyle and dietary changes can be initiated that will be an important part of her long term health maintenance.

Women who come to be evaluated for any of the above symptoms should be given a complete exam and work-up to rule out illnesses that might be the source of symptoms. A careful history is crucial to any diagnosis of PMS. Particular attention needs to be made to the timing of symptoms. Women who have symptoms occurring primarily during the menstrual flow or during the first two weeks of the menstrual cycle do not have PMS as defined in the literature.

RISK FACTORS

According to Lichtman and Papera (1990), a woman is at increased risk of having PMS if she

- is older than 30 years of age. The most severe symptoms occur in women 30–40 years of age.

- is under a great deal of emotional stress.

- has poor nutritional habits.

- has experienced side effects from birth control pills. Women who do not tolerate the pill are more likely to get PMS.

- is a married woman. Statistically, married women have more symptoms of PMS than their unmarried counterparts.

- has had children.

- had toxemia during pregnancy.

WHAT CAUSES PMS?

Medical researchers have not yet found an answer to the question of what causes PMS.

Cause and Symptom Clusters or Subgroups of PMS

Lichtman and Papera (1990) have summarized early research findings, that attempt to clarify the complex symptom picture with PMS, noting that four main symptom clusters have been defined in the early research literature. Each may have a different cause, requiring a unique approach to treatment. This classification system for PMS was developed by one of the pioneering researchers in the field of PMS—Guy Abraham, former clinical professor of obstetrics and gynecology at the University of California, Los Angeles.

The four main symptom clusters mentioned earlier are as follows:

1. **Type A** ("anxiety"): Mood swings, irritability, anxiety, nervous tension

2. **Type H** ("hyperhydration"): Edema, abdominal bloating, breast tenderness, weight gain

3. **Type C** ("cravings"): Sugar craving, headaches, fatigue

4. **Type D** ("depression"): Memory loss, depression, confusion

In addition, Lark (1984) describes two subgroups:

1. **Acne:** Oily skin and hair, worsening skin blemishes

2. **Dysmenorrhea:** Cramps, lower back pain, nausea, vomiting

Each of these groups is discussed in more detail below.

Type A

The following overview of, as well as suggestions for treatment of PMS symptoms in, the type A PMS symptom cluster is based on a description of PMS by Lichtman and Papera (1990). They cite several helpful statistics and results of research on PMS, which have been included in this commentary.

Type A is the most common type of PMS, being reported by 80% of women in studies. Women with type A PMS have high serum estrogen levels combined with low serum progesterone levels. Estrogen and progesterone both affect the chemistry of the brain and therefore mood and emotion. They have opposite effects. Estrogen is a stimulant—too much leads to anxiety. Progesterone is a tranquilizer—too much causes depression. The balance of estrogen and progesterone depends on both how much are produced and how they are eliminated from the body. The liver is the site of breakdown for both hormones, and the byproducts are excreted through the kidney and bowel. Deficiency of B vitamins and magnesium and excess fat and sugar in the diet, all impair the ability of the liver to break down hormones.

Treatment recommendations center around providing nutrients that are involved in optimizing liver function and balancing brain chemistry and hormone function. In general, a diet low in animal protein and fat (including dairy products) is recommended, with elimination of sugar, caffeine, and spicy foods—all of which put added stress on the liver's detoxifying functions. Chemicals, preservatives, pollutants, and drugs also have an impact on the liver and should be avoided.

Fresh fruits and vegetables, whole grains, and legumes should form the basis of the diet. These are high in vitamins and trace minerals essential for balancing the body's functions. Fiber helps the body get rid of excess estrogen and balance elimination. A good multiple vitamin–mineral supplement that has all the nutrients in balanced proportions is advised. Vitamins should not be substituted for improvements in the diet. In addition, exercise is very important. Study findings have shown that exercise causes the brain to produce hormones called endorphins, which give a feeling of well being.

Type H

The following description on the type H PMS symptom cluster, with citation of pertinent research results, is gleaned from Lark (1984).

Type H PMS is characterized by weight gain of 1–3 pounds. It can be accompanied by fluid shifts, causing a bloated feeling in the abdomen, swelling of hands and feet, and breast tenderness. Retention of sodium and water occurs because of high levels of the hormone aldosterone. The excess of this hormone could be triggered by stress, deficiency of magnesium, too much estrogen, or other imbalances. Study results have

shown that vitamin B^6 helps bring the fluid balance back to normal levels. Vitamin B^6 is one of the most important vitamins given for PMS symptoms because it is involved in so many functions in the body.

Dietary recommendations for type H PMS are the same as those for type A PMS. Water is a natural diuretic, and intake of at least 6–8 glasses a day is recommended.

Type C

Fuchs and Winograd (1985) note that women whose symptoms fall into the subgroup of type C PMS crave sweets, especially chocolate. A high sugar intake leads to headaches, fatigue, heart palpitations, shakiness, dizziness, and sometimes fainting, all of which are symptoms of low blood glucose. An interesting clue to why this happens is that during the week before the period, a woman's body is more responsive than usual to the hormone insulin, which allows cells to take up glucose from the blood stream. This tends to lower the blood glucose level because it allows more glucose to enter the cells. One of the first places in the body that is affected is the brain, which relies on glucose for its functions. The brain records this drop in glucose as stress, and the body begins to respond as if it is threatened. This sets off a vicious cycle that makes symptoms worse.

Fuchs and Winograd (1985) report further that chocolate is thought to be desired because it has a high magnesium content. Magnesium levels are commonly low in women with PMS. Magnesium is essential to breaking down sugars and helps decrease the craving for sugar. Chocolate also contains chemicals that have an antidepressant effect.

Fuchs and Winograd (1985) also report that dietary recommendations are the same as those described earlier for type A PMS. The trace mineral chromium is often recommended as it is involved in regulation of blood glucose.

Type D

Fuchs and Winograd (1985) note that type D PMS is almost always accompanied by type A. Thus the woman's moods tend to swing from irritable to depressed, often accompanied by confusion, forgetfulness, crying, insomnia, low energy, difficulty finding the words to express what she wants to say, and, in more severe cases, suicidal thoughts. Women with suicidal thoughts need to be referred for evaluation for underlying clinical depression.

According to Fuchs and Winograd (1985), type D PMS is thought to be related to an imbalance of hormones with low estrogen and abnormally high progesterone levels. Why this imbalance of hormones occurs is not known. Again magnesium and vitamin B[6] are thought to be involved because they play such a central role in brain chemistry and blood glucose balance. Dietary interventions would be the same as those already described for the other types of PMS.

Acne

Lark (1984) indicates that a worsening of acne, pimples, and oily skin and hair is thought to be due to an increase in male-type hormones called androgens. Androgens are produced by the adrenal glands, and they cause changes in the acid-base balance of the skin as well as stimulate secretion of oil by the skin. The decreasing of fat in the diet and addition of foods or supplements (or both) containing beta carotene, vitamin E, vitamin C, and zinc help improve the condition of the skin.

Painful Periods (Dysmenorrhea)

DeMarco (1996) indicates dysmenorrhea may be due to an imbalance in the local tissue factors that control contractions of the uterus. These local hormones, called prostaglandins, are produced in the uterus and many other parts of the body. They act locally, producing contraction or dilation of local smooth muscles and blood vessels in the uterus.

DeMarco (1996) reports that a number of nutrients are involved in synthesis of the "good" relaxation-producing prostaglandins, including magnesium, zinc, vitamins B[6] and C, and essential fatty acids. High intake of animal fats may cause an overabundance of the "bad" prostaglandins to be produced, resulting in uterine cramping. Dietary interventions, which help normalize periods and reduce cramping, include reducing intake of animal fats and supplementing with oils that provide the essential fatty acids that help the body synthesize the "good" prostaglandins. These oils include flax seed oil, safflower oil, evening primrose oil, black currant seed oil, and borage seed oil.

DeMarco (1996) also notes that painful periods can have other causes, such as fibroids, endometriosis, or infection. Women with dysmenorrhea should have a complete pelvic examination and evaluation.

Other Theories on Cause

Some researchers have proposed that women who experience PMS have low levels of progesterone during the second half of the menstrual cycle (Keye & Keye, 1998).

Another theory currently under investigation links hormonal changes during ovulation with changes in brain chemistry, particularly with the neurotransmitter serotonin. Decreased serotonin levels have been associated with depression, irritability, carbohydrate cravings, and insomnia (Parker, 1994).

Additional theories implicate elevated prolactin levels, hypoglycemia, calcium or magnesium deficiency, as well as a deficiency in vitamin B or E. None of these potential causes has yet been confirmed (Keye & Keye, 1998).

DIAGNOSIS

There are four steps that are generally recommended to evaluate a woman who is experiencing symptoms of PMS (Keye & Keye, 1998):

1. Complete medical history

2. Physical examination

3. Blood tests

4. Two-month record of symptoms

The purpose of these steps (Keye & Keye, 1998) is to determine

1. whether the symptoms correspond to the cyclic pattern of PMS.

2. whether there are any possible underlying physical, mental, or emotional conditions.

3. to what degree symptoms interfere with the woman's quality of life.

TREATMENT

Once the diagnosis of PMS has been made, the first step in treatment is to validate the woman's experience and reassure her that her symptoms are real and have a physiologic base. This simple validation can be a great source of relief and healing for women who have concerns about their sanity (Lichtman & Papera, 1990). Many women find measurable relief from their symptoms by instituting changes in their dietary patterns and exercise; supplementation with selected vitamins, minerals, and herbs; and changes in lifestyle and sources of stress. A small percentage of women will not find adequate relief from these measures and may need some form of drug therapy (DeMarco, 1996).

Health Promotion

Most women with mild to moderate symptoms of PMS will respond well to simple health promotion. The first step in counseling women with PMS symptoms is to reassure them that they are not crazy. There has been so much distortion of PMS by the media that many women still do not realize that symptoms of PMS are physiologic changes that are real.

Research findings affirm that simple dietary and lifestyle interventions have a profound impact on PMS symptoms (DeMarco, 1996). This is an area in which women can feel very encouraged. Health care providers need to help guide women in making the long-term changes necessary to improve their symptoms.

Getting clients to make dietary changes is a very creative and challenging process for health care providers. Longstanding habits and often cultural patterns have to be addressed. Women need support and inspiration for making these changes. Health care providers would be wise to learn about the resources for nutritional guidance available in their community, such as nutritional counselors and cooking classes.

There are six areas in particular that health care providers can focus on in counseling and assisting clients with PMS: foods to avoid or include in the diet; exercise; vitamins, minerals, and other nutrients; herbs; relaxation techniques, including massage, yoga, meditation, and biofeedback; and Asian medicine.

Detrimental and Beneficial Foods for PMS

Clients should be aware of foods that can worsen as well as help their symptoms of PMS:

1. Foods that worsen PMS (Gladstar, 1993):

    *   Foods high in

        — refined sugars

        — animal fat, including dairy products

        — salt. (Beware of the "hidden" sodium in most packaged and processed foods.)

    *   Foods that are processed and full of chemicals

    *   Caffeinated beverages

- Alcoholic beverages

This list includes cola drinks, alcohol, chocolate, candy, ice cream, hamburgers, hot dogs, hard cheese, beef, pork, and pizza. Most women who have PMS crave one or more of these foods.

2. Foods that help PMS (DeMarco, 1996):

   - Foods made from whole grains, which could include breads, pasta, pancake mix, and crackers

   - Nuts and seeds

   - Fresh fruits and vegetables

   - Oils, especially safflower, sesame, olive, corn, and flax

   - Seaweeds

   - Seafood and skinless natural poultry (no hormones or growth factors)

   - Legumes, including soy products such as tofu

Exercise

Exercise is another key to PMS self-help. Results of many studies have proven its merit in alleviating symptoms of PMS. Regular aerobic exercise three or four times per week has many physiologic and psychologic benefits (Keye & Keye, 1998).

Vitamins, Minerals, and Other Nutrients

General Recommendations: According to DeMarco (1996), diet is always the first and best source of nutrients. Vitamins and minerals as they are found in food are better absorbed and assimilated and balanced. Those nutrients can be lost in cooking and preparation. Thus in addition to recommending types of food, health care providers should guide clients in how to prepare the food to maintain its nutritional value. For example,

- *steaming vegetables* instead of boiling them in water preserves many of the more delicate nutrients such as vitamin C.

- *including raw foods* at each meal is a great way to maximize nutritional value.

- *eating a wide variety of fruits and vegetable* ensures more nutrient balance. Encourage clients to be brave and try a new fruit or vegetable each week.

- *eating seasonal fruits and vegetables,* organically grown if possible, provides the best chance of clients ingesting foods that have not been stored for long periods or irradiated, which diminishes the nutritional value of these foods.

- *substituting whole grains* and whole grain breads, pasta, and pancake mixes for these products made with white flour gives these foods hundredfold more nutritional value.

- *encouraging the use of vegetable oils,* especially in helping clients from cultures that use lard as part of the cuisine, as they make the transition to a more healthful diet.

   A positive, enthusiastic, and experimental approach with specific suggestions can help women get behind the program.

Specific Recommendations: The following seven nutrients are recommended specifically for women with PMS. Please refer to the resource guide at the end of this course for books that contain specific, safe guidelines for nutritional supplementation.

- *Beta carotene:* Beta carotene is useful in improving the condition of the skin.

- *B complex vitamins:* Fuchs and Winograd (1985) note that the B complex vitamins include choline and inosotol, two B vitamins that help the liver break down fatty foods and hormones and also calm the nervous system. Soybeans, wheat germ, bran, and corn are high in these nutrients.

   Fuchs and Winograd (1985) also report that vitamin B^6 is one of the key nutrients in PMS therapy because it is essential for many metabolic functions, including brain chemistry, glucose metabolism, and liver function. B^6 can help alleviate mood swings. Good sources include wheat germ, brewer's yeast, whole grains, legumes, brown rice, chicken, tuna, salmon, and sunflower seeds.

- *Vitamin E:* DeMarco (1996) indicates that study findings have shown that vitamin E helps to improve cystic breast symptoms and also protect cells from harmful effects of chemicals. Sources include sunflower, corn, sesame, and walnut oils; nuts and seeds; broccoli; and corn (DeMarco, 1996).

- *Calcium:* Adequate calcium intake helps with menstrual cramps and balances nervous system function. Sources include tofu, broccoli, sesame seeds, greens, and yogurt (DeMarco, 1996).

- *Magnesium:* Keville and Korn (1996) report that menstrual cramps are also improved with adequate magnesium intake. Magnesium is involved in glucose metabolism and helps stabilize moods. It also enhances the absorption of calcium. Sources of magnesium include legumes, dark leafy greens, carrots, corn, nuts and seeds, and whole grains (DeMarco, 1996).

- *Zinc:* Zinc, a trace mineral, acts along with vitamins C and A to promote healthy skin. Sources include pumpkin seeds, legumes, and whole grains (DeMarco, 1996).

- *Essential fatty acids:* According to Keville and Korn (1996), essential fatty acids are a type of oil that the body cannot make and must be obtained from food. They are involved in the body's production of the good prostaglandins described earlier. Sources of these nutrients include flax seed oil and evening primrose or borage oil (often taken in supplement form). They are also found in certain types of fish (Keville & Korn, 1996).

Herbs

Keville and Korn (1996) indicate that there are a number of safe herbal medicines that have been used throughout history by women to help with PMS symptoms. They can be taken as teas or tinctures. These include herbs that are very high in vitamins and minerals, such as nettle and alfalfa, and herbs that support healthy liver function, such as burdock root, dandelion root, and milk thistle.

Gladstar (1993) reports that helpful herbs also include ones that tone the uterus, such as red raspberry leaf; those that relieve cramps, such as cramp bark and wild yam; and hormone-balancing herbs, such as chaste berry, black cohosh, and licorice. The leaf of the common dandelion is a safe and effective diuretic. Please refer to the resource guide for more information on the use of herbs.

Relaxation Techniques, Massage, Yoga, Meditation, and Biofeedback

Relaxation techniques, massage, yoga, meditation, and biofeedback practices, when done consistently, have great benefit in a PMS self-help program. Again, please refer to the resource guide for more specific information.

Asian Medicine

The healing approach in Asian medicine has much to offer for women who suffer from PMS symptoms. The Asian perspective is very different from that of Western medicine. All the seemingly disconnected symptoms make sense in the Asian model of how PMS occurs. Premenstrual syndrome is seen as an energetic imbalance, a blockage and stagnation of vital energy, or "chi," which normally flows through the body and enlivens it. When this energy is blocked in the pelvic region it can manifest in many of the symptoms described earlier. The Asian approaches aim to rebalance the energetics of the body, thereby allowing the hormone and nervous systems to return to a balanced function.

Drug Therapy

Many drug therapies are available, but only a few have been shown to be beneficial when subjected to scientific study (Keye & Keye, 1998):

- **Natural progesterone:** Natural progesterone is synthesized in the laboratory, but unlike the synthetic "progestins," its chemical structure is identical to the form naturally synthesized by the body. Natural progesterone has been used successfully in the treatment of PMS in the form of oral micronized progesterone (Keye & Keye, 1998), as well as in a topical cream form, which is available without prescription (DeMarco, 1996).

- **Antidepressants:** Some success has been achieved with the use of a new type of antidepressant called selective serotonin re-uptake inhibitor (SSRI) (Keye & Keye, 1998).

- **Medroxyprogesterone acetate (Depo-Provera):** Depo-Provera is a contraceptive that suppresses ovulation. (See chapter 5 for additional information.)

- **Allergy desensitization therapy:** Lichtman and Papera (1990) report that some women have exhibited an allergic response to their own hormones. Allergy desensitization therapy aims at eliminating or decreasing the level of this response. This is accomplished by giving graded doses of the hormones (the allergen).

- **Bromocriptine therapy:** Lichtman and Papera (1990) note that bromocriptine mesylate suppresses the body's production of the hormone prolactin, which is also produced by the pituitary gland and connected with the hormones of the menstrual cycle. They indicate that too much prolactin can cause an imbalance in the serum levels of estrogen and progesterone. Bromocriptine has been effective in decreasing breast tenderness, bloating, and depression in women with PMS (Lichtman & Papera, 1990).

- **Diuretics:** For some women, diuretics are prescribed (Lichtman & Papera, 1990).

- **Prostaglandin inhibitors:** Ibuprofen has been used successfully to control painful menstruation and may relieve breast tenderness as well (Lichtman & Papera, 1990).

CONCLUSION

Premenstrual syndrome in some form is common to the lives of the large majority of women in the United States. Although still not well understood, symptoms have been grouped and classified in an attempt to find common causes. A woman's stressful lifestyle—which seems customary—with its repercussions from inconsistent diet and exercise patterns as well as lack of rest and play time takes its toll. In turn, the body has its way of letting the woman know.

For most women, making simple changes can dramatically improve PMS symptoms. Health care providers can be a tremendous source of information and support.

EXAM QUESTIONS

CHAPTER 8
Questions 57–65

57. Supplementation with vitamin E is useful in alleviating which symptom or symptoms of premenstrual syndrome?

    a. High blood pressure

    b. Fluid retention and weight gain

    c. Cystic breast

    d. Mood swings

58. Increasing the amount of zinc in the diet is useful for which symptom of premenstrual syndrome?

    a. Migraine headaches

    b. Mood swings

    c. Skin problems

    d. Fluid retention

59. The nutrient that is one of the keys to improving symptoms of premenstrual syndrome because of its broad range of action in the body is

    a. vitamin D.

    b. calcium.

    c. vitamin A.

    d. vitamin B^6.

60. If a woman tells you that she experiences dramatic mood swings during her period and for the first week after she stops bleeding, her symptoms are

    a. characteristic of premenstrual syndrome.

    b. not characteristic of premenstrual syndrome.

    c. psychologically induced.

    d. caused by excessive bleeding during her period.

61. A client describes to you feelings of anxiety and frequent fits of anger, alternating with thoughts of suicide. You would

    a. simply let her know that she has symptoms of type A and type D premenstrual syndrome.

    b. help her make changes in her diet and exercise patterns.

    c. advise her to supplement her diet with vitamins and minerals.

    d. immediately refer her to a qualified mental health professional for further evaluation.

62. An herb that might be helpful for women with type H premenstrual syndrome is

    a. cramp bark.

    b. wild yam.

    c. dandelion leaf.

    d. chaste berry.

63. A good source of magnesium in the diet is

    a. meat.

    b. chicken.

    c. legumes.

    d. citrus fruit.

64. Magnesium helps relieve symptoms of

    a. diarrhea.

    b. nausea.

    c. sugar craving.

    d. poor muscle tone.

65. Vitamin B^6 helps with symptoms of

    a. constipation.

    b. mood swings.

    c. acne.

    d. dry skin.

CHAPTER 9

PREVENTIVE HEALTH CARE

CHAPTER OBJECTIVE

After completing this chapter, the reader will be able to identify the components of health maintenance and good preventive health care for women. The reader will also be able to discuss factors that make health care an individual matter, including age, risk factors, and personal history.

LEARNING OBJECTIVES

After studying this chapter, the reader will be able to

1. identify common components of a well-woman examination.

2. identify individual factors that influence choice and frequency of tests and evaluation.

3. discuss components of a good health history.

Key Words

- Bimanual examination
- Breast self-examination (BSE)
- Clinical breast examination
- Integrated medical therapies

INTRODUCTION

An annual examination provides an opportunity to develop and nurture the ongoing relationship that providers have with their clients. It also presents an opportunity to teach health-promotion skills. Most practitioners advise beginning annual exams whenever a woman becomes sexually active, or in the absence of sexual activity, by approximately age twenty. Nurses find themselves in a variety of roles, depending on the setting. They have varying levels of responsibility, ranging from assessing vital signs, history taking, counseling and assisting with office procedures to providing health education and referrals. One of the first rules of thumb is not to assume that the health care providers that clients may have in other settings are providing comprehensive care for those clients. It is very common to find errors and inconsistencies in care because of one provider not being informed about what another is doing. The responsibility of keeping each provider fully informed needs to be shared between providers and clients.

Health History

A thorough history will lead the health care provider to gold. History taking is an art. Guided listening is an important skill, and it can be practiced by

- allowing the client to tell what she wants to be known about why she came in for evaluation.

- eliciting from the client what needs to be known to plan her care.

To elicit the chief complaint allow the client to tell her story without interruption, helping her stay on track. Being heard is often the beginning of the healing process for the client.

According to Stenchever (1996), the history should also include at least the following components:

- **Menstrual history**—typical cycle, including quality, duration, and problems

- **Pregnancy history**—each pregnancy, with details regarding miscarriages, abortions, ectopic pregnancies, and any complications

- **Gynecologic history**—infections, sexually transmitted infections (STIs), surgeries, diagnostic procedures, and history of Pap smear findings

- **Sexual history**—current and past partner history, STI testing and results, and sexual function

- **Contraceptive history**—past and current use of methods, type; why the client stopped using a method (e.g., side effects, problems)

- **General health history**—review of systems, illnesses, hospitalizations, and surgeries

- **Medications**—past and current

- **Allergies**

- **Family history**—genetic diseases, serious illnesses, cause of death in family members, pregnancy problems, and use of drugs during pregnancy

- **Lifestyle history**—current and past use of alcohol, cigarettes, and social drugs; diet and exercise habits and patterns; living situation; partner habits; occupation and possible hazards and exposures; and travel

- **Psychiatric history**—including emotional and psychologic illness, abuse and trauma, and weight issues

The above-listed information should be updated each year during the annual examination.

Physical Examination

An annual examination should include the components of a general physical examination, including evaluation of thyroid gland, heart, lungs, extremities, and reflexes. A gynecologically oriented health maintenance examination should include the following six components as well:

1. Complete pelvic examination, including

   - observation of the

     — external genitalia for evidence of infection, abnormal coloration or growths, irritation, or discharge

     — vagina for evidence of inflammation or discharge

     — cervix for lesions, discharge, and signs of irritation

   - a Pap smear with a sampling of the outer and inner portions of the cervix

   - a bimanual examination, determining the size, shape, position, and consistency of the uterus and ovaries *(see Figure 9-1)*

   According to Stenchever (1996), current guidelines set forth by the American College of Obstetricians and Gynecologists recommend an annual Pap smear for women at risk for cervical cancer and one every 2–3 years for women with negative findings on two consecutive Pap smears and who are at low risk. Special considerations that may warrant more frequent Pap smears include exposure to diethylstilbestrol, history of abnormal Pap smear findings, or risk of STI. In light of the widespread prevalence of the human papillomavirus (HPV), which can be asymptomatic for many years and is now associated with most abnormal Pap smear findings, most women might be considered at moderate risk. Thus an annual Pap smear might be a good recommendation.

2. For women older than 40 years, screening for colon cancer, including (Stenchever, 1996)

   - a rectal examination to check for masses,

FIGURE 9-1
Bimanual Examination

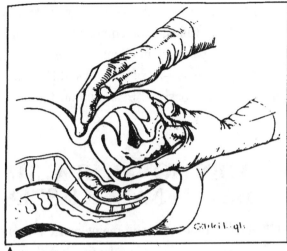

A

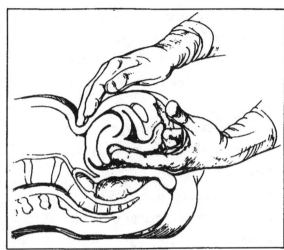

B

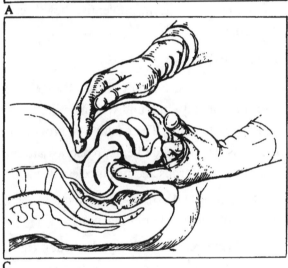

C

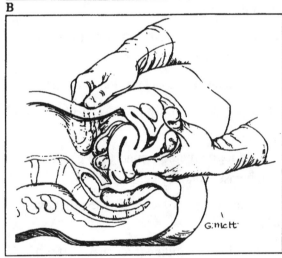

D

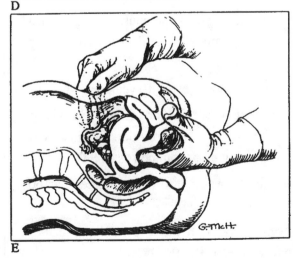

E

Bimanual pelvic examination. A. Palpation of cervix and fundus. B. Anteflexion of fundus with palpation of fundus; consistency of lower uterine segment. C. Palpation of fundus with retroversion. D. Approximate internal and external fingers lateral to uterus and above adnexa. E. Move internal and external fingers toward examiner to palpate adnexa.

Source: Niswander, K. R. (Ed.). (1981). *Obstetrics: Essentials of clinical practice* (2nd ed.). Boston: Little, Brown.

as well as to palpate the uterus and pelvic structures for masses not detectable with the bimanual examination

- a stool sample to check for blood in the stool. The best method is to use a "take-home-mail-back" kit with specific dietary instructions and tools for sampling the stool.

- a sigmoidoscopy every 3–5 years for women with a strong family history of colon cancer

- a sigmoidoscopy every 3–5 years in addition to an annual rectal examination for women older than 65 years regardless of family history

3. Screening for breast cancer, including (Stenchever, 1996)

- yearly clinical breast examination (CBE)

- teaching of monthly breast self-examination (SBE)

- mammography/ultrasound (See chapter 12 on breast health for guidelines.)

4. Screening for STIs as needed (Stenchever, 1996)

5. Immunizations, including (Stenchever, 1996)

- vaccines against the causative agents for rubella, measles, and polio for young women

- tetanus booster every 10 years

- hepatitis B vaccination (three injections)—advised by some providers because it is becoming more common as an STI

- influenza vaccine for women older than 60 years

6. Screening for other health conditions, including (Stenchever, 1996)

- hematocrit or complete blood cell count to screen for anemia, especially in young women

- a lipid panel to screen for heart disease risk factors in women older than 35 years

- tests to evaluate possible thyroid disease; diabetes; possible occupational exposure to body fluids, toxic chemicals, and radiation; and parasites in clients who travel to high-risk areas—all of which would be indicated on the basis of examination findings and history

ADDITIONAL HEALTH MAINTENANCE ISSUES

Three additional health maintenance issues may come into play in preventive health care for women.

Grief and Loss

Grief and loss are part of life. They may come into focus at any time in a woman's life, but especially so with aging. The health care provider needs to assess whether the client's reactions are normal and provide referrals and resources as needed.

Stenchever (1996) describes some of the components of abnormal grief reactions:

- **Delayed reaction:** Delayed reaction can occur when grieving has been postponed for some reason, often until recovery from a serious injury. Because time has elapsed, the grieving may seem to be out of context with the current life situation.

- **Distorted reaction:** In a distorted reaction the woman may take on characteristics of the lost one, including symptoms the person may have experienced before death.

- **Psychosomatic symptoms:** The woman in grieving may experience psychosomatic symptoms for which there is no identifiable disease or pathologic cause at the time, such as colitis or asthma.

- **Severe alterations in ability to function:** The client's inability to function may affect her relationships, and she may manifest severe depression or agitation as well as insomnia.

- **Referral for counseling** may be advised.

Weight Issues

For many women of all ages in American society, concerns about weight, body image, ideals of beauty, and self-esteem are central in their lives and form a core of self-concern that has very destructive consequences. This is a broad consideration and beyond the scope of this course. However, it is an area of women's health that requires careful assessment and consideration because it has an impact on women's motivation and ability to carry out good health care behaviors and develop healthy living habits. These issues will be highlighted in other chapters.

Transitions

Major changes in women's lives require mobilization of their personal resources, and they often tax women's coping abilities. Changes that are positive, such as new careers, childbirth, and marriage, are stressors, nonetheless. These events often occur at a time when women need extra support, both emotional and physical. Menarche and menopause represent two ends of the spectrum for women, marked by major shifts in hormone levels as well as shifts in self-perception. Special attention to health maintenance during major transitions can help women come through the period of stress with a decreased chance of experiencing illness or emotional trauma. This is often a time when diet and exercise patterns fall by the wayside, and support systems may be ignored to "get by." Health care providers can help women keep on track with their self-care habits. Health education for transitions could include the following:

- **Diet:** Specific dietary suggestions during stress include intake of fresh fruits and vegetables; tips for healthy snacks; supplementation of diet with vitamins and minerals; and herbal remedies called adaptogens, which help the body cope with stress.

- **Exercise:** Regular exercise is one of the best stress reducers, and it often can be implemented free of charge.

- **Massage therapy**

- **Support groups and other resources**

INTEGRATED MEDICAL THERAPIES

When health care providers think about health care, they most often think of Western medicine because it is currently the predominant form of health care in the United States. This was not always the case. Other forms of healing, such as herbal medicine and homeopathic medicine, were once widely available and broadly accepted. Various political forces shaped the course of health care in America, and these forms of medicine lost credibility.

In the past decade there has been a resurgence of interest in forms of health care other than the Western medical model, especially with the failure of Western medicine to provide cures or causes for many chronic health conditions. People are becoming more informed, and there is an explosion of information exchange worldwide. Health care providers are learning about health care systems from all over the world that have been effective in maintaining and restoring health. In China, where Chinese herbal medicine and acupuncture have been practiced for several thousand years, it was common for the practitioner to be paid for maintaining health. If a patient did get sick, the practitioner stopped getting paid. Many of these other forms of healing have a whole-systems approach to understanding and describing how the body and mind interact and function and have much to offer in the way of health maintenance, as well as therapies for healing specific ailments.

The following is a list of non-Western medical systems of healing that can be of benefit for health promotion. Integrated health modalities include

- Western herbal medicine.
- homeopathy.
- Asian medicine and acupuncture.
- ayurvedic medicine.
- massage techniques.
- color therapy.
- water therapy.
- energy-healing techniques.
- therapeutic touch.
- healing with sound.
- nutritional medicine.
- osteopathic and chiropractic manipulation.
- living foods.
- macrobiotic diet.
- psychic healing.
- traditional native healing practices from around the world.

Along with this explosion of other health care systems and practices comes the danger of lack of discrimination and unsubstantiated claims. It is often up to the consumer to wade through the muddy waters and try to make health care choices among all these options. Many organizations are forming to self-regulate. The government has licensing programs and requirements for acupuncturists, naturopaths, chiropractors, and other providers. Regulations vary from state to state.

The other danger is that the consumer can become too casual with the use of widely accepted and available remedies. Herbs and vitamins are very powerful substances and need to be used knowledgeably and with caution. They are wonderful allies, but they need to be respected as medicine.

It is the hope of many health care providers, both Western and non-Western, that there will be a mutual respect for and integration of Western medical theory and practice with other forms of health care. With this integration, clients will benefit from all that humanity has developed in the realm of health maintenance and healing.

It is beyond the scope of this course to provide detailed information about all other health care options. I hope that this brief description has piqued your interest to do more reading. Clients are increasingly asking their providers for more information and resources in this area. Please refer to the resource guide and recommended reading list at the end of the course.

CONCLUSION

There is much that women can do to maintain the quality of their health throughout the life cycle. This includes regular health maintenance examinations, which should be thorough and accomplished with attention to the individual needs of each woman, including age-appropriate health screening. Ultimately, it is the responsibility of each woman to engage in self-care behaviors that enhance her well-being. There are a number of healing traditions and modalities that might be recommended by a woman's health care practitioner for the woman to use to promote health and augment and enhance therapy for specific illnesses.

EXAM QUESTIONS

CHAPTER 9
Questions 66–68

66. In response to a significant personal loss, the presence of psychosomatic symptoms

    a. indicates a normal response to grief and loss.

    b. indicates problems that do not require treatment but will go away on their own.

    c. may signal an abnormal response to grief.

    d. is always a sign of a serious psychiatric disorder.

67. In addition to a pelvic examination, all women older than 40 years of age should have a yearly

    a. check for sexually transmitted infections.

    b. complete blood cell count.

    c. rectal examination and stool test for blood.

    d. sigmoidoscopy.

68. A bimanual examination is done primarily to

    a. assess the cervix.

    b. assess vaginal discharge.

    c. determine the size, shape, position, and consistency of the uterus and ovaries.

    d. check for uterine cancer.

CHAPTER 10

ABNORMAL CERVICAL PAP SMEAR FINDINGS AND THE HUMAN PAPILLOMAVIRUS

CHAPTER OBJECTIVE

After completing this chapter, the reader will be able to specify problems associated with Pap smears and identify new methods of Pap smear screening and evaluation that increase the accuracy of Pap smear results. The reader will also be able to recognize the link between the presence of certain strains of human papillomavirus and cervical cancer.

LEARNING OBJECTIVES

After studying this chapter, the reader will be able to

1. identify risk factors for cervical cancer.

2. discuss the problems with Pap smear accuracy.

3. identify ways to increase the accuracy of a Pap smear.

4. describe technologic advances in Pap smear screening and evaluation.

5. discuss issues in educating clients who have been exposed to the human papillomavirus.

6. describe treatments for abnormal conditions identified with the use of Pap smears.

7. discuss some of the myths and facts about the human papillomavirus.

Key Words

- Colposcopy
- Columnar epithelium
- Cryotherapy
- Endocervical canal
- Squamocolumnar junction
- Squamous epithelium
- Transformation zone

INTRODUCTION

This chapter on abnormal cervical Pap smear findings and human papillomavirus (HPV) has been included in this course on women's health because of the growing concern of the coexistence of cervical cancer and HPV infection in women and the suggestive link between the two. In addition, the quality of the Pap smear—the test historically used to screen for cervical cancer, among other conditions—has been a subject of attention in the media in the past several years. The presence of certain strains of HPV has recently been firmly linked to cervical cancer ("Human

Papillomavirus—An Initiator of Cervical Cancer," 1997). Although infection with HPV is a rising epidemic in the United States, information on this infection available from both the medical literature and the news is often outdated and disparate. It is hoped that the information presented here—on cervical cancer, Pap smears, and the HPV—will provide a resource to readers and health care providers in women's health.

CERVICAL CANCER

Although an in-depth discussion of cervical cancer is beyond the focus of this chapter, some background information is important to the discussion of this disease, Pap smear screening, and the HPV and its association with cervical cancer.

Cervical Cancer and Pap Smear Screening

An article in the June 1997 issue of *Women's Health Forum* ("Did You Know?," 1997) provides some interesting statistics on cervical cancer and Pap smear screening. Before the 1940s when the Pap smear was first developed, cervical cancer was the most common cause of cancer death in women in the United States. Today, invasive cervical cancer occurs at about one third the rate it did before widespread use of the Pap smear. Even though the rate of death for this disease has decreased dramatically, 5,000 women still die of cervical cancer each year. This cancer is largely preventable by regular screening and timely treatment.

Risk Factors

Although the exact progression of cervical cancer is unknown, a number of key contributing factors have been identified. The term *risk factors* refers to certain behaviors or personal history that may increase an individual's vulnerability to a particular disease problem. Health care providers should consider with their patients whether any of

the following risk factors apply, regardless of how long ago these events may have occurred ("Cervical Cancer Risk Factors," 1997):

- Smoking *(doubles the risk)*
- Early onset of sexual activity (before age 18 years)
- Multiple sexual partners (three or more in a lifetime)
- A sexual partner who has had
  — multiple partners
  — genital warts
- Contraction of a sexually transmitted disease, especially HPV (only certain viral types are associated with progression to cervical cancer)
- Other sexually transmitted diseases, including herpes and HIV (however, these other viruses in and of themselves *do not cause cervical cancer)*
- History of abnormal Pap smear findings
- Exposure to diethylstilbestrol during fetal development
- Possible nutritional deficiencies especially of folic acid, a B vitamin important for normal cell growth
- Immunosuppression

The Older Woman and Cervical Cancer

Cervical cancer has been perceived by the public as a young woman's disease, but one fourth of all cervical cancers develop in women older than 60 years of age ("The Older Woman and Cervical Cancer," 1997). Therefore, it is important for older women at risk to be screened with Pap smears.

Although only one quarter of all cervical cancers develop in women older than age 60 years, 41% of all deaths from cervical cancer occur in this age group ("The Older Woman and Cervical Cancer," 1997). This is not clearly understood. It may be due in part to the fact that screening for older women is recommended much less often by physicians. Women should undergo regular screening throughout life.

The more that is being discovered about the HPV, the more health care providers are realizing that many women thought to be at minimal risk are in fact at great risk. This is because HPV can be asymptomatic and remain in the body for life. For example, an older woman who may have been in a monogamous relationship for many years may have acquired the HPV at an earlier phase of life. Lifestyle factors that have an impact on the immune system, such as smoking, illness, or stress, could increase the risk of a recurrence of viral activity. Health care providers should not assume that because a woman is older her risk is low. Careful assessment needs to be done for each individual.

CERVICAL PAP SMEARS

In ironic contrast to its eventual success, the Pap smear was initially met with skepticism and resistance from the scientific community ("Did You Know?," 1997). Nationwide acceptance and use of the test lagged decades behind its introduction until large-scale studies began to be conducted in the early 1950s and the government began to reimburse for wide-scale screening ("Did You Know?," 1997).

How Is a Cervical Pap Smear Normally Obtained?

The Pap smear samples two sites on the cervix: (1) the junction between the squamous cells and the endocervical cells and (2) a sample of endocervical cells. Various sampling devices are used. Some facilities use a wooden spatula to obtain the first sample, sweeping in a circular motion around the outside surface of the cervix and then using a small plastic cytobrush to sample the cells inside the cervical canal. A newer tool called a "cytobroom" may be used. It obtains both samples simultaneously. The vaginal wall is usually not sampled unless the woman is nearing menopause. In this case, a second slide may be done to evaluate the hormonal effects on vaginal tissue.

Problems with Screening and Initial Solutions

Problems

According to the article "Addressing the Issue of Undetected Abnormalities on Pap Smears" (1997), two major problems exist with Pap smear screening. The first is that a large percentage of women are still not having Pap smears because of lack of awareness or motivation, fear, and cost or access problems. Results of a recent survey revealed that of 2,500 women 35% had not had a Pap smear within the past year ("Addressing the Issue of Undetected Abnormalities on Pap Smears," 1997).

As reported in the article "The Pap Smear: Success in Cervical Cancer Screening" (1997), the second problem has to do with the accuracy of Pap smears. Because this test is a relatively simple and low-cost test, health care providers and patients alike have come to accept it as an integral part of gynecologic care. Unfortunately, more than four decades of reliance on this tool has quietly elevated the status of the Pap smear in the public perception from general screening procedure to foolproof diagnostic test. The test was never expected to have a 100% accuracy rate.

Also (as reported in the article "Addressing the Issue of Undetected Abnormalities on Pap Smears" [1997]), because early-stage cervical cancer usually progresses slowly a woman should have a Pap smear performed regularly to ensure a higher accuracy rate over the course of multiple tests. In addition, according to this article, the false-negative rate is fairly high: 5%–28% of women have abnormalities that are not detected by the Pap smear and show a negative result.

According to the article "Should Women Be Informed of Screening Options?" (1997), the above findings are further confused by differences in how slides are assessed by those doing the evaluation. One of five abnormalities may be missed. This means that both low-grade abnormalities, which probably would not progress to cervical cancer by the next Pap test, and higher grade abnormalities, which could become cancer within a year, can be missed. This is not a new problem, but it has received more attention recently, resulting in new regulations for Pap smear laboratories. According to this same article, now by law cytology laboratories are required to do a primary screen and to rescreen a random selection of 10% of the slides showing negative results. All slides with negative findings are to be archived for 5 years, and all laboratories are subject to regular inspections. In addition, technologists are limited to reading a maximum of 100 slides per day.

Initial Solutions

The article "The Pap Smear: Success in Cervical Cancer Screening" (1997) provides several solutions to the problems with Pap smear screening. The discussion that follows highlights those solutions, along with several statistics and research findings pertinent to the topic (which have been gleaned from this article).

Initial solutions for Pap smear inaccuracy start with the client. Ideally, Pap smears should be collected midcycle, with no intercourse or douching for 48 hours before collection. Any localized vaginal infection such as a yeast infection can interfere with the results because of the presence of inflammation. Any over-the-counter creams, gels, or suppositories used within 24–48 hours before the Pap smear is obtained will also impair the collection of a good sample.

The next crucial step is the collection process. The quality of the smear depends on how well the health care provider collected and preserved the sample. Results of a recent study showed that up to two thirds of false-negative findings could be accounted for by sampling errors. In addition, there are problems with current methods of obtaining the Pap smear. Approximately 300,000 cells are collected onto the collection tool, but only 50,000–200,000 of these cells actually get transferred onto the slide. Any cells that show abnormalities could be easily lost in this transfer process.

The last step is the reading by the cytotechnologist. The average slide that reveals a positive finding may have only a few abnormal cells among hundreds of thousands of normal cells. It is not surprising that some abnormal cells will be overlooked.

Current Developments

In response to the need for more accuracy in Pap smear screening, a number of new sampling and screening technologies have been developed and are becoming more widely available. Some insurance companies are starting to reimburse the costs associated with these new tests, and efforts are being made to obtain reimbursement for clients under federal and state health care programs as well. Five such tests are described below.

1. **Cervicography:** According to Winegardner (1998), cervicography is a process whereby acetic acid (vinegar) is applied to the woman's cervix. After several minutes, a specially designed camera is used to take a photograph of the area. Then the photograph is mailed to a laboratory for analysis.

2. **Speculoscopy:** According to Winegardner (1998), speculoscopy uses a light source and magnifier attached to the speculum to view the cervix after vinegar has been applied. If any whitened lesions or unusual areas are found, the client is referred for colposcopy.

3. **"Papnet":** According to Bonfiglio and colleagues (1996), Papnet is the name for one of the new computer-assisted Pap smear screening

technologies. It has recently been approved by the Food and Drug Administration (FDA). Some laboratories that evaluate Pap smears are using this system to evaluate 100% of their Pap smear slides. The computer optically scans each slide, creating 128 different images, and evaluates them against normal cell configurations. The data gathered from each slide and stored in the computer are evaluated by the cytotechnologist. Images that contain large deviations from normal are then selected for a manual review by a cytotechnologist.

4. **"Autopap 300 QC System":** As reported by Bonfiglio and colleagues (1996), the Autopap 300 QC System is similar to Papnet and has also received FDA approval. The Pap smear slide is scanned optically and analyzed by the computer. This system is being used for quality assurance by some laboratories that evaluate Pap smears, where 100% of the Pap smears are rescreened after being viewed by a cytotechnologist. Each slide receives a score based on how far it deviates from norms, and the computer selects approximately 10% of the slides for a second evaluation by a cytotechnologist. A large number of false-negative findings are picked up by this rescreening system. Rescreening is also performed for clients identified as being at high risk for abnormal Pap smear findings or who have a previous history of an abnormal Pap smear finding.

5. **"Thin Prep":** The new sampling technique called Thin Prep has been approved by the FDA. The Pap smear is taken as usual with spatula and cytobrush or with cytobroom. Rather than being placed on a slide, the sample is put into a fluid fixative medium and sent to the laboratory for processing. At the laboratory, the liquid is centrifuged and filtered. This removes a great deal of debris, blood, and inflammatory cells, called artifact, which tend to obscure the cells. The cells collected on the filter are transferred to a slide, which now has cells only a single layer thick for viewing by the technologist. There is a better chance of getting a representative sample of cells, and the thousands of cells that normally end up being thrown away on the collection devices have not been lost. In addition, the sample is cleaner and better preserved.

Results of studies with the use of this collection method have revealed up to a 50% increase in the detection of high-grade abnormalities (Bonfiglio et al., 1996). This is an exciting and sizeable improvement in Pap smear accuracy.

Understanding the Cervix

To understand normal and abnormal Pap smear findings, health care providers should first consider the makeup of the cervix.

The surface of the cervix and the canal that leads into the uterus (the endocervical canal) are made up of the following two types of cells:

1. **Squamous epithelium:** Squamous epithelium covers the vagina and the outside surface of the cervix. It generally looks pink and smooth (Seibert & McMullen, 1996).

2. **Columnar epithelium:** According to Seibert and McMullen (1996), columnar epithelium is found in the endocervical canal, and in young women it also can be seen on the outer surface of the cervix around the external cervical opening (os). They note that this type of tissue looks rough and is dark pink. Women who take birth control pills also tend to have this type of cell on the outer surface because of the effects of the hormones in the pills.

The area in which the squamous epithelium and the columnar epithelium come together on the cervix is called the squamocolumnar junction or transformation zone. This is a site in which there is a lot of cell growth and replacement. The squamous type of cell is replacing the columnar type in a constant cycle of cell turnover, which is influenced by the female hormones. The term for this process is *squamous metaplasia*. Metaplasia is a word that may appear on a Pap smear reading and is not to be confused with abnormal cell growth. It is a normal process of cell turnover. It occurs most rapidly during adolescence and pregnancy.

Seibert and McMullen (1996) report that cervical cancer usually develops in the area of this rapid cell division. The immature cells undergoing this process are especially vulnerable to events that can change the genetic material of the cells. These changes, or mutations, result in premalignant changes or cancer.

Mild abnormalities on Pap smear readings may have a number of causes including a mild injury or irritation to the cervix resulting from intercourse or tampon use, or due to bacterial or yeast infection. After appropriate treatment, a repeat of the Pap smear (recommended intervals range from 6 weeks to 3 months) most often results in a return to normal. According to Seibert and McMullen, researchers have now come to a point of agreement that mutations in the cells of the cervix which can lead to cervical cancer are due to infection with certain strains of the HPV virus in combination with other cancer-promoting cofactors. As we will discuss later in this chapter, most strains of the HPV virus rarely progress to cervical cancer.

What Should Women Be Told About Their Pap Smear Findings?

Informing women of Pap smear results is a hot topic among health care providers as increasing legal action is being seen for false-negative errors that resulted in a delayed detection of advanced disease ("Should Women Be Informed of Screening Options?," 1997). For their own legal protection, as well as for the protection of clients, health care practitioners are being advised to inform all women about the limits of Pap smear accuracy, including the following information ("Should Women Be Informed of Screening Options?," 1997):

- Annual Pap smears are the best means now available for early detection of cervical cancer.

- No guarantee exists, however, that a particular Pap smear will pick up diseased cells that may be present.

- New enhanced screening techniques are becoming available. It is not yet clear what the benefit will be for any individual.

- Rescreening will add to the cost of the Pap smear. This may or may not be covered by insurance, whether funded by private, state, or federal sources.

After receiving this information, all women should be given the option to have their Pap smear, which showed a negative finding, rescreened as a protective measure.

Classification

According to Seibert and McMullen (1996), the classification system for reporting Pap smear results has undergone several major changes in approach and terminology in attempts to standardize reporting systems worldwide and provide more information about what was actually seen in the sample. These changes can result in confusion for clients who may remember words (e.g., dysplasia) that are no longer being used.

Seibert and McMullen (1996) note that the new reporting format gives a determination of the adequacy of the specimen and a description of any infectious process that may be indicated. It also reports on indications of the presence of infection with HPV and grades the various stages of abnormal cell growth.

It is beyond the scope of this course to include a detailed discussion of the Pap smear grading system. Please refer to a text in the bibliography for more specific information.

Further Evaluation

Depending on the result of the Pap smear, further evaluation or treatment (or both) may be advised (Seibert & McMullen, 1996). The first step in this process is generally referral for a colposcopic examination:

Colposcopy: As reported by Seibert and McMullen (1996), the colposcope is essentially a low-powered binocular microscope with a powerful light source, mounted in such a way as to allow visualization of the vagina and cervix during a pelvic examination. It is essentially a way of taking a closer look at the cervix and surrounding tissue for evaluation. The area is typically painted with acetic acid (vinegar). This has a dehydrating effect on HPV lesions, which causes them to turn white (acetowhite) and allows better visualization. Training in colposcopic technique involves learning to identify other specific features of abnormal cell growth such as blood vessel patterns and to interpret these findings. Biopsies are performed on any suspicious areas, and the biopsy samples are evaluated. A sample of tissue is also taken from the endocervical canal to be sent to the pathologist for evaluation. Examination of this sample will determine whether HPV lesions are found inside the canal, an important determinant in what type of treatment will be recommended (Seibert & McMullen, 1996).

Client preparation: Colposcopy is often a source of anxiety for clients because they are unfamiliar with the procedure and concerned about what will be discovered. The procedure should be explained thoroughly beforehand. It is advisable for the client to take a mild pain reliever such as ibuprofen 30 minutes to 1 hour before the procedure because the client may experience mild to moderate cramping when the biopsy and endocervical samples are taken.

The client should be encouraged to bring a support person with her.

Treatment for Abnormal Pap Smear Results

There are a variety of ways to treat the lesions identified in a colposcopic examination; the treatment depends on the location and severity of the lesions. Five such treatments are described below.

1. **Cryotherapy:** Cryotherapy is done in an office setting. This technique freezes the top layer of cells of the cervix, thereby destroying abnormal tissue. Clients need to have the procedure explained beforehand, including discomfort involved. Cramping can be managed by having the client take ibuprofen beforehand. Vasovagal reactions can occur, and the client can expect a discharge for 2–4 weeks after the procedure as the sloughing and healing process proceeds. Clients should wait to have sex for 2 weeks until their follow-up examination.

    One of the complications observed with this procedure is that the squamocolumnar junction (described earlier)—in which the two different cell types—associated with the surface of the cervix and endocervical canal meet on the cervix—migrates upward into the cervical canal after cryotherapy (Stenchever, 1996). The consequence of this could be the need for a more invasive procedure in the future if lesions recur and are not visible with the colposcope because they extend up inside the canal. Cryotherapy can also cause some scarring of the cervix.

2. **Laser:** The advantages of laser treatment are rapid healing (3 weeks), minimal scarring, and no retraction of the transformation zone (Stenchever, 1996).

3. **Laser cone biopsy (conization):** If the lesion is found on colposcopy to be deeper in the endocervical canal and cannot be fully seen, a cone biopsy is needed to ensure that the entire

lesion is removed. A conelike section of the cervix is removed for evaluation (Stenchever, 1996).

4. **Electrocautery:** Electrocautery is comparable to cryotherapy and laser except more discomfort is involved. In addition, cervical stenosis (inability of the cervix to dilate) can result (Stenchever, 1996).

5. **Loop electrosurgical excision procedure (LEEP):** With LEEP, the cervix is anesthetized with a local anesthetic, and a fine wire loop is used to remove a portion of the cervix. The advantage of this technique over cryotherapy, laser, and elecrocautery is that the tissue is removed, not destroyed. Thus the tissue is available for evaluation by a pathologist (Stenchever, 1996).

Follow-up Pap smears after these procedures are advised every 3–4 months for a year. Protocols for the second year vary from every 3–4 months to every 6 months (Stenchever, 1996).

Guidelines in Pregnancy

According to Stenchever (1996), management of abnormal Pap smear results during pregnancy presents some difficulties. Considerations include the duration of the pregnancy, desire to maintain the pregnancy, and degree of abnormality. Colposcopy is used for diagnosis. Usually with low-grade lesions, a rescreening by Pap smear or colposcopy (or both) is advised every 2–3 months. If the abnormality is severe, conization may be advised.

Treatment Specific to Cervical Cancer

According to Sifton (1994), treatment for cervical cancer depends on the stage of the cancer; that is, whether it is localized or has spread to surrounding tissues or distant organs. Preinvasive cancer (i.e., carcinoma in situ), if left untreated, usually develops into an invasive cancer. A conization procedure is usually recommended, but hysterectomy may also be advised, depending on the individual situation.

Sifton (1994) notes that for invasive cancer, radiation can be used alone or in combination with some form of surgery. Surgery options range from conization of the cervix to a radical hysterectomy, in which the cervix, uterus, upper portion of the vagina, and lymph nodes in the area are removed. Two forms of radiation are used: radioactive implants placed directly at the cancerous site or external radiation. The former option destroys less of the healthy tissue and is associated with fewer side effects. Implants usually require a hospital stay of 2–3 days. External radiation is an outpatient procedure, usually 5 days a week for several weeks. Side effects include diarrhea, nausea and vomiting, bladder irritation, loss of appetite, fatigue, and the long-term effect of destruction of the ovaries, resulting in premature menopause. Cervical cancer, when detected at an early stage, has a high rate of cure (Sifton, 1994).

HUMAN PAPILLOMAVIRUS

Cervical cancer, rarely found among women in celibate religious orders, has long been associated with sexual activity (Stenchever, 1996). It is on the rise again in association with the rising epidemic of the sexually transmitted HPV infection. According to the article "The Older Woman and Cervical Cancer" (1997), the average age of women with abnormal Pap smear findings is declining steadily. In addition, the HPV is most prevalent among the younger population of women, although it does occur with some frequency in older women as well. Thus it seems that this association of HPV with cervical cancer may change the landscape of women's health care. Indeed, it seems that most sexually active women are at some risk.

As noted in "Human Papillomavirus—An Initiator of Cervical Cancer" (1997), the HPV is responsible for the most common sexually transmitted viral disease in the United States. Estimates are that approximately 24 million Americans are infected. Results of studies have shown that certain strains of the HPV are found in almost every case of cervical cancer. More than 70 different strains of the virus have been identified, and most are quite specific in the sites they can invade and the disease they can cause. The good news is that only a few of these 70 strains tend to initiate cervical cancer. External genital warts are caused by several other strains that are virtually never found in cervical cancer and do not, in and of themselves, increase the risk of cervical cancer.

The article on "Human Papillomavirus" (1997) notes further that with most HPV infections there are no symptoms, and a woman may discover that she has been exposed to the virus only after undergoing a routine Pap smear. This can be a shocking and emotionally difficult experience. Currently there is no simple reliable way to detect who is infected and what strain or strains of the HPV people may have.

As reported in "HPV: Myths and Misconceptions" (1998), the HPV is an elusive virus. It is difficult to culture and therefore hard to study. Many questions remain about its life cycle. Controversy exists about whether the virus stays in the body for life. Results of recent studies show that HPV may eventually be cleared in people with well-functioning immune systems ("HPV: Myths and Misconceptions," 1998). At least in some cases, however, the virus apparently does persist in the body. For most people, with time the immune system seems to gain mastery over the virus, making recurrences less frequent. As noted in "HPV: Myths and Misconceptions" (1998), until further research clarifies these issues, HPV-infected women have to consider themselves potentially contagious even if they have no current symptoms or have completed a form of treatment.

As described in "HPV: Myths and Misconceptions" (1998), there is no test to find out whether a woman has been exposed to HPV or has the virus in her system in the absence of symptoms. What triggers the virus to activate and cause abnormal cell growth, as well as why some lesions heal on their own and others become precancerous, is not known. The strains most strongly associated with cervical cancer are types 16, 18, 31, and 45 and a few others to a lesser degree. In most women with high-risk types of HPV on the cervix, cervical cancer will not develop.

According to "Human Papillomavirus" (1997), researchers are examining other factors that promote the development of cervical cancer. Some known factors that play a role are smoking and the health of the immune system. Stenchever (1996) notes that results of studies have shown that HPV infection in women who are seropositive for HIV and have abnormal Pap smear findings can progress rapidly to cervical cancer. Women who have had organ transplants and are receiving immunosuppressive drugs are also at a higher risk (Stenchever, 1996). For women with a healthy immune system it may take decades for cervical cancer to develop from an initial exposure to high-risk viral types.

Myths and Misconceptions

The overall topic of genital HPV is complex and confusing to everyone, lay person and scientist alike. Unfortunately, myths and misconceptions about genital HPV abound. Inaccurate information can cause a person to suffer tremendous anxiety unnecessarily, to doubt a partner's faithfulness, or even to undergo painful and expensive treatment that could have been avoided. Because of fear it can also lead a woman to avoid a simple Pap smear that could save her life.

One of the best sources for accurate information on HPV is the newsletter published by the American Social Health Association. In its Spring

1998 issue of *HPV News* the association discussed common misconceptions about the HPV ("HPV: Myths and Misconceptions," 1998). Some of these myths and misconceptions, as well as relevant statistics and research findings, have been gleaned from this issue and are reviewed below. (See the resource guide at the end of the course for information on how to contact this organization.)

Myth: I'm the only one with HPV.

Fact: According to an article published in the *American Journal of Medicine* in 1997, about 74% (nearly three of four) of Americans have been infected with genital HPV at some point in their lives. Because most often genital HPV produces no symptoms or illness, a person who has been infected may never know about it.

Myth: Only people who have casual sex get HPV.

Fact: It is true that the greater the number of sexual partners a woman has the higher her risk of exposure. Most women during the course of their lives do have more than one partner, or they get together with a partner who has already had other partners himself. This has nothing to do with casual sex. Sexually transmitted diseases can be passed along as readily in a loving, long-term relationship as in a one-night stand. Results of one study of middle-class, middle-aged women, most of them married with children, showed that 21% were infected with cervical HPV. One researcher stated that about 80% of people who have had as few as four sexual partners have been infected with HPV.

Myth: An HPV diagnosis means one partner has not been monogamous.

Fact: The virus can remain in the body for months or years without symptoms. An HPV diagnosis means only that the infection was contracted at some point in the person's life. Most people infected with HPV never know they have it.

Myth: Genital warts lead to cervical cancer.

Fact: Many women do have signs in the form of fleshy growths on the external genital area. In most cases these do not lead to or predispose a woman to cervical cancer. As discussed earlier, there are many different viral types of HPV, and the types causing genital warts are not the same as those predisposing a woman to cervical cancer.

Myth: An abnormal Pap smear finding means a woman is at high risk for cervical cancer.

Fact: An abnormal Pap smear result can be due to infection, local irritation, a low-risk HPV type, or a higher risk HPV type. Depending on the degree of abnormality, further evaluation or follow-up Pap smear obtained 3 months later may be recommended. For minor abnormalities, repeating of the smear in a few months helps weed out short-lived problems. Even if a second smear shows abnormal results, this is usually a premalignant change, not cancer, and it can be easily monitored and treated. Only one in four cases of cervical lesions, if left untreated, will progress to cancer, and treatment is almost always successful in preventing cancer if the cells are found in time. According to the National Cancer Institute, about half of women with newly diagnosed cervical cancer have never had a Pap smear, with another 10% having no Pap smears in the past 5 years. Clearly it is a good idea for women to have Pap smears obtained and evaluated regularly.

Prevention

There are no easy answers in the realm of prevention, given the long-term and often asymptomatic nature of HPV infection. Limiting the number of sexual partners is one of the keys to HPV prevention. Health practices that enhance the strength of the immune system—such as quitting smoking; limiting use of alcohol; eating a healthful, high-nutrient diet; and avoiding chemical and environmental exposures—help the body fight any current infections with HPV as well as help prevent recurrences after initial infection. Whether these practices actually help decrease the potential for initial infection remains an area for research.

Hatcher and colleagues (1994) report that although male condoms provide effective protection for many sexually transmitted diseases, they are less effective for HPV and herpes, which spread through skin-to-skin contact. This is because condoms do not cover the entire genital area of either sex. They note that condom use does provide some protection, however, and it is better than no barrier at all. Female condoms are somewhat more effective in that they offer a broader area of protection. Results of laboratory studies of spermicides have failed to show effectiveness (Hatcher et al., 1994).

Typing

Testing for HPV types is now available through some laboratories that evaluate Pap smears. These tests can distinguish between the more benign strains of the virus and those that have been found to be more aggressive in promoting cervical disease and cervical cancer. These tests are new and expensive. However, they hold promise, as they become more available and cost effective, in helping clinicians plan follow-up care and treatment for women with HPV-related abnormal Pap smear findings. Information about viral type can potentially save clients needless worry and invasive procedures with the accompanying financial burden.

Current Research

According to another article in the *HPV News* ("Vaccine Update," 1997), research is proceeding on several fronts. Several companies in the United States and Europe are working on different types of vaccines for prevention of HPV infection and also to treat existing HPV infection. One potential candidate is currently undergoing human trials in the United States. Vaccines for the treatment of cervical dysplasia and cervical cancer are also in development. The vaccines act by stimulating the body's immune system to develop antibodies and other immune defenses against specific strains of the virus.

CONCLUSION

The prevalence of the HPV and its link to cervical cancer are changing the way health care providers approach health care for women. These providers have to realize that most women are at risk to one degree or another and thus need to educate women with this in mind. The major co-factors and risk factors now known to influence cervical cancer risk can be changed by personal behavior choices. This is true for all women, but especially so for young women just beginning their sexually active life. In addition, women of all ages need to be educated about the benefits and limitations of Pap smear screening and encouraged to get Pap smears at regular intervals. It is also the task of health care providers to give accurate and up-to-date information about HPV infection and compassionate and sensitive care to those struggling with a new diagnosis or ongoing life issues resulting from exposure.

EXAM QUESTIONS

CHAPTER 10
Questions 69–84

69. The Pap smear has a false-negative rate of

    a. 2%–15%.

    b. 20%–30%.

    c. less than 10%.

    d. 5%–28%.

70. Although there are many factors which increase a woman's risk of contracting cervical cancer, a more rapid progression of this disease is characteristic of women who

    a. have a compromised immune system.

    b. are older than 40 years of age.

    c. have had multiple sexual partners.

    d. have a history of sexually transmitted infections.

71. The "Thin Prep" sampling technique

    a. allows computer reading of pap slides.

    b. results in a greater recovery of cells from the sampling tools.

    c. is a way of speeding up the amount of time it takes to get pap smear results back to the office.

    d. use new sampling tools to take a sample from the cervix.

72. Most cells that are lost during the Pap smear sampling process are lost

    a. during shipping of the slide to the laboratory.

    b. in the process of putting the fixative on the slide.

    c. in the process of transferring the sample to the slide.

    d. during processing by the laboratory.

73. "Papnet" is a new technology that provides

    a. a better sample of cervical cells than that obtained with standard technology.

    b. a more complete analysis of cells on the Pap slide.

    c. a magnified view of the cervix.

    d. analysis of photographs taken of the surface of the cervix.

74. Cervicography is a technique that

    a. uses acetic acid on the cervix and a magnifier to view the cervix.

    b. uses a computer to scan the cervix.

    c. uses vinegar on the cervix and takes a picture of the cervix.

    d. takes a sample of abnormal areas seen on the cervix.

75. In young women, the squamocolumnar junction of the cervix is usually

   a. inside the cervical canal.

   b. visible on the outer surface of the cervix.

   c. not seen with the naked eye.

   d. seen where the vaginal tissue meets the cervical tissue.

76. Pap smears normally sample the

   a. squamocolumnar junction and the vaginal wall.

   b. vaginal wall and the neck of the cervix.

   c. neck of the cervix and the canal of the cervix.

   d. canal of the cervix and the squamocolumnar junction.

77. An abnormal Pap smear finding is

   a. always associated with the human papillomavirus.

   b. not always related to viral infection.

   c. always associated with a sexually transmitted infection.

   d. always associated with a history of multiple sexual partners.

78. A definite link has been confirmed between cervical cancer and infection with

   a. the human papillomavirus.

   b. anaerobic bacteria.

   c. the human immunodeficiency virus.

   d. the herpes simplex virus.

79. Transmission of the human papillomavirus primarily occurs through

   a. contact with blood or other body fluids.

   b. skin-to-skin contact.

   c. oral sex.

   d. anal sex.

80. The viral types of human papillomavirus that cause external genital warts

   a. are the same viral types that cause cervical cancer.

   b. do not increase the risk of cervical cancer.

   c. increase the risk for cervical cancer.

   d. cause noncancerous changes on the cervix.

81. If a 60-year-old woman comes to your office for an annual exam and evaluation, you

   a. can assume that her risk of cervical cancer is low.

   b. cannot assume from just this information what her risk of cervical cancer is.

   c. can assume that she would already be informed if her risk of cervical cancer was high.

   d. cannot assume her risk of cervical cancer is high.

82. Your client just received the results of her Pap smear, which are abnormal and show infection with human papillomavirus. What would be the most important health intervention you would recommend among the following list?

   a. Eat more fresh fruits and vegetables.

   b. Have your partner examined for the presence of genital warts.

   c. Use condoms every time you have intercourse.

   d. Quit smoking.

83. Rescreening of negative Pap smear results should be

    a. recommended only for women who have had a previous abnormal Pap smear result.

    b. recommended for young women with multiple sexual partners.

    c. offered to all women regardless of known risk.

    d. advised for women older than 40 years of age.

84. If an abnormal Pap smear result requires further evaluation, which procedure is recommended first?

    a. Cryotherapy

    b. Colposcopy

    c. Speculoscopy

    d. Cervicography

CHAPTER 11

COMMON GYNECOLOGIC DISORDERS

CHAPTER OBJECTIVE

After completing this chapter, the reader will be able to recognize common gynecologic problems and treatments, including self-care and prevention.

LEARNING OBJECTIVES

After studying this chapter, the reader will be able to

1. list common gynecologic disorders and treatments.

2. discuss health maintenance and prevention related to gynecologic problems.

3. discuss diagnostic and therapeutic procedures for common gynecologic disorders.

Key Words

• Endometrioma

• Endometrium

• Fomite

• Laparoscopy

• Lesion

INTRODUCTION

It is important to keep in mind that the body is a whole system. A gynecologic problem may seem to be confined to the pelvic area, but it actu-

ally may be sourced by many other influences, activities, and imbalances. For example, amenorrhea can be caused by excessive exercise, dietary factors can influence the balance of organisms in the vagina and lead to infections (Stenchever, 1996), and thyroid disorders can influence the menstrual cycle (Lichtman & Papera, 1990).

Many gynecologic problems are not well understood by practitioners of Western medicine and have no effective therapy that is free of side effects. Women have a strong emotional response to gynecologic disorders because these problems can profoundly affect the quality of life and a woman's ability to function. Even minor problems often have a strong emotional component. The health care provider needs to be sensitive to these broader dimensions of gynecologic care.

It is beyond the scope of this course to consider each topic in great detail. Please refer to the resource guide and bibliography for a more in-depth consideration of each topic. Although abnormal Pap smear findings is one of the common gynecologic disorders seen in women, this subject is discussed in detail in chapter 10.

MENSTRUAL DISORDERS

There are four menstrual disorders that health care providers commonly encounter as they care for clients with gynecologic disorders: amenorrhea, irregular bleeding, dysmenorrhea, and premenstrual syndrome. The first three of these four are discussed briefly below. Please refer to chapter 8 for a discussion of premenstrual syndrome.

Amenorrhea

The normal menstrual cycle depends on the integrated functioning of the hypothalamus, pituitary gland, ovaries, uterus, cervix, and vagina or outflow tract. Lack of menstruation, or amenorrhea, may result from abnormalities of structure or function of any of these organs.

Amenorrhea is further defined as primary or secondary (Hatcher et al., 1994):

Primary:

- No period by age 15 years in the absence of secondary sex characteristics
- No period by age 16½ years regardless of the appearance of secondary sex characteristics

Secondary:

- Absence of 3 or more periods (or amenorrhea for 6 months) in a woman who has been menstruating

The first step in evaluating a woman for amenorrhea is to test for pregnancy. According to Stenchever (1996), after pregnancy has been ruled out there is a long list of potential causes, possibly requiring an extensive workup. He notes that a thorough history can often lead the health care provider to the cause. For example, the cause can be simply excessive exercise, inducing lack of menses. Alternatively, a complex hormone imbalance or tumor of the pituitary gland may be the culprit.

Irregular Bleeding

Stenchever (1996) notes that a host of possible diagnoses fall under the general heading of bleeding disorders. A number of factors play a role in determining whether a menstrual pattern is normal.

According to Stenchever (1996), one of the first considerations is age. He reports that in ado-

lescence it takes an average of 20 cycles before ovulation occurs regularly. Irregular bleeding, in both timing and amount, is the rule rather than the exception in early adolescence. Similarly, older women often experience an increased variation in menstrual interval and quantity during the 5 years preceding menopause.

As with amenorrhea, causes range from simple to complex. Evaluation for a woman with abnormal bleeding requires a careful and thorough history and workup, including physical examination and laboratory tests and possibly ultrasound (Stenchever, 1996).

Dysmenorrhea

Dysmenorrhea is the term used to describe painful menses, and it is further divided into two types: primary and secondary (Stenchever, 1996).

Primary: Primary dysmenorrhea usually begins in adolescence, with onset of menses and no apparent disease involved.

Secondary: In secondary dysmenorrhea pain is related to illness or disease, such as endometriosis or fibroids.

With regard to cause, Sifton (1994) reports that results of studies have revealed altered levels of local tissue chemicals. These local hormones, called prostaglandins, are found in tissues all over the body. They control local functions, such as vasodilation or vasoconstriction. When the normal levels of prostaglandins are out of balance in the uterus, cramping can result. Dietary factors and stress are known to influence prostaglandin levels as well.

According to Sifton (1994), before prostaglandins were discovered painful periods were ignored and considered to be a psychologic problem. Fortunately, dysmenorrhea is currently recognized as a physiologic problem.

Sifton (1994) notes that prostaglandin inhibitors such as ibuprofen are very effective in controlling dysmenorrhea. According to Gladstar (1993), historically women have known about the use of safe local herbs (that is, herbs that grow in the area in which the woman lives), such as cramp bark, wild yam, and raspberry leaf, to ease menstrual cramps. In addition, essential fatty acids (discussed in chapter 8) increase production of the "good" prostaglandins, which help the uterus relax.

VAGINAL INFECTIONS

The vaginal environment is an ecosystem much like a forest or a pond. It maintains a fairly constant state as it interacts with the environment outside the vagina. A number of organisms normally reside in the vagina, including various species of bacteria and yeast. Stenchever (1996) reports that usually 5–10 different types of microorganisms are present at any one time. He notes that the dominant bacteria, *Lactobacillus* species, help keep the balance in the vagina by producing byproducts, such as lactic acid and hydrogen peroxide. These byproducts maintain a fairly constant acidic pH of less than 4.5, preventing the overgrowth of less desirable vaginal residents (Stenchever, 1996). When the complex balance of microorganisms is upset, the potentially pathogenic "minor residents" can proliferate to a concentration that causes symptoms.

Mechanisms

Vaginal infections occur through primarily two mechanisms:

1. Imbalance and overgrowth of organisms that normally inhabit the vagina but overgrow and cause symptoms when the normal balance is altered

2. Introduction of organisms from outside the vagina, usually from intimate sexual contact

Causes of an Altered Vaginal Environment

Several events or factors may cause the normal vaginal environment to be altered and thus set the scene for infection. These include the following:

- Stress
- Douching
- Use of feminine hygiene products
- Use of harsh soaps for washing or as laundry detergent
- Dietary changes such as increased consumption of sugar or caffeine
- Sexual intercourse
- Use of barrier contraceptive methods, such as condoms and diaphragms
- Spermicides
- Wearing of synthetic underwear or tight-fitting pants
- Illness
- Chronic metabolic diseases such as diabetes
- Immunosuppression or illness that weakens the immune system
- Some medications
- Pregnancy

Health Education

According to Stenchever (1996), many women do not realize that they have a normal vaginal discharge. The discharge changes throughout the menstrual cycle, becoming clear, thin, and stretchy in response to estrogen and then thicker and tacky in response to progesterone. The quantity of this normal discharge differs from woman to woman.

Health practitioners can explore ways to help clients maintain a balanced vaginal environment through changes in lifestyle and habits, diet, and choice of birth control method. The possibility of exposure to a sexually transmitted infection (STI) should be discussed with any client who comes in for evaluation of vaginal symptoms even if the primary diagnosis is an imbalance in normal flora.

Douching in general has a drying effect on the vagina and disrupts normal vaginal flora. It can actually cause an increase in the amount of discharge (Stenchever, 1996). Findings in recent studies on douching have shown an association between douching and serious infection of the upper reproductive tract, (i.e., pelvic inflammatory disease [PID]) (Stenchever, 1996).

Common Infections

Seven infections or conditions involving the vaginal environment are commonly encountered in women with gynecologic disorders: bacterial vaginosis, candidiasis, infections that fall under the general category of STIs, cervicitis, PID, vaginal carcinoma (primary [rare], secondary [because of the cancer spreading to the vagina from another site], or related to exposure to diethylstilbestrol [DES] in utero), and toxic shock syndrome. With the exception of STIs, cervicitis, and PID, each is discussed briefly below. The reader is referred to chapter 7 on STIs, as well as to the specific section in that chapter on PID. Cervicitis may be accompanied by a purulent cervical discharge, which is often produced in gonorrhea and chlamydial infection. Both of these infections are discussed in chapter 7.

Bacterial Vaginosis

Bacterial vaginosis is the most common vaginal infection, and it is considered in general not to be transmitted sexually.

Causes: Bacterial vaginosis occurs because of a dramatic overgrowth of the vaginal resident bacterium *Gardnerella vaginalis* and anaerobic bacteria, often from ten to one hundred times the amount usually present. Anaerobic bacteria live in a low-oxygen environment.

Signs and symptoms: Characterized by a thin, milky discharge with a "fishy" amine odor, this odor is often worse after intercourse and menses. Bacterial vaginosis may be present without evident signs or symptoms.

Diagnosis: According to Stenchever (1996), diagnosis is made on the basis of a positive finding on the "whiff" test. (The characteristic amine odor is produced when a sample of the discharge is combined with a 10% solution of potassium hydroxide.) Microscopy reveals the presence of "clue" cells; that is, epithelial cells from the vagina with bacteria clinging to their edges, giving the cells a characteristic appearance. *Lactobacillus* species are rarely seen, and the pH of the vagina is above the typical 4.5.

Treatment: DeMarco (1996) reports that if bacterial vaginosis is found on a routine examination but the client has no symptoms, it is not usually treated unless the client is undergoing an invasive surgical procedure, such as abortion, hysterectomy, or insertion of an intrauterine device. DeMarco notes further that these procedures increase the risk of pelvic infection. Bacterial vaginosis is also associated with complications of pregnancy, including prematurity of the fetus and infection after cesarean section.

As reported by Hatcher and colleagues (1994), for women who do have symptoms the standard treatment is metronidazole (Flagyl®), given either orally or vaginally. Flagyl should not be used in women with a history of seizures. No alcohol is to be ingested 24 hours before or after taking this medication. It causes an "Antabuse"-like reaction, producing severe nausea. Hatcher and colleagues note further that the most common side effect of Flagyl is nausea, so it is best to take it with food. Its use is somewhat controversial during the first trimester of pregnancy. Pros and cons should be weighed in consultation with the client's health care provider.

Stenchever (1996) reports that clindamycin

orally or as a vaginal cream is also used in treating bacterial vaginosis. In addition, in my clinical practice experience some providers have reported success in clients who have used a douche of hydrogen peroxide and water half strength every other day for 10 days. Self-help treatments include

- vinegar and water douche (1–2 tablespoons per quart)
- garlic suppository (peeled and wrapped in cheesecloth with a tail for retrieval and changed every 12 hours) (Lichtman & Papera, 1990)
- douche with goldenseal, bayberry
- increased intake of vitamins C and B complex (Boston Women's Health Book Collective, 1992)

Hatcher and colleagues (1994) note that treatment of male partners has no effect on the recurrence rate in female partners.

Candidiasis

Causes: Commonly known as a yeast infection, candidiasis is generally caused by *Candida albicans*. Other related yeast species, however, can be causative agents as well.

Signs and symptoms: Candidiasis classically produces a characteristic itching and irritation of the vulva and often a thick, white, cheesy-type vaginal discharge that can have a sour odor. Symptoms can be more subtle.

Diagnosis: Diagnosis can be made on the basis of microscopic examination. A vaginal smear, which has been fixed and stained, reveals budding yeast or hyphae. The pH of the vagina may be unaltered or slightly more acidic than normal.

Treatment: Many over-the-counter treatments are currently available for candidiasis. These are usually fungistats—they inhibit the organisms from reproducing, so the woman's immune system can take over to kill the yeast. According to Stenchever (1996), boric acid, 600 mg twice a day for 14 days, is quite effective. Clients can sometimes obtain the 600-mg capsules from the pharmacist. Alternatively, clients put together their own capsules by purchasing boric acid powder and size 00 gelatin capsules from the pharmacist. The client pours enough powder into the capsule to fill it (roughly equivalent to 600 mg), pierces a hole in the end of the capsule, and then inserts the capsule into the vagina for the twice-a-day, 14-day regimen. Another effective product is a suppository containing an acidophilic bacteria. The suppository can be purchased in health food stores (Stenchever, 1996).

Stenchever (1996) also notes that stronger antifungals are available in creams or suppositories by prescription, as is a one-time oral dose of the antifungal fluconazole (Diflucan®). Fluconazole can have side effects, including nausea, vomiting, diarrhea, abdominal pain, or headache—even with one dose—but it is well tolerated by most women.

According to Stenchever (1996), study findings have shown that eating yogurt, which contains live bacterial cultures, is effective in reducing recurrences. Reducing sugar and caffeine intake in the diet can favorably affect the vaginal flora and restore balance. Any woman with recurrent yeast infections should be evaluated for diabetes and infection with HIV.

Stenchever (1996) also reports that yeast infections during pregnancy should not be treated with oral medication or boric acid. The topical antifungals have limited systemic absorption and are considered safe during pregnancy.

Vaginal Carcinoma

Lichtman and Papera (1990) describe that vaginal cancer can be primary, secondary, or related to

DES exposure in utero. Vaginal cancer often is asymptomatic. Clients with a history of cervical or vulvar cancer are at a higher risk for this cancer. For these clients, the Pap smear should include a vaginal sample.

Lichtman and Papera (1990) note that DES is a nonsteroidal synthetic estrogen that was used between 1940 and 1971 to prevent miscarriage in high-risk pregnant women. It was taken off the market when study results revealed that DES was linked to abnormalities in both male and female offspring of women who received this drug during pregnancy. Clear cell carcinoma of the vagina, formerly a rare disease, was seen in young women who were exposed to DES in utero.

Lichtman and Papera (1990) report further that structural changes as well as changes in the tissue of the vagina and cervix are commonly seen, and DES exposure has also been linked to infertility. Women exposed to DES should be evaluated with a colposcopic examination. In addition, daughters of women who received DES during pregnancy should have regular vaginal samples included with their Pap smears.

Toxic Shock Syndrome

According to Lichtman and Papera (1990), toxic shock syndrome is not well understood. It seems to be associated with tampon use. Although women of any age can be affected, it seems to occur more frequently in women younger than 30 years of age, especially in 15- to 19-year-olds, during or just after the menstrual period. Although it is a rare disease (occurring in 1–17 of 100,000 women), it is life threatening.

Causes: As noted by Lichtman and Papera (1990), researchers believe that the bacteria *Staphylococcus aureus* is responsible. Use of superabsorbent tampons that are often left in place for a number of hours can lead to the growth of bacteria, which then enter the blood stream, causing septicemia. Toxic shock syndrome has also developed in women who were not menstruating. Thus the causes are not completely understood.

Signs and symptoms: According to Lichtman and Papera (1990), signs and symptoms include acute illness with high fever (38.8°C [102°F] or greater), hypotension, tachycardia, abdominal pain, diarrhea, and nausea. The skin has a characteristic sunburn red appearance, or a rash may develop. Toxic shock syndrome may also present with flulike symptoms of malaise, sore throat, and aching muscles. This condition can be life threatening; coma or death may result.

Diagnosis: Diagnosis is made on the basis of physical examination findings and symptoms, along with results of a complete blood cell count. The latter often shows an elevated white blood cell count, indicating an acute infectious process (Lichtman & Papera, 1990).

Treatment: Treatment for toxic shock syndrome is immediate hospitalization with fluid replacement and aggressive antibiotic therapy (Lichtman & Papera, 1990).

Health teaching: Women should be taught to avoid use of superabsorbent tampons, change tampons frequently (at least every 6 hours), and alternate sanitary pads with tampons, especially during the night (Lichtman & Papera, 1990). If any symptoms develop as described above, the tampon should be removed, and help should be sought immediately (Lichtman & Papera, 1990).

URINARY TRACT INFECTIONS

The following discussion on urinary tract infections, including citation of several statistics and research findings, is gleaned from Marchiondo (1998).

Urinary tract infections occur more commonly in women than in men because of the shorter route from the external environment to the bladder in women and the close proximity of the urethra to the vagina and anal area.

Normally, the flow of urine keeps bacteria flushed from the tract, and the entire urinary system remains sterile. The bladder wall has antibacterial properties, and the urine is usually acidic, designed to inhibit growth of bacteria.

Infection of the lower urinary tract can extend upward to include the bladder, ureters, or kidneys. Therefore the infection can become increasingly serious as it extends upward.

Causes

Up to 90% of uncomplicated urinary tract infections are due to the bacterium *Escherichia coli*, a common inhabitant of the intestine that causes infection in this case only when introduced into the urinary tract. Sexually transmitted infections can cause symptoms of urinary tract infection, so testing for chlamydial infection and gonorrhea should be done if the woman is at risk.

Risk Factors

Extremes of age, altered immunity, diabetes, obstructions, pregnancy, sexual activity, and diaphragm use head the list of risk factors for urinary tract infection. Irritation of the urethra during sexual activity can cause bacteria to migrate up into the urinary tract. Spermicide use can change the vaginal pH and decrease levels of normal protective bacteria, allowing more bacteria to grow in the vagina. In turn, these bacteria can migrate to the bladder.

Signs and Symptoms

Common signs and symptoms include dysuria (pain with urination); frequency; urgency; discomfort in the area above the pubic bone; and cloudy, foul-smelling urine. If the infection has ascended to the kidneys, the lower back region where the vertebrae and ribs meet can be tender or extremely painful, and fever may be present.

Diagnosis

Diagnosis varies according to the location and extent of the infection. For uncomplicated infection of the lower urinary tract, diagnosis is made on the basis of symptoms and urinalysis, including microscopic examination of a clean catch urine sample for the presence of white or red blood cells (or both) and bacteria.

Treatment

New approaches for uncomplicated lower urinary tract infections include antibiotic therapy as a single-dose treatment or 3- to 5-day course:

Single-dose therapy: Two double-strength tablets of co-trimoxazole (sulfamethoxazole-trimethoprim) (Bactrim®, Septra®, TMP-SMX®).

Three-day regimen: Nitrofurantoin, 50–100 mg four times a day; can also use Bactrim twice a day.

The single-dose therapy is not as effective in eliminating bacteria, but it can be effective and useful when patient compliance is an issue. The listed antibiotics are the most common and cost effective ones used. (See Marchiando [1998] for other medication options.)

Prevention/Health Teaching

Urinary tract infections can often be prevented by increasing clients' awareness of the causes, as well as by implementing simple health-promotion measures (Marchiando, 1998):

- Void frequently (every 2–4 hours).
- Empty the bladder before and after intercourse.
- Drink plenty of water (6–8 glasses per day).
- Drink liquids before and after having sex.
- Avoid harsh soaps, powders, and sprays.
- Avoid tight-fitting underwear and pants.
- Use cotton underwear.

- Take vitamin C regularly to inhibit bacterial growth.

- Drink cranberry juice/take cranberry capsules, which prevent bacteria from adhering to the bladder wall.

- Wipe urethral meatus and perineum from front to back after voiding.

- Take the full course of any antibiotics prescribed.

ENDOMETRIOSIS

Endometriosis is the presence of tissue that is similar in structure and biologic function to that of the inner (endometrial) lining of the uterus but is found in other locations in the body. Other common sites include the ovaries, fallopian tubes, lining of the inside of the pelvic cavity, cervix, bladder, bowel, and even the liver and lungs.

According to Stenchever (1996), among infertile women it is estimated that 30%–60% have this disease. Why endometriosis is associated with infertility is not understood.

Causes

Endometriosis is not well understood. There are a number of theories about how this tissue wound up outside the uterus and was able to implant, none of which provide a full enough explanation to be broadly accepted. There may be an autoimmune component to the picture as well.

Signs and Symptoms

The misplaced accumulations of tissue, as does the uterine lining, respond to stimulation by estrogen and progesterone during the course of each menstrual cycle. Signs and symptoms of endometriosis include pelvic pain during menses, pain with intercourse, painful periods, and abnormal uterine bleeding.

Diagnosis

A laparoscopy is needed to give a certain diagnosis, although endometriosis would be suspected on the basis of symptoms. Symptoms of the disease do not always correspond to the actual volume of lesions that might be found during a laparoscopy. Some women with extensive endometriomas (as they are called) have mild symptoms, and women with more severe symptoms may have fewer lesions.

Treatment

Stenchever (1996) notes that because endometriosis can persist during the entire reproductive life of the woman, any treatment plan needs to be holistic. Many factors in the life of the woman and her significant others have to be taken into account, including the woman's desire to bear children, family size, and lifestyle factors.

Stenchever (1996) notes further that there are no ideal treatments; each has pros and cons and associated side effects.

Drug Therapy

The following five drug therapies are currently in use (Stenchever, 1996):

1. Low-dose oral contraceptives to suppress ovulation

2. Progestogens

3. Danazol therapy, a drug that is a testosterone derivative

4. Hormone treatments that suppress the hypothalamus and pituitary gland

5. RU486. Preliminary trials are underway. RU486 is an antiprogestin. It binds to progesterone receptors. It produces anovulation and amenorrhea and has fewer side effects than those associated with other treatment regimens.

All these drug regimens may help control symptoms, but none are curative.

Surgery

Laparoscopic surgery is the only way to diagnose and determine the severity of the lesions of endometriosis. During this procedure, the lesions can be removed or destroyed by using thermal cautery or laser (Stenchever, 1996).

Natural Healing

The premise of all systems of natural healing is that given the right tools, the body heals itself. The goal of natural therapies for endometriosis is to reduce estrogen levels in the body and regulate hormone production. The focus is on the liver and the endocrine system.

The first step is to eliminate foods that tax the liver's detoxification pathways, such as caffeine; alcohol; and foods that are high in fat, contain chemicals, and may contain hormones and growth factors. Examples are meat and dairy products. These foods can be replaced with foods that have high nutritional value and thus support liver function, such as fruits, nuts, seeds, legumes, and vegetables. Foods high in fiber help eliminate excess estrogen. Shitake mushrooms can be added to the diet, which inhibit the growth of abnormal tissue in the body (Gladstar, 1993). Exercise is important because it increases blood flow to the pelvis and also reduces estrogen levels. Finally, there are a number of safe herbs that support liver function and help balance hormone levels. (Please see the resource guide at the end of this course for more information.)

Natural therapies take time to work. A program of dietary change, with herbs and nutritional support, may take 4–6 months to be effective in controlling symptoms. However, it does not "cure" endometriosis (McIntyre, 1995).

FIBROIDS (LEIOMYOMATA)

Lichtman and Papera (1990) comment that fibroids, or myomas, are the most common tumors of the pelvis. They arise from the multiplication of smooth muscle cells of the uterus. They are almost always benign or noncancerous.

Lichtman and Papera (1990) note further that fibroids may be located at a number of different places in and around the uterus. The most common fibroids form within the uterine wall. Some protrude into the uterine cavity, some bulge outward through the uterine wall into the pelvic cavity, and some form a stalk (called a pedicle) and are attached at the narrow base.

Fibroids occur more commonly in Black than in White women. They also occur more frequently with increasing age and regress after menopause (Lichtman & Papera, 1990).

Causes

What causes fibroids is not well understood. Evidence suggests that estrogen stimulates their growth (Lichtman & Papera, 1990).

Signs and Symptoms

In most women, fibroids can be present without any awareness of their existence. They are often discovered on a routine bimanual pelvic examination. For women who do have signs and symptoms, the following three are the most common (Lichtman & Papera, 1990):

1. **Abnormal bleeding:** With fibroids there tends to be an increased flow and duration of menses. Bleeding between periods or irregular bleeding is usually not seen.

2. **Pressure:** Depending on the location of the fibroid, pressure may be experienced on the bladder or rectum. The former causes urinary frequency or incontinence, and the latter causes constipation and feelings of heaviness.

3. **Pain:** With fibroids there may be heavier cramping with menses, but pain is not typical of fibroids. If chronic pain is present, the health care provider should look for a co-existing problem. Acute pain could indicate a twisting of a fibroid that is on a stalk.

Diagnosis

On examination, the uterus may feel enlarged or irregularly shaped (or both). Pregnancy should always be suspected (Lichtman & Papera, 1990). A sonogram should be done to confirm and provide baseline measurements, with a follow-up sonogram performed in 3–4 months (Lichtman & Papera, 1990).

Treatment

Clients are usually seen at 6-month intervals after the initial and second visits as long as no signs or symptoms are occurring. If heavy and prolonged bleeding occurs, clients should be referred to a specialist for further evaluation and intervention. This could include the following:

- **Drug therapy:** Progesterone, or medications that inhibit ovulation and induce a pseudomenopause, can be prescribed. Side effects include hot flashes and, with long-term use, compromised bone density. Drug therapy is most commonly used to shrink fibroids before surgery (Lichtman & Papera, 1990).

- **Dilation and curettage:** Dilation and curettage can be used to control bleeding. According to the article "Fibroids and Abnormal Uterine Bleeding" (1998), a small electrode is inserted through the hysteroscope, and electrical energy is used to vaporize the fibroid.

- **Hysteroscopy:** A hysteroscopy may be done for removal of the fibroids through the cervical canal.

- **Myomectomy:** Removal of the fibroids (myomectomy) can be accomplished during a laparotomy. The uterus (and therefore child-bearing potential) is preserved.

- **Hysterectomy:** Removal of the uterus (hysterectomy) may be a treatment of choice if bleeding cannot be controlled by other means.

- **Fibroid embolization:** According to the article "Fibroid Surgery Alternative" (1998), fibroid embolization is a nonsurgical technique that is still undergoing experimentation. A catheter is introduced into the groin by way of a small incision. The catheter is guided to the uterus. A radiologist injects small plastic particles into the artery supplying blood to the fibroid to cut off the blood flow to it.

Complications

Fibroids can interfere with fertility, depending on their size and location. If excessive bleeding occurs, anemia may result. Surgical intervention may be necessary.

Health Promotion

Several changes in diet and lifestyle can help reduce symptoms due to fibroids, as well as help curb further growth. Consider the following, with the first two recommended by Lichtman and Papera (1990) and the remaining eight noted by Gladstar (1993):

- Do not use an intrauterine device.

- Do not use estrogen-containing birth control products.

- Perform aerobic exercise (decreases excess estrogen).

- Avoid meat, chicken, and dairy products, which may contain hormones.

- Eat food high in fiber (helps the body get rid of excess estrogen).

- Avoid chemicals and drugs that place stress on the liver. (The liver is responsible for breaking down excess estrogen in the body.)

- Minimize intake of alcohol.

- Eat a low-fat diet.

- Keep weight moderate. (Excess fat causes the body to have higher estrogen levels.)

- Have a program of stress reduction. (Stress causes the body to increase production of estrogen.)

ABNORMAL OR EXCESSIVE UTERINE BLEEDING

The following information has been gleaned from an article in the June 1998 issue of the *National Women's Health Report* ("Abnormal Uterine Bleeding, Treatment Options").

Heavy bleeding is a common problem for women in the perimenopausal period between the ages of 40 and 50 years. There are two types of abnormal bleeding: dysfunctional and structural.

1. Abnormal bleeding related to dysfunctional causes: Dysfunctional bleeding is most commonly caused by hormone imbalances, being implicated in approximately 75% of women with excessive bleeding. As ovulation becomes more erratic during the perimenopausal period, progesterone levels decrease. Progesterone stabilizes the uterine lining. Without progesterone, bleeding may become unpredictable, excessive, or prolonged. Heavy bleeding can also be due to thyroid or adrenal gland disorders, clotting disorders, liver or kidney disease, leukemia, or medications such as anticoagulants.

2. Abnormal bleeding related to structural causes: Structural causes of excessive bleeding include fibroids, polyps, or infection. (Fibroids are commonly present without causing abnormal bleeding.) Precancerous or cancerous conditions of the uterus or cervix can also cause abnormal bleeding.

Diagnosis

Diagnostic tests used in evaluating women for abnormal or excessive uterine bleeding include hysteroscopy, hysterosalpingogram or sonohysterography, and endometrial biopsy.

Treatment

Current treatment options include the following:

- **Drug therapy:** Medications used for abnormal or excessive bleeding include low-dose birth control pills, progestins, nonsteroidal antiinflammatory drugs, and insertion of the Progestasert intrauterine device.

- **Surgery:** Three surgical procedures are available to treat abnormal or excessive bleeding:

  1. Dilation and curettage (D&C). The D&C was once a mainstay of treatment, but new options are more effective.

  2. Hysteroscopic endometrial ablation. With the hysteroscopic endometrial ablation procedure the uterine lining is viewed through a hysteroscope. An electrosurgical tip or laser is used to burn away the uterine lining. Fertility is not preserved.

  3. "Thermachoice" uterine balloon therapy. The Thermachoice therapy is safer than ablation. A flexible balloon attached to a thin probe is inserted through the cervix and inflated in the uterus with sterile fluid. The fluid is heated and thereby destroys the uterine lining. Fertility is not preserved.

HYSTERECTOMY

Hysterectomy was discussed briefly in other chapters. However, mention of it here is important because it affects large numbers of women in midlife, often inducing an abrupt premature menopause.

According to DeMarco (1996), hysterectomy is the most common major surgery performed in the

United States. DeMarco notes that only about 10% of hysterectomies are done for life-threatening reasons. The remainder are elective surgeries, with 63% being performed on women younger than 45 years of age. Frequently, the ovaries are removed, inducing premature menopause with its associated increased risk for heart disease and osteoporosis. Even if the ovaries are left intact, they often fail prematurely.

Findings from several studies show an estimated 30%–50% of hysterectomies are performed unnecessarily for medical conditions such as fibroids, which could have been treated in other ways. New techniques to remove fibroids or control excessive bleeding offer alternatives to hysterectomy ("Abnormal Uterine Bleeding, Treatment Options," 1998). Women should always seek a second opinion when faced with recommendations for hysterectomy (DeMarco, 1996).

It is beyond the scope of this course to consider the issues surrounding hysterectomy in more detail, but much has been written on the subject. Please see the resource guide for further information. The Internet is a good resource for information on this subject as well.

OVARIAN TUMORS

Because the ovary is made up of so many different tissue types, growths or tumors involving this structure can be of many different types. More than 50 different types of tumors of the ovary have been identified (Lichtman & Papera, 1990). Two of the most common types will be discussed here: Follicular cysts and corpus luteal cysts.

Follicular Cysts

A follicular cyst is the most common growth that occurs on the ovary, and it is formed during the first half of the menstrual cycle, the follicular phase. It forms when ovulation does not occur, and the developing dominant follicle continues to grow and becomes a large fluid-filled cyst containing a high concentration of estrogen. This type of cyst can also form from one of the other follicles that failed to regress when the dominant follicle took over.

Signs and Symptoms

According to Lichtman and Papera (1990), with a follicular cyst there may be no symptoms, or they can create a heavy, achy feeling in the pelvis. Because of the excess estrogen collecting in the cyst, the client may have irregular periods.

Diagnosis

Diagnosis may be made on the basis of symptoms and confirmed with an ultrasound. Pregnancy should always be suspected and ruled out (Lichtman & Papera, 1990).

Treatment

As noted by Lichtman and Papera (1990), usually watching and waiting, with another examination performed in 6–10 weeks, is the "treatment" of choice unless symptoms worsen. They note further that most follicular cysts go away on their own without intervention.

Corpus Luteal Cysts

Lichtman and Papera (1990) reports that a corpus luteal cyst forms from the corpus luteum during the second half, or luteal phase, of the menstrual cycle. Again, menstrual irregularity, especially delayed menstruation, may result. Lichtman and Papera note further that these cysts usually contain blood. Most often they regress and disappear spontaneously. Less commonly they rupture, and they can cause severe abdominal pain from the bleeding. Surgical removal of the cyst may then be necessary.

ECTOPIC PREGNANCY

The following discussion, statistics, and research findings on ectopic pregnancy are

FIGURE 11-1
Etopic Pregnancy

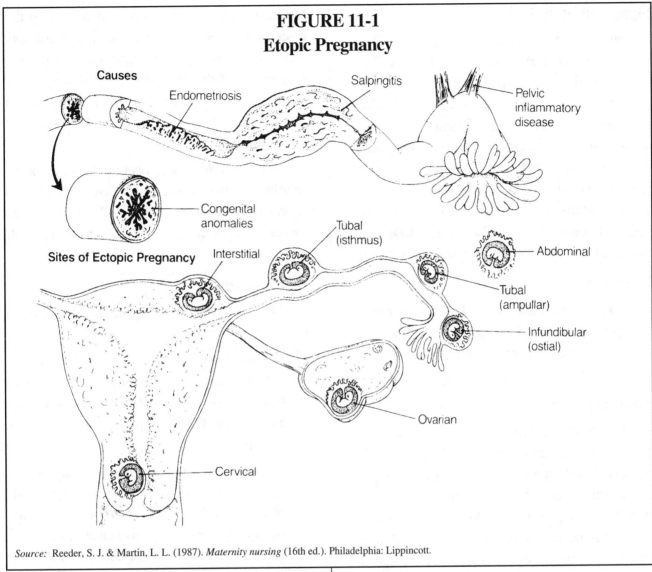

Causes

Endometriosis

Salpingitis

Pelvic inflammatory disease

Congenital anomalies

Sites of Ectopic Pregnancy

Interstitial

Tubal (isthmus)

Abdominal

Tubal (ampullar)

Infundibular (ostial)

Ovarian

Cervical

Source: Reeder, S. J. & Martin, L. L. (1987). *Maternity nursing* (16th ed.). Philadelphia: Lippincott.

based on the report of Hatcher and colleagues (1994).

A failure of the fertilized egg to implant in the uterus results in implantation elsewhere in the pelvis (see *Figure 11-1*). Ninety-seven percent of ectopic pregnancies occur in the fallopian tubes. Rarely the egg will implant on the ovary or the cervix or in the abdomen outside the uterus. The implanted fertilized egg, located most often in the tiny fallopian tube, grows until it can no longer be contained in the small space, and it spontaneously ruptures. This can cause severe bleeding into the abdominal cavity, leading to shock and death if no intervention occurs.

Risk Factors

The leading single predisposing factor in ectopic pregnancy is a history of infection in the fallopian tube (salpingitis or PID) usually caused by an STI, especially chlamydial infection. Partial obstruction or narrowing and twisting of the tubal canal usually results from infection, damaging the small hairs (cilia) inside the tube and leaving pockets in which an egg can get trapped on its way to the uterus. The incidence of ectopic pregnancy is on the rise in the United States, probably coincident with the rise in STIs.

Signs and Symptoms

An unruptured ectopic pregnancy is difficult to diagnose in the early stages because it is often asymptomatic. Signs and symptoms that may be present include lack of menses, lower abdominal pain, slight vaginal bleeding, and a mass in the area of the ovary. A ruptured ectopic pregnancy usually presents with severe abdominal pain, referred shoulder pain as a result of abdominal bleeding, dizziness, fainting, and shock. This is an emergency situation, and immediate hospitalization is essential for stabilization and surgical intervention.

Diagnosis

Diagnosis is made on the basis of examination, pelvic ultrasound, and a blood test for levels of the pregnancy hormone human chorionic gonadotropin.

Treatment

An unruptured early ectopic pregnancy is treated in some facilities with the drug methotrexate, traditionally used in treating cancer, psoriasis, and a number of other conditions. Methotrexate stops the growth of rapidly dividing cells. It thus stops the growth of an early embryo. Surgical intervention may be needed for larger ectopic pregnancies and those that have ruptured.

Long-Term Complications

Only about half of clients with an ectopic pregnancy eventually achieve a normal intrauterine pregnancy. Ten percent may have another ectopic pregnancy, and 40% experience infertility.

OVARIAN CANCER

The following description, statistics, and research findings on ovarian cancer are gleaned from Lichtman and Papera (1990).

Because the pelvis contains not only reproductive organs but also major components of the gas-trointestinal and urinary tracts, determining the cause of a pelvic mass requires careful evaluation, including evaluating for the possibility of ovarian cancer. Any of the different cell types in the ovary can give rise to cancerous growth. It is beyond the scope of this course to discuss the many different forms of ovarian cancer.

Most ovarian cancer occurs in women at or shortly after menopause. Sixty percent of ovarian cancer is found in women age 40–60 years. This cancer is one of the leading causes of cancer death in women.

Risk Factors

There are several factors that place women at risk for ovarian cancer:

- **Family history:** If two or more first-degree relatives or many second-degree relatives had ovarian cancer, the risk may approach 50%, especially for a woman who is post-menopausal.

- **Age:** The risk for ovarian cancer increases 12 times for women who are postmenopausal, compared with that in women age 20–29 years. For women who are premenopausal there is a 13% risk that an ovarian mass is malignant. This increases to 45% after menopause.

- **Never having children** (nulliparity)

- **Early menarche**

- **Late menopause**

- **Talc, asbestos, and diet high in animal fat:** Preliminary research findings show possible association with these factors.

- **Obesity**

Signs and Symptoms

Signs and symptoms are often vague. Ovarian cancer should be considered whenever any woman older than 40 years of age has complaints of vague abdominal or pelvic discomfort, sense of bloating, or flatulence.

Screening and Evaluation

Four procedures are used in screening and evaluation for ovarian cancer:

1. **Ultrasound:** Ultrasound can be used to determine size, location, and quality (i.e., fluid filled, solid, complex) of the mass.

2. **Genetic screening:** BRCA1 is a genetic marker for ovarian cancer. Clients can be screened during genetic counseling and testing to determine whether they carry the cancer susceptibility gene BRCA1.

3. **Serum Ca-125 antigen levels:** The test to determine the serum Ca-125 antigen levels was originally used to monitor the course of epithelial ovarian cancer. It is often used currently in preoperative decision making about managing pelvic masses. False-positive results can be caused by other conditions, including nongynecologic cancers and active endometriosis. There can also be false-negative results: 82% of known ovarian cancers were associated with elevated serum levels of Ca-125 antigen, leaving an 18% false-negative rate.

4. **Laparotomy:** Laparotomy can be performed for surgical confirmation of the cancer.

Treatment

Usually a total abdominal hysterectomy with removal of the ovaries and fallopian tubes is performed, followed by some combination of radiation or chemotherapy (or both).

Prevention

Women with a strong family history of ovarian cancer may want to consider the use of oral contraceptives, which have been shown to reduce substantially the risk of ovarian cancer. Results of some studies have shown a protective effect of vitamin A supplementation. Avoidance of exposure to talc and asbestos, as well as reducing dietary fat intake, is also advised.

UTERINE CANCER

Once again, the following information, including pertinent statistics and research results, on uterine cancer is gleaned from Lichtman and Papera (1990).

There are a number of different types of cancer of the uterus, depending on the site and the type of tissue involved. Most arise within the inner lining of the uterus, the endometrium, and are cancers of the glandular tissue. Most uterine cancer is found in women age 50–70 years old.

Causes

There is a relationship between unopposed estrogen (i.e., estrogen not balanced by progesterone, which causes the cells that estrogen stimulates to grow and mature) and uterine cancer. Estrogen may be a tumor promoter. Progesterone inhibits the growth of cells that estrogen stimulates by causing them to go into a more mature secretory state. Women who receive estrogen replacement therapy without progesterone have much higher rates of uterine cancer. Progesterone is now added to any hormone replacement therapy for women who have a uterus. (See chapter 13 for more information.) The exact cause of uterine cancer is not known.

Risk Factors

Nulliparity or low parity, early menarche, late menopause, and obesity are risk factors for uterine cancer. Study findings have shown that women who are 40% overweight are five times more likely to develop uterine cancer. A form of estrogen is produced by the fat cells. Normally this production takes over when the ovaries start to decrease their hormone output. However, for women who are greatly overweight, this overproduction of estrogen puts them at increased risk for cancer.

Signs and Symptoms

Any woman around the age of 50 years (i.e., the age at which menopause usually begins) with abnormal bleeding should be evaluated for uterine cancer. Ninety percent of women with uterine cancer have painless irregular bleeding.

Diagnosis

A biopsy of the endometrium is taken to evaluate the uterine lining for diagnosis. If the biopsy results are positive, a dilation and curettage would be done for the purpose of staging the cancer.

Treatment

The cancer is staged on the basis of its location and extension into surrounding tissue and distant metastasis. Treatment involves total abdominal hysterectomy, along with removal of the ovaries and fallopian tubes. This is followed by radiation or chemotherapy (or both), depending on the individual case. The most common uterine cancer, adenocarcinoma, usually remains localized for a long time, and 5-year survival rates approach 80%. Survival rates depend on the stage of disease.

DISEASES OF THE VULVA

The following introduction and background information on diseases of the vulva; highlighted information that follows on vaginal infections, Bartholin's gland or Skene's gland duct abscess, and vulvar warts; and brief comments on other vulvar diseases, such as systemic diseases, premalignant lesions, and Paget's disease, are gleaned from Stenchever (1996). In addition, the information on parasites and molluscum contagiosum is a summary from descriptions by Lichtman and Papera (1990). Again, any pertinent statistics and research findings noted here are taken from these sources as well, and the reader is referred to both sources for more expanded information on diseases of the vulva.

Vulvar tissue is richly supplied with sweat and sebaceous glands. Hair follicles are present in some areas as well. It is a moist environment with increased concentrations of skin bacteria.

Symptoms on the vulva can be caused by any one of a number of different problems, ranging from something benign such as contact dermatitis to vulvar cancer. A careful history is important in any diagnosis. However, common symptoms include itching, burning, a "lump," a sore, vaginal discharge, rash, and pain.

Interestingly, study findings have shown that women who have chronic symptoms with negative clinical findings have a higher incidence of depression and anxiety than women with similar complaints who do have diagnostic findings. Thus a definite mind-body connection is at work. Five specific vulvar diseases are described in more detail in the following sections.

Vaginal Infections

Vaginal infections can cause symptoms on the vulva. Candidiasis or yeast infection is the most common infection causing itching and irritation. Women who are immunocompromised, have diabetes, or are overweight or receiving antibiotics on a long-term basis are particularly susceptible to yeast infections of the vulva that may be resistant to treatment. Further testing is indicated, because infection in these cases may be due to other forms of yeast or combination infections, including bacterial ones.

Bartholin's Gland or Skene's Gland Duct Abscess

The Bartholin's gland or Skene's glands are located just inside the vaginal opening on either side. They can become blocked, leading to formation of a cyst behind the blockage. These cysts may cause no symptoms, or they may become infected and painful. In the latter case, incision and drainage is required. Antibiotics may be given. Rarely, this abscess is caused by gonorrhea. In women who are postmenopausal, this problem is rare, and cancer should be suspected.

Parasites

Lice or mites may infect the vulva. Itching of the skin that contains hair follicles is characteristic. With scabies (a dermatitis caused by the itch mite, *Sarcoptes scabiei),* excoriated areas are found, and they are also evident on the wrists and webs of the fingers. Lice often leave eggs that are adhered to the hair shaft.

Molluscum Contagiosum

The lesions of molluscum contagiosum are caused by a poxvirus. They are not necessarily transmitted sexually but are easily passed from one person to another. They are small, pearly looking umbilicated papules and usually produce no symptoms. They usually infect the skin of the lower abdomen, inner thigh, and external genital area. Removal of the central core with a needle will cause them to heal and resolve.

Vulvar Warts

Vulvar warts are caused by certain strains of the human papillomavirus, but they are not the same types as those that produce lesions on the cervix. They can appear as small warty growths or large cauliflower-like masses on the vulva or perineum or in and around the anus. They can be treated with chemicals, cryotherapy, or laser, but the chemical method is the most common for an office procedure.

None of the treatments have been highly successful, and recurrence is common. Even if the lesions are removed, the normal-appearing area around them still has the human papillomavirus. There is no guarantee that removing the warts will prevent transmission of the virus. Vulvar warts are not always attributable to sexual contact and can be passed by fomites (see chapter 7).

Other Vulvar Diseases

The health care worker may encounter vulvar disease in clients related to one of three additional conditions:

1. **Systemic diseases:** Diseases such as Crohn's disease can cause vulvar symptoms.

2. **Premalignant lesions:** Vulvar intraepithelial neoplasia can occur in women of all ages. However, it occurs most commonly in women in their late 20s and early 30s, as well as in immunosuppressed women. The most common symptom is persistent itching, usually at multiple sites. The area is often pigmented. The likelihood of these lesions progressing to vulvar cancer is low. Biopsy is needed for diagnosis.

3. **Paget's disease:** Paget's disease is a rare neoplasm that is often confused with a yeast infection. It occurs more commonly in elderly women, often with persistent redness of the vulva. Diagnosis is made on the basis of biopsy results.

Health Promotion

The following health-promotion measures can help women maintain a healthy vulvar environment and decrease the chance of irritation and infection (Stenchever, 1996):

- Wear cotton underwear.

- Keep the vulvar area clean and dry.

- Avoid
  - use of perfumed or colored toilet paper.
  - douches.

- Notice if certain soaps or laundry detergents cause allergic reaction.

- Be aware that
  - lubricants, spermicides, or barrier birth control methods may provoke reactions.
  - food allergies can also cause skin reactions.

CONCLUSION

The most common disorders affecting a woman's reproductive system have been highlighted in this chapter. It is disturbing to find that the causes and cures for many chronic gynecologic problems elude modern medicine. Many of these problems have become increasingly prevalent in modern society. Perhaps health care workers have to look for broader explanations. What are human beings putting into their bodies, what chemicals are they being exposed to, and what stresses are constantly altering their internal chemistry? Teaching women general health-promotion measures is the best prevention strategy health care providers can implement for many of these "diseases of imbalanced hormones," including dietary recommendations, exercise, and stress reduction techniques.

CHAPTER 11
Questions 85–91

85. Uterine balloon therapy is a technique developed to

   a. open blocked fallopian tubes.

   b. treat infertility.

   c. treat excessive uterine bleeding.

   d. treat uterine cancer.

86. Which of the following is not considered to be a sexually transmitted infection?

   a. Gonorrhea

   b. Bacterial vaginosis

   c. Hepatitis B

   d. Hepatitis C

87. Ectopic pregnancy

   a. is always accompanied by one-sided pain.

   b. can be life-threatening.

   c. can resolve spontaneously if left untreated.

   d. results in infertility.

88. Exposure to diethylstilbestrol in utero has been linked to

   a. vaginal cancer.

   b. fibroids.

   c. endometriosis.

   d. dysmenorrhea.

89. Clients with uncomplicated lower urinary tract infection will usually not report

   a. tenderness above the pubic area.

   b. foul-smelling urine.

   c. intense lower back pain.

   d. urgency and frequency.

90. A bimanual pelvic examination often can be used to detect

   a. ovarian cancer.

   b. fibroids.

   c. endometriosis.

   d. ectopic pregnancy.

91. Ovarian cancer

    a. occurs at a higher rate in women who have taken birth control pills than in women who have not taken these pills.

    b. occurs at a higher rate in young women than in older women.

    c. has a strong genetic component.

    d. has a weak genetic component.

CHAPTER 12

BREAST HEALTH AND DISEASE

CHAPTER OBJECTIVE

After completing this chapter, the reader will be able to describe the anatomy of the breast, and discuss breast self-examination techniques and teaching points. The reader will also be able to identify abnormal breast examination findings, as well as diagnostic techniques, statistics, and risk factors associated with breast cancer. The reader will also be able to discuss ways in which risk for breast cancer can be reduced through changes in lifestyle and diet.

LEARNING OBJECTIVES

After studying this chapter, the reader will be able to

1. describe the anatomy of the breast.

2. describe how to teach breast self-examination to clients.

3. discuss recommendations for mammography and breast self-examination.

4. discuss techniques available for diagnosing abnormalities of the breast.

5. discuss risk factors for breast cancer.

6. describe diet and lifestyle factors that may be potential agents in breast cancer, as well as changes that can decrease breast cancer risk.

7. identify treatments for breast cancer.

Key Words

- Adjuvant
- Fine needle aspiration
- In situ
- Mammotome
- Metastasis
- Microcalcifications
- Node negative
- Node positive
- Open biopsy
- Staging

INTRODUCTION

Stenchever (1996) reports that the prevalence of breast cancer has been increasing in the United States at the rate of 1%–1.5% every year. Current statistics indicate that 1 in every 9 women will get breast cancer at some point in her life. He notes further that most of the women who get breast cancer have none of the known risk factors except for being female and advancing age.

Breast cancer is an epidemic for which no known cause has been clarified, and women understandably feel frightened and helpless about its elusiveness. Women often do not check their breasts because of confusion about what to look for and fear of what they might find.

Kradjian (1994) notes that because the question of cause still eludes scientific proof, the current approach to breast cancer by the medical community is based on early detection. However, he reports that there is a growing body of evidence that points to dietary and environmental influences as causative or contributing factors. By their very nature, these influences are difficult to isolate and study in human populations, and therefore causation is difficult to prove. Some of these issues are discussed in more detail later in the chapter.

Weed (1996) points out that an increasing number of health care providers are taking the approach of making specific recommendations regarding diet, lifestyle, and environmental exposure, believing that while waiting for proof thousands of women are losing their breasts and thousands are dying. She comments further that changes in diet, lifestyle, and environmental exposure are aspects of health that human beings have control over, and the general health benefits of such changes have been proved. Prevention strategies such as these, combined with early detection, are clearly the best approach.

NORMAL BREAST ANATOMY

According to Stenchever (1996), breast tissue normally feels lumpy. Adipose tissue lies just under the skin, overlying tissue that is fibrous and glandular. The fatty tissue is thicker in some areas and thinner in others, and there is often a distinct ridge of tissue under the breast. The underlying fibroglandular tissue has ridges and indentations as well.

Stenchever (1996) notes that the breasts are composed of milk-secreting glands; ducts; and fatty, connective, and lymphatic tissue. Lobules are the glands that produce milk. Ducts are the small passages connecting the milk-producing glands or lobules to the nipple. When health care providers teach a client breast self-examination (SBE) it is important to show pictures of breast tissue and talk about the normal lumpiness of breasts. This will do much to ease women's fears about checking their breasts.

BREAST SELF-EXAMINATION

Before instructing clients about SBE techniques, the health care provider should find out the following from the client:

1. What the client already knows about doing SBE

2. Whether she does SBE on a regular basis

3. How she does her SBEs

4. How she feels about checking her breasts

Breast self-examination is often very emotionally charged, and women feel embarrassed to confess that they have not been doing their examinations. Health care providers can do much to allay women's fears and make SBE a more life-positive experience:

• Try to put clients at ease.

• Be nonjudgmental and compassionate.

• Remind clients that the purpose of SBE is to get to know their breasts.

Women are not expected to diagnose themselves. Even a professionally trained examiner cannot tell by palpation whether an abnormal-appearing area is cancer. What women can do is notice changes that persist and come in for evaluation if they find something that feels different to them, just as they would for any other part of their body.

Components

The SBE has two components: visual inspection and palpation (see *Figure 12-1*):

FIGURE 12-1 *1 of 2*
Breast Self-Examination: A New Approach

Breast Self-Examination
A   N e w   A p p r o a c h

All women over 20 should practice regular monthly breast self-examination (BSE). Regular and complete BSE can help you find changes in your breasts that occur between clinical breast examinations by a health professional, and mammograms.

Women should examine their breasts when they are least tender, usually seven days after the start of the menstrual period. Women who have entered menopause, are pregnant or breastfeeding, and women who have silicone implants should continue to examine their breasts once a month. Breast feeding mothers should examine their breasts when all milk has been expressed.

If a woman discovers a lump or detects any changes, she should seek medical attention. Nine out of ten women will not develop breast cancer and most breast changes are not cancerous.

How Often?

American Cancer Society Guidelines for breast cancer detection.

Breast self-exam
Age 20 + ...Monthly

Clinical breast exam
Age 20 - 40 . . . . .Every 3 years
Age 40 + ...Yearly

Mammography
Age 40 + ...Yearly

1 Positions

Visual Inspection: Standing

In each position, look for changes in contour and shape of the breasts, color and texture of the skin and nipple and evidence of discharge from the nipples.

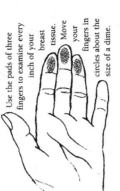
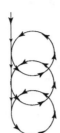

arms raised above head

hands on hips

arms relaxed at side

bending forward

Palpation: Flat and Side-lying

Use your left hand to palpate the right breast, while holding your right arm at a right angle to the rib cage, with the elbow bent. Repeat the procedure on the other side. The side-lying position allows a woman, especially one with large breasts, to most effectively examine the outer half of the breast. A woman with small breasts may need only the flat position.

Side-lying Position: Lie on the opposite side of the breast to be examined. Rotate the shoulder (on the same side as the breast to be examined) back to the flat surface. Use the side-lying position to examine the outer half of your breast.

Flat Position: Lie flat on your back with a pillow or folded towel under the shoulder of the breast to be examined.

2 Perimeter

The exam area is bounded by the line which extends down from the middle of the armpit to just beneath the breast, continues across the underside of the breast to the middle of the breast bone, then moves up and along the collar bone and back to the middle of the armpit. Most breast cancers occur in the upper outer area of the breast (shaded area).

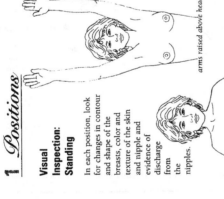
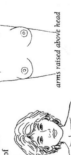
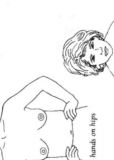
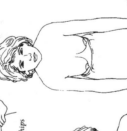
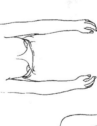
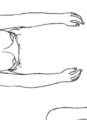

3 Palpation with Pads of Fingers

Use the pads of three fingers to examine every inch of your breast tissue. Move your fingers in circles about the size of a dime.

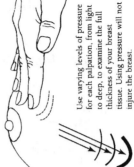
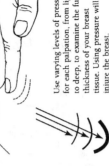

Do not lift your fingers from your breast between palpations. You can use powder or lotion to help your fingers glide from one spot to the next.

4 Pressure

Use varying levels of pressure for each palpation, from light to deep, to examine the full thickness of your breast tissue. Using pressure will not injure the breast.

Source: American Cancer Society. (1997). *Breast self-examination: A new approach.* Oakland, CA: American Cancer Society.

FIGURE 12-1 *2 of 2*
Breast Self-Examination: A New Approach

5 *Pattern of Search*

Vertical Strip:

Use the following search pattern to examine all of your breast tissue. Be sure to palpate carefully beneath the nipple. Any incision should also be carefully examined from end to end. Women who have had any breast surgery should still examine the entire area and the incision. Start in the armpit, proceed downward to the lower boundary. Move a finger's width toward the middle and continue palpating upward until you reach the collarbone. Repeat this until you have covered all the breast tissue. Make at least six strips before the nipple and four strips after the nipple. You may need between 10 and 16 strips to cover all of your breast tissue.

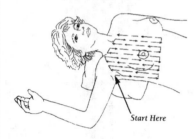

Start Here

Remember the seven P's for a complete BSE:

1 Positions   **5** Pattern
2 Perimeter   **6** Practice with Feedback
3 Palpation   **7** Plan of Action
4 Pressure

Axillary Examination:

Examine the breast tissue that extends into your armpit while your arm is relaxed at your side.

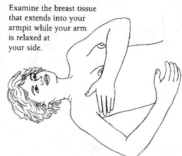

6 *Practice with Feedback*

It is important that you perform breast self-examination (BSE) while your instructor watches to be sure you are doing it correctly. Practice your skills until you feel comfortable and confident.

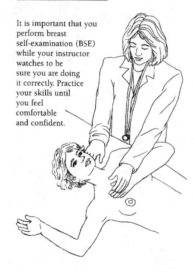

7 *Plan of Action*

Every woman should have a personal breast health plan of action:

Discuss the American Cancer Society's breast cancer detection guidelines with your health professional.

Schedule your clinical breast exam and mammogram as appropriate for your age.

Perform monthly breast self-examinations (BSE). Ask your health professional for feedback on your BSE skills.

Report any breast changes to your health professional.

AMERICAN CANCER SOCIETY
SANTA ROSA UNIT
(707) 545-6720
PETALUMA
(707) 766-8066

AMERICAN CANCER SOCIETY

For more information please call

1 (800) ACS-2345

Website: www.cancer.org

The American Cancer Society's materials and programs are provided free of charge and are supported by public contributions.

Revised 10/97

6438.39

Source: American Cancer Society. (1997). *Breast self-examination: A new approach.* Oakland, CA: American Cancer Society.

1. **Visual inspection:** Visual inspection consists of observing for indentations, puckering, or dimpling of the skin (not for lumps protruding from the skin, which would be a very advanced sign). The changes that are being watched for occur more subtly, such as minor skin retraction or pulling of the nipple to one side. Breasts that are different sizes are usually not of concern unless it is a new development.

    The visual examination should be done with the client facing a mirror, first with arms raised overhead. Then arm, hand, and body movements should progress—and visual examination should take place at each position change—to hands squeezing the hips; then body leaning forward; and, finally, arms relaxed at the sides. The nipples should be observed for symmetry, discharge, or discoloration. The skin should be observed for changes in color or texture.

2. **Palpation:** The entire breast needs to be palpated, in a section defined by the axillary area, which contains lymph nodes; to the brassiere line and breast bone; and, finally, up to the collar bone. Nipples should be palpated for internal thickening or lumps as the woman simultaneously looks for signs of spontaneous nipple discharge. The key word is spontaneous. Many women can elicit some discharge by squeezing the nipples, especially women who have had children. Discharge that is of concern is most often spontaneous.

The examination is best done with the woman lying down, especially for women with large breasts, but it can be done while the woman is standing in the shower. *Figure 12-1* illustrates different patterns that can be used for checking the breasts. It is up to the woman to find a pattern that is most comfortable. The main point is to be systematic and cover all the areas noted.

By using the pads of the fingers, small circles are made just on the surface and then deeper. The fingers are then walked to the next spot, and the circular pattern is repeated. Because menstruating women often have increased discomfort and lumpiness in their breasts during the second half of the menstrual cycle, the ideal time for SBE is during the week after menstruation. More than 75% of breast cancers are found by women themselves. Breast self-examination is a simple yet powerful self-help behavior that can save lives (Sifton, 1994).

Self-Massage

Weed (1996) points out that in American culture touching one's own breasts is somewhat taboo. Doing SBE can seem like a somewhat foreign activity to some women. Women should be encouraged to take off their brasierres when they get home from work. Brasierres can restrict the blood and lymph flow into the area of the body the brasierre fits. Women would not think of binding up other parts of their body in this way. Use of sports brasierres should be encouraged because they can be less binding.

Weed (1996) comments further that doing breast self-massage is a way of introducing a pleasurable way of keeping in touch with what is happening in this part of the body. The woman can use a little lotion or oil and massage from the axilla toward the center of the body. This increases the blood flow and helps the lymphatic system remove excess fluid. Partners can also get involved. After the woman becomes accustomed to massaging the breast, SBE will often be less intimidating.

BREAST DISEASE

When health care providers evaluate clients for breast disease, what may come to mind almost immediately is the breast tumor. Indeed, there are many types of breast tumors, and fortunately most are benign, not cancerous. Refer to *Figures 12-2* and *12-3* for descriptions of noncancerous lumps.

However, what should also come to mind is the complexity that centers around the terms *cyst* and *tumor* and how this complexity pertains to both breast disease and breast health when the normal texture and landscape of the woman's breast is taken into consideration. In addition, other processes besides the formation of cysts can lead to breast disease. These include inflammatory or infectious processes as well as trauma or injury to the breast. All three manifestations of breast disease—cysts, inflammation or infection, and changes due to trauma or injury—need to be considered in evaluating women for breast disease and breast health. The discussion that follows, with pertinent statistics and research findings related to breast disease, is gleaned from Stenchever (1996).

FIGURE 12-2
Noncancerous Lumps

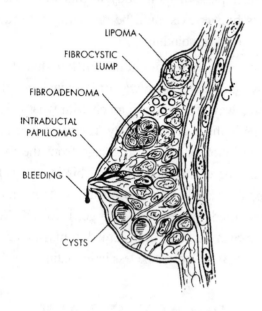

If you feel a lump, chances are it's a false alarm. Four out of five lumps are the harmless growths illustrated here:

- Fibrocystic lumps, which tend to swell in rhythm with the menstrual cycle, and diminish after menopause

- Cysts, which generally are found in both breasts and appear most often between the ages of 35 and 50

- Fibroadenomas, solid, round, and rubbery, which are found more often in younger women

- Lipomas—painless lumps the size of a coin—which develop slowly, primarily in older women

- Intraductal papillomas, small nodules underneath the edge of the nipple, which typically appear during your 40s

Even if you feel certain that a lump is just one of these growths, you should still see your doctor. Diagnostic tests are needed to conclusively rule out cancer.

Source: Sifton, D. W. (Ed.). (1994). *The PDR family guide to women's health and prescription drugs.* Montvale, N.J.: Medical Economics Data Production Company.

FIGURE 12-3
Is It a Lump…Or a Gland?

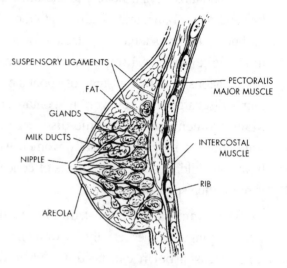

Distinguishing a lump from a normal milk gland during your breast self-exam may be difficult at first. There's always a possibility, too, of overlooking a lump amid all the glandular tissue of the breast. Your doctor can help you learn to feel the difference; and regular monthly self-exams will quickly make you familiar with your breasts' own unique textures.

Source: Sifton, D. W. (Ed.). (1994). *The PDR family guide to women's health and prescription drugs.* Montvale, N.J.: Medical Economics Data Production Company.

Cysts

It is common for a client to say she has "cystic breasts." However, this is often a misinterpretation by the client or the practitioner of normal irregularities of the breast; that is, large fatty lumps or ridges and troughs. Often, there has never been any actual documentation or diagnosis—on the basis of biopsy or ultrasound results—that the client has cysts.

There are a number of different types of cysts, and each has certain defining characteristics:

- **Fluid-filled sacs:** Fluid-filled sacs are often tender and fluctuate in size with the menstrual cycle.

- **Fibroadenomas:** Fibroadenomas are solid cysts. They are composed of fibrous and glandular tissue, usually movable, and not usually tender.

- **Papillomas:** Papillomas are small wartlike growths that can occur in the lining of milk ducts near the nipple. They may produce a clear or bloody discharge from the nipple.

- **Breast cysts:** Breast cysts are usually smooth, round lumps, which may be soft or firm and rubbery.

It is rare for a fluid-filled cyst to be cancerous. Cysts do not necessarily increase one's risk for breast cancer. High-risk clients would be women whose mothers have (or have had) breast cancer. More research needs to be done in this area to determine what is occurring in women with cysts, as well as whether this process of cyst formation is at all related to breast cancer.

Research is being done on the fluid found in cysts to determine what it is composed of. It is a complex fluid containing hormones, growth factors, and other biologic compounds that may influence the growth of breast tissue and yield information about breast cancer.

Mastitis

Mastitis is an infection of the breast that occurs when bacteria enter the mammary ducts through a nipple. This occurs most often during breast-feeding. Localized pockets of infection appear as tender warm lumps. Mastitis is usually treated with antibiotics and warm compresses.

Trauma or Injury to the Breast

Trauma or injury to the breast may result in an accumulation of blood at the site (hematoma) or a destruction of the fatty tissue, which can appear as a lump. There is no evidence that injury causes cancer.

EVALUATION OF BREAST ABNORMALITIES

No one would argue that the fear-inducing and ominous—as well as potentially benign—finding of a lump in the breast needs to be evaluated, and a decision-tree approach among available and emerging diagnostic tools is helpful in that process. Other common breast abnormalities that should be evaluated as well are discharge from the nipple, changes in the skin overlying the breast, and breast pain. All four breast abnormalities need to be evaluated to determine cause, appropriate treatment, and likelihood of their being associated with, or a precursor to, breast cancer.

A Lump Is Found: What Then?

If an area of abnormal breast tissue is found on examination, unless it feels suspicious the client is typically advised to return for a second evaluation after the next menses. The client may also be advised to have a mammogram at this time. An ultrasound may be done at the time of the mammogram to determine whether the lump is solid or fluid filled.

If the lump persists after the next menses or any abnormality is found on mammogram or ultrasound, further testing is recommended. If the ultrasound reveals that the lump is solid, a biopsy is the next step. If the lump is fluid filled, a needle aspiration biopsy is indicated. If a distinct palpable lump persists, even with normal mammographic findings, immediate follow-up is recommended.

Mammograms are not diagnostic. Some form of biopsy is needed to provide a sample of tissue for analysis, so that a definitive diagnosis can be established (Stenchever, 1996). Tests for progesterone and estrogen receptors may also be indicated.

Biopsy

According to Stenchever (1996), with current practice diagnosis and treatment of breast abnormalities is a two-step procedure in which some form of biopsy is done and then decisions are made regarding treatment on the basis of findings on biopsy.

Stenchever (1996) notes further that in earlier years a biopsy was done with the woman under general anesthesia. She remained on the operating table and under anesthesia while the tissue sample was evaluated. If cancer was found, the procedure continued with surgical removal of the breast. The woman would awaken not knowing whether or not her breast would be intact. This approach is rarely recommended today.

Stenchever (1996) also notes that palpation cannot determine that an abnormal area is not cancer, nor can clinical examination or available technology provide definitive proof that a tissue or structure is not cancerous. It can be said only that no evidence of cancer is found. Confirmation of cancer can be made only by examining the suspected tissue.

Four biopsy procedures used to obtain a sample of breast tissue or fluid within that tissue for evaluation are described next: fine needle aspiration, core needle aspiration, and surgical or open biopsy, as well as a newly developed technique known as mammotome.

Fine Needle Aspiration: The technique of fine needle aspiration uses a thin needle, which is guided into the area of concern while the practitioner feels the lump. This is usually done as an office procedure. If the abnormality is too small to feel, ultrasound or a stereotactic biopsy can be used to help locate and ensure sampling of the suspect tissue. In the latter technique, the biopsy is guided with the aid of mammography. The needle is guided to the area by computer-assisted x-ray, which can help the examiner control the placement of the needle precisely. Suction is applied to the needle. This procedure is used to determine whether the lump is a fluid-filled cyst or a solid tumor.

According to Sifton (1994) if fluid is aspirated, the procedure may eliminate the lump altogether and provide a preliminary diagnosis. Further testing may be done on the fluid as well if it is dark colored, if the fluid-filled cyst has recurred several times, or if the sample has been obtained from a woman who is postmenopausal and thus not expected to have cysts because of low estrogen levels. Clear fluid usually indicates a benign cyst, whereas cloudy or bloody fluid may be present in benign or cancerous tumors.

Sifton (1994) notes further that if no fluid is aspirated or a residual thickened area remains after fluid is aspirated, the next step is a core needle biopsy.

The false-positive rate for needle aspiration is almost zero. False-negative results occur frequently, however, because the needle may have missed abnormal tissue.

If no abnormalities are found with aspiration, a follow-up mammogram or ultrasound is recommended in 2–4 months to check for recurrence of the cyst (Sifton, 1994).

Core Needle: A core needle biopsy uses a large needle, and a small cylinder of tissue is removed. The needle placement is often guided as in the fine needle aspiration procedure. Core needle biopsy can be done as an office procedure with the use of local anesthesia (American Cancer Society, 1997).

Surgical or Open Biopsy: According to the pamphlet *Breast Cancer* (American Cancer Society, 1997), removal of all or a portion of the lump for microscopic analysis may be required. In this case a number of decisions need to be made about how much tissue to take. The aim is to have the surgical margins free of possible cancerous tissue.

The article "Breast Cancer" (American Cancer Society, 1997), notes further that an open biopsy is done with the woman under general anesthesia. The surgeon removes as much of the suspicious breast area as possible. Because these excisions leave a scar and can disfigure the breast, the incision is usually made near the areola of the nipple to hide the scar.

The surgical or open biopsy is considered the most accurate biopsy technique for large masses or large areas of suspicion. (See the next section on mammotome regarding small masses.) Radiation may be advised as follow-up therapy (American Cancer Society, 1997).

Mammotome: As described in the report *Mammotome Biopsies: More Accurate, Less Invasive* (1997), a new breast biopsy technique is available called mammotome. It uses a tiny hollow needle probe, which is guided to the abnormal area by using either computer images projected on two screens or ultrasound. The needle is inserted into the breast tissue. A vacuum is created to withdraw the tissue, which has been excised by a high-speed rotating cutter. A much larger sample of tissue can be obtained than with a core needle biopsy. Therefore there is a better chance of reducing false-negative reports, because of cancer cells being missed in needle biopsy.

Mammotome biopsy has been shown to be as accurate as a surgical biopsy for small breast masses that cannot be felt. It is not advised for larger abnormalities that can be palpated. In this case, the surgical or open biopsy remains the most accurate.

Tests for Estrogen and Progesterone Receptors

According to the pamphlet *Breast Cancer* (American Cancer Society, 1997), an important step in evaluating a person with early breast cancer is to test for the presence of hormone receptors. This provides important information about future hormone therapy, which can affect the prognosis of a woman's breast cancer. A sample of the cancerous tissue is evaluated for hormone receptors.

Nipple Discharge

The following information on nipple discharge is gleaned from the pamphlet *Breast Cancer* (American Cancer Society, 1997).

Any spontaneous nipple discharge needs to be evaluated. There are a number of different causes for this discharge.

A spontaneous milky discharge is termed *galactorrhea,* and it can occur in response to a stimulus, such as seeing a baby or taking a hot shower. If it occurs more than once, it should be evaluated.

Metabolic disorders and pituitary tumors can cause nipple discharge and should be part of the workup for spontaneous discharge. A smear of the discharge should be sent to the laboratory for analysis; mammography should be done as well. In addition, a special radiographic procedure may be performed by injecting contrast material into the ducts from which the discharge is coming. If the discharge is bloody, a biopsy is in order.

Skin Changes

As reported by Stenchever (1996), there are many causes for reddening of the skin. Infection is the most common cause in young women, and with this infection the skin can be very tender. Antibiotic therapy will usually resolve the infection. If not, further evaluation is needed to determine the cause.

Stenchever (1996) notes further that reddening of the end of the nipple could be Paget's carcinoma, and a biopsy is needed for diagnosis. A discoloration of the skin, called peau d'orange (which looks like orange peel), is an indication of a type of inflammatory cancer and warrants immediate evaluation.

Breast Pain

As described by Stenchever (1996), the most common type of breast pain occurs cyclically and is associated with the time before menses. No one knows exactly why this occurs, but it is suspected that it may be related to hormone imbalances. Pain can occur in one breast or both breasts.

Stenchever (1996) notes that results of some studies have revealed an association between the group of chemicals called methylxanthines (found in coffee, tea, colas, and chocolate) and premenstrual breast pain. Vitamin E, 400–600 mg taken orally each day, is often helpful in alleviating this type of cyclic pain.

Stenchever (1996) comments further that in general, breast pain does not indicate breast cancer. This is not to say that breast cancer does not exist if there is pain. The kinds of discomfort that are more often associated with breast cancer are a localized tightening or pulling sensation or a localized burning or itching.

MAMMOGRAPHY

One of the most controversial subjects in the field of women's health is the issue of mammographic screening recommendations for women age 40–49 years. Experts disagree and study results are not definitive. In addition, the consequences of frequent mammographic screening on long-term health are not known.

The Mammogram Controversy

In February 1997 *Newsweek* presented an excellent feature article, "The Mammogram War" (Begley, 1997). The controversy over whether to recommend regular mammographic screening for all premenopausal women age 40–49 years was reviewed. The article also included interviews of a number of different experts in the field of breast cancer, and stories of individual women's varied experience with how mammography affected their breast cancer diagnosis are also told. Much of the following discussion is excerpted from this article.

Results of studies have clearly established that annual mammography for women age 50 years and older decreases mortality from breast cancer up to 30%. The controversy over the benefits of mammography centers around women in the age group of 40–49 years. Analysis of the major studies of women in this age group shows a marginal benefit in decreasing the death rate from breast cancer. Many reasons for these findings have been proposed, including the following:

- Some of the older studies may be flawed because mammography was much cruder 20 years ago.

- Breast cancer in women age 40–49 years is rare (16 per 1,000 women).

- Mammography in premenopausal women is not that accurate because of the dense breast tissue of women in this age group, as compared with breast tissue in postmenopausal women. Mammograms miss as many as 25% of invasive cancers in women age 40–49 years, compared with 10% in women age 50 years and older.

- Some tumors, even if detected early, are not curable. Results of a 1996 study showed that women in their 40s had much faster growing tumors than older women. Possible explanations are higher levels of estrogens in the blood and tissues of premenopausal women that can stimulate tumor growth or genetic predisposition that becomes expressed in this age group.

In January 1997 the National Institutes of Health (NIH) convened an expert panel to determine recommendations for mammographic screening for women age 40–49 years. The American Cancer Society had already been advising women in this age group to obtain yearly mammograms, even though the body of scientific evidence had not shown a clear benefit in decreased mortality. After hearing 32 expert presentations, the panel concluded that breast cancer mortality was only marginally lower in women who received regular mammograms in their 40s than in women who did not. The newest data showed a reduction in deaths of about 17% (National Cancer Institute, 1998). The panel advised women and their physicians to make their own decision on an individual basis. A number of the panel members did not agree with the recommendations, but other respected breast specialists across the country did agree. One notable physician among those in agreement was Susan Love, coauthor of a definitive work on breast cancer, *Dr. Susan Love's Breast Book*. She was quoted in the *Newsweek* article as saying, "So it makes doctors feel somewhat impotent to say, 'We don't know,' but it's about time we started telling women the truth" (p. 56).

The National Cancer Advisory Board was convened in February to review the NIH decision (Brenner, 1997). The board's recommendations were that women between the ages of 40 and 49 years who are at an average risk for breast cancer get screening mammograms every 1–2 years (National Cancer Institute, 1998). (Women who may be at higher risk need to confer with their health care practitioners regarding screening recommendations.) The complexity and controversial nature of this issue is clearly illustrated by the fact that two different bodies of distinguished scientists examining the same body of evidence came to different conclusions.

Mammograms are an imperfect screening tool. To illustrate this, the *Newsweek* article (Begley, 1997) tells the stories of two women in their 40s. One woman's life was saved by a mammogram, results of which picked up abnormalities in time for effective treatment. The other woman had a negative mammographic finding at age 41 years. A few months later she found a lump that was cancerous. She expressed the concern, echoed by a number of health care providers and researchers, that mammograms may seem to offer women a false sense of security, giving women reason to slack off on breast self-examinations. Women need to be educated about the limitations of mammograms. A clear mammogram does not mean a woman is cancer free. For women in their 40s, because of their dense breast tissue, a tumor may not show up on the x-ray film and could still be detected through self-examination or clinical breast examination. Manual examinations pick up about 75% of tumors in women age 40–49 years, as compared with about 50% in women age 50 years and older.

The false-positive rate for mammograms is quite high, especially for women age 40–49 years. Ninety-five percent of "abnormal" mammograms did not turn out to be malignancies, according to figures reported in the *Newsweek* article (Begley, 1997). The diagnostic workup for these false-positive findings is costly in terms of its toll on the women and their families emotionally, the physical stress and risks of invasive diagnostic procedures, and the financial costs involved. But then again, these are all statistics. If you are the one for whom mammography was effective as a lifesaving tool, wouldn't you personally advise in favor of mammography? There are no easy answers.

It is important to remember that mammography is a detection tool, an imperfect one with some potential risks of its own. It offers nothing in the way of cure or prevention. It is my opinion that energy and resources need to be focused on finding the causes of breast cancer, and therefore ways to prevent this disease, as well as on the development of better screening devices and techniques that provide more accuracy than mammography now affords without radiation exposure.

Not Definitive in Diagnosis

As emphasized by Stenchever (1996), a negative finding on mammography in no way guarantees that there is no cancer. Cancers are not made of cells that are a new type of tissue in the breast. They consist of alterations of cells normally found within the breast, so cancerous cells do not stand out. Stenchever notes further that one investigator describes that looking for a cancer on the basis of an abnormal shadow in a mammogram of a dense breast is like looking for a polar bear in a snowstorm. A sizeable cancer can be present but not evident, and microscopic evaluation of the tissue is the only definitive way of determining whether cancer is present.

Stenchever (1996) notes that the earliest indicators of cancer on mammograms are tiny white dots, which are calcifications. These dense microcalcifications are found in 60%–70% of breast cancers and tend to occur within the milk ducts (Stenchever, 1996). According to the pamphlet *Breast Cancer* (American Cancer Society, 1997), calcifications can also be present in noncancerous tissue. Microcalcifications are not usually detected with ultrasound.

Several types of breast cancer are not generally detectable with an examination, but they can be seen on a mammogram. Certain rare types of cancers cannot be detected by examination or mammogram (American Cancer Society, 1997).

Risks of Radiation

According to the pamphlet *Breast Cancer* (American Cancer Society, 1997), large reductions in radiation exposure with mammography have been made in the past 20 years as more rigorous criteria have been established. Women should ensure that the facility they use for screening has been accredited by the American College of Radiology. Women can call their state or local chapter of the American Cancer Society or the

National Cancer Institute at 1-8-4-CANCER for information about accredited facilities in their area.

DeMarco (1996) notes that although the dose of radiation received with mammography through an accredited facility is generally considered safe, health care providers need to understand that this has not been proved, especially in the long term. In general, breast tissue in young women is more sensitive to radiation than is the tissue in women who are postmenopausal. Although radiation doses with mammography have been greatly reduced, the risks of radiation exposure are cumulative. In addition, no minimum dose has been proved safe.

DeMarco (1996) points out that confounding the problem is that many women have a history of exposure from past injury or disease that needs to be taken into account. Radiation may also interact with hormones or other factors. In a subset of women, there is a genetic sensitivity to radiation, and exposure can increase their risk more so than in the general population. There is no way of testing for this genetic sensitivity. These are all concerns and need to be weighed with the benefits afforded by early detection by mammography.

DeMarco (1996) comments further that there is no other part of the body in which radiation is recommended on a yearly basis for a large population of healthy individuals. If a woman starts at age 40 years with yearly mammograms, by the time she is 80 years old she will have had 40 mammograms. Many health care practitioners are concerned about the unknown risks of such exposure. This subject needs to be addressed to assure women that yearly mammography is the best way to deal with the issue of breast cancer detection.

No one can deny, however, that mammography does detect cancers that could not be detected through examination. In addition, it detects other cancers at an earlier stage than would have been discovered (or discovered later) without the use of mammography (DeMarco, 1996).

NEW TECHNIQUES FOR CANCER DETECTION

Three new techniques hold promise for early detection of breast cancer or cancer in general, as well as play a role in predicting recurrence and selecting treatments for breast cancer: thermography, digital mammography, and Oncor® INFORM® HER-2/neu gene detection system.

Thermography

The following information on thermography is gleaned from an Internet online article by Emerson (1997).

Thermography is a noninvasive test that measures infrared (or heat) patterns of the breast. A picture is taken of the breasts with the use of sophisticated infrared cameras linked with computers. Heat and blood vessel patterns are compared between right and left breasts, with any differences indicating a potential disease process or possible anatomic variation. When a thermogram reveals a positive finding, other tests such as mammography, ultrasound, and biopsy, can provide further information.

Thermography has been approved by the Food and Drug Administration (FDA), but it is not widely available. One of its best potential uses is with premenopausal and young women whose breast tissue is dense.

Thermography is a test of physiology, whereas mammography is a test of anatomy. Thermography can detect possible abnormalities long before a tumor has grown to the size where it can be detected by mammography. This technique has not been widely accepted, nor used, by the medical community as yet, but it holds great potential. The accuracy and usefulness of thermography in breast cancer detection need to be researched and tested among a wide client population. (Contact the "Breast Cancer Action," as listed in the resource guide, for more information.)

Digital Mammography

According to Cowley (1997), digital mammography is currently under development at the University of Toronto. It uses digital code to distinguish a range of subtle differences in tissue density. As with x-ray, it exploits the fact that tissues of different densities absorb different amounts of radiation. X-ray films show only gross variations; digital imaging gives much more resolution. In addition, these images can be transmitted easily between computers, enabling consultation over long distances. Large studies need to be done to show how rates of tumor detection compare with those in standard mammography.

Oncor® INFORM® HER-2/neu Gene Detection System

According to Degen and Wilkinson (1998), the Oncor® INFORM® HER-2/neu gene detection system is used to detect the HER-2/neu gene in human breast tissue, and it was recently approved for use by the FDA. It measures the number of HER-2/neu genes per cell. It is believed that this gene prompts the production of a protein that helps cancer cells reproduce.

Degen and Wilkinson (1998) note further that the test can be used to predict breast cancer recurrence, as well as to determine the types of treatments that would be most effective. (Contact the "Breast Cancer Action" for more information.)

BREAST CANCER

Breast cancer is probably every woman's worst fear. All women have one or more risk factors for breast cancer. Most of these risks are at such a low level that they do not explain the high frequency of this disease among women.

Statistics

The following statistics provide a foundation to the pervasiveness of breast cancer in women's lives and American culture (American Cancer Society, 1997):

- Excluding skin cancer, breast cancer is the most common cancer among women.

- Breast cancer is the second leading cause of cancer death in women, exceeded only by lung cancer. It is the leading cause of cancer death among women age 40–55 years.

- In 1998, estimates were that
  — 178,700 new cases of invasive breast cancer would be diagnosed among American women.
  — 43,500 women in the United States would die of breast cancer.

- Seventy-seven percent of women with new diagnoses of breast cancer each year are older than age 50 years.

- Young women age 20–29 years account for 0.3% of breast cancer.

- One in nine women will contract breast cancer in her life.

The last statistic in the previous list is somewhat misleading. Women of different ages have different risks of breast cancer. Risk increases with age and only rises greatly as a woman reaches old age.

Risk Factors

Known risk factors for breast cancer can be divided roughly into four categories: those that are related to demographics, history, or lifestyle, as well as factors classified as possible risks or that are currently considered less of a risk than some but nonetheless in the breast cancer risk equation.

1. **Demographics and history** (American Cancer Society, 1997):

   - **Age.** Age is the single most important risk factor. Seventy-seven percent of cases occur in women older than 50 years of age. However, more breast cancers are occur-

ring in young women.

   - **Sex.** Breast cancer is more prevalent in women than in men. However, men do get breast cancer.

   - **Personal history.** Women who have (or have been diagnosed with) breast cancer are at 3–4 times the risk of developing new cancer in the other breast as their counterparts who do not have breast cancer.

   - **Family history.** History of breast cancer in the family increases risk, especially if the relative has premenopausal breast cancer.

   - **Previous breast biopsy** results showing particular types of cell changes.

2. **Lifestyle** (American Cancer Society, 1997):

   - **Alcohol.** Results of some studies have shown a link between alcohol use and increased risk.

   - **Smoking.** Smoking increases risk for other forms of cancer and affects overall health.

   - **Obesity and high-fat diet.** Obesity and high-fat diet are currently under study, but preliminary indications are that they increase risk.

   - **Exposure to radiation.** Exposure to radiation is known to increase cancer risk in general.

   - **Race or culture.** White women of European extraction are at a greater risk than other women.

3. **Possible risk factors:**

   - **Hormone replacement therapy.** This is an area of intense controversy. (See chapter 13 for discussion of this issue.)

   - **Oral contraceptive use.** Study results are contradictory. However, a recent analysis, with the use of data obtained from most of the larger, well-designed studies, showed that women who are currently using oral contraceptive pills have a slightly greater risk than nonusers. Women who stopped using oral contraceptives more than 10 years ago do not seem to have increased risk (American Cancer Society, 1997).

- **Environmental exposure.** Research on environment and breast cancer is currently underway (American Cancer Society, 1997).

- **Exposure to electromagnetic fields** (DeMarco, 1996).

- **Genetics.** Some breast cancer is hereditary and linked to genetic mutations of the BRCA1 and BRCA2 genes. These genes normally produce substances protective against breast cancer (American Cancer Society, 1997).

4. **Lesser risk factors** (American Cancer Society, 1997):

   - Early menarche

   - Late menopause

   - No children or first child after age 30 years

Most currently known risk factors for breast cancer are those that are generally not under a woman's control. However, it is important to note that the great majority (75%) of women who get breast cancer have none of the known risk factors (Stenchever, 1996). This gives women hope that health-promotion measures, which have been shown to be generally preventive for other cancers, will decrease the risk for breast cancer as well (Weed, 1996).

Two factors in particular warrant close monitoring regarding a woman's risk for breast cancer:

1. History of development of breast cancer before menopause in a first-degree relative (mother, sister, or daughter) (Stenchever, 1996): In comparison with nonhereditary breast cancers, hereditary breast cancers usually occur at earlier ages. They occur most often when women

are in their 40s, but they can occur when women are in their 20s as well. They are more likely than nonhereditary breast cancers to occur in more than one location. Approximately 15% of women diagnosed with breast cancer have hereditary factors.

Recommendations for high-risk women (i.e., women with a hereditary risk of breast cancer) are as follows (Stenchever, 1996):

- Breast self-examination at age 20 years and older with annual clinical breast examination

- Clinical breast examination every 6 months in the late 20s until age 30 years; then annually

- Baseline mammogram at 25 years and every 3 years until age 30–35 years; then annually. Biopsy advised for any abnormality

- Genetic counseling

2. Biopsy results revealing a lobular carcinoma in situ (LCIS) (Stenchever, 1996): With an abnormal finding on biopsy, the woman often has what is called lobular carcinoma in situ. Sometimes called lobular neoplasia, this condition is not considered a true cancer. It is, however, a premalignant condition that puts a woman at an increased risk of developing breast cancer elsewhere in the same breast or in the opposite breast at a later time. This condition is localized to the milk-producing glands or lobules and does not invade surrounding tissue.

Women with this diagnosis should have a physical examination 2–3 times a year and a yearly mammogram.

According to Stenchever (1996), health care providers also need to be aware of the risk for breast cancer in young women, in view of both the statistics of breast cancer and the prognosis with breast cancer that occurs before menopause. Ninety percent of breast cancers in women younger than age 35 years are first detected as a palpable lump. In young women, there is often a delay in diagnosis because providers expect lumps found in young women to be benign. Premenopausal breast cancer is often more aggressive, and by the time the lump is found the cancer is often in a more advanced stage. In addition, compared with the broader population, women age 25–35 years with breast cancer are 3–4 times more likely to have a first-degree family member with breast cancer.

Types

There are many different types of breast cancer that arise in the various tissue types of the breast. It is beyond the scope of this course to discuss this in detail. Most breast cancers are a type of adenocarcinoma. This means a cancer of the glandular tissue. Four subtypes account for most breast cancers. Each is reviewed briefly next, and the information has been gleaned from the pamphlet *Breast Cancer* (American Cancer Society, 1997).

Ductal Carcinoma In Situ (DCIS)

Ductal carcinoma in situ is a noninvasive cancer of the ducts. It has not spread through the walls of the ducts into the fatty tissue. This type of cancer can rarely be detected by examination, although it can usually be seen with mammography. Nearly 100% of women diagnosed at this early stage can be cured (American Cancer Society, 1997).

Invasive or Infiltrating Ductal Carcinoma (IDC)

Invasive or infiltrating ductal carcinoma breaks through the duct wall and invades the surrounding fatty tissue where it can also metastasize to other parts of the body by way of the lymphatic or circulatory system. This type of cancer accounts for 80% of malignancies (American Cancer Society, 1997).

Infiltrating Lobular Carcinoma (ILC)

Infiltrating lobular carcinoma arises in the milk-producing glands. It has spread into the fatty tissue and can metastasize. Infiltrating lobular carcinoma accounts for 10%–15% of invasive cancers (American Cancer Society, 1997). It is often difficult to detect by examination or mammography.

Inflammatory Breast Cancer

Only 1% of all breast cancers are of the inflammatory type (American Cancer Society, 1997). It is usually aggressive and metastasizes rapidly. It often makes the skin over the breast appear inflamed—red and warm and thickened—and resembling an orange peel.

Staging

The American Joint Committee for Cancer Staging uses the TNM system of staging to determine how widespread the cancer is (American Cancer Society, 1997): "T" = tumor size, "N" = extent of spread to lymph nodes, and "M" = distant metastasis. Treatment decisions are based largely on staging. The cancer is further staged by using the following system (American Cancer Society, 1997):

Stage 0: Ductal carcinoma in situ. This is the earliest stage of diagnosis. Cancer cells are in the milk duct but have not escaped into surrounding tissue. Cure for this stage is nearly 100%. Mammograms can detect this type of cancer at this early stage. With the increased use of mammograms, this diagnosis is becoming more frequent.

Stage I: The tumor is less than 2.0 cm (about 0.75 inch) in diameter and does not appear to have spread.

Stage II: The tumor is either larger than in stage I or has spread to the lymph nodes under the arm on the same side (or both). The lymph nodes are not attached to each other, nor to the surrounding tissue.

Stage III: More advanced. The tumor is either larger than 5 cm (greater than 2 inches) in diameter or the lymph nodes are attached to one another or to the surrounding tissue (or both of these findings are present). No signs of further spread. This stage also applies to cancers of any size that have spread to the skin, chest wall, or internal mammary lymph nodes beneath the breast and inside the chest.

Stage IV: Metastases have occurred to distant organs.

Treatment

Considerable progress has been made in the treatment of breast cancer. There are many brave women and their surgeons, both male and female, to thank because they chose to go against the traditional radical mastectomy, which was the standard of care for so many years, in favor of more breast-conserving procedures.

Breast-conserving surgical procedures involve removal of the malignant tissue and a clear margin of normal tissue. This may also involve removal of lymph nodes, with the intention to preserve as much of the breast as possible. Some form of adjuvant therapy is usually recommended, depending on the individual case.

In 1990, the NIH held a conference on the treatment of early stage breast cancer (Latour, 1993). The conclusion drawn from that conference was that breast conservation for appropriate candidates should be considered equivalent in terms of survival to any other treatment. However, this was not considered a statement against mastectomy. The option of mastectomy depends on many factors, such as size of tumor in relation to breast size, extent of lymph node involvement, and other factors that need to be considered on an individual basis (Monohan, 1997). An encouraging note in the treatment equation is that the earliest forms of breast cancer are almost 100% curable.

It is beyond the scope of this course to detail the treatment options for each stage of breast cancer. Combinations of surgery, followed by radiation, chemotherapy, or hormone therapy, are advised, depending on the stage of the cancer and its characteristics.

According to the pamphlet *Breast Cancer* (American Cancer Society, 1997), it was once thought that metastases could be controlled by extensive surgery at the primary site of cancer, but it is now believed that cells may break away from the primary tumor and begin to spread through the blood stream even in the early stages of the disease. These stray cancerous cells cannot be detected by any of the diagnostic tools available, and they cause no symptoms. The goal of adjuvant therapy is to kill hidden cells, that may have gained access to other parts of the body, by using systemic therapy. Not everyone needs systemic therapy, especially if the cancer was caught at an early stage and is considered to be a slow-growing or localized type of tumor.

Adjuvant Treatment Options

Four adjuvant treatment options are currently available for women with, or at high risk for, breast cancer.

Chemotherapy. According to the pamphlet *Breast Cancer* (American Cancer Society, 1997), combinations of drugs have been shown to be more effective than single drugs. Chemotherapy is given in cycles, with rest periods in between, usually for 4–9 months. New medications are being given to reduce the nausea and vomiting traditionally associated with chemotherapy. Other side effects can include change in appetite, loss of hair, mouth or vaginal sores, suppression of the immune system leading to increased chance of infection, anemia, fatigue, menstrual cycle changes, and infertility. With the exception of infertility, most of these side effects are temporary.

High-Dose Chemotherapy. According to the article "Bone Marrow Transplants" (1997), high-dose chemotherapy is under investigation for use in women with either high risk of recurrence of breast cancer or advanced breast cancer. Before chemotherapy is begun, stem cells are removed from the patient. Stem cells are a kind of a "starter cell" from which red blood cells, white blood cells, and platelets are formed. Because high-dose chemotherapy poses a great risk in killing these cells and thus crippling the immune system, these cells are removed. They are taken from either the bone marrow or the blood, preserved, and reinfused back into the patient after chemotherapy. The bone marrow is reseeded and restores the body's immune system.

This process takes from about 10 days to 4 weeks, depending on facility protocol. The procedure is nonsurgical, does not require general anesthesia, and is usually less expensive than the traditional bone marrow transplant. The great danger to the patient occurs during the period when there is no immune defense. Life-threatening infections and bleeding are constant threats until the immune system recovers. Studies are underway to determine who would benefit most from this type of therapy ("Bone Marrow Transplants," 1997).

Radiation therapy. As described in the pamphlet *Breast Cancer* (American Cancer Society, 1997), radiation uses x-rays to kill cancerous cells locally around the affected area. It may be used preoperatively or postoperatively to reduce the size of the tumor. Lumpectomy is usually followed by radiation therapy. Common side effects include fatigue, heaviness or swelling in the breast, and "sunburn" of the affected skin.

Hormone Therapy. Hormone therapy is a form of chemotherapy in which a drug is used to reduce the effects of estrogen on breast tissue by interacting with estrogen receptor sites. This class of drugs, termed *selective estrogen receptor modulators* (SERMs), acts like estrogen in some tissues of the body, such as the uterus and bones, but blocks the effects of estrogen in other tissues such as the breast.

The earliest and most widely used SERM is tamoxifen citrate, which was approved for use by the FDA in 1978 only for treating breast cancer. However, it is available for use by any woman who wants to take it and has a physician who will prescribe it. Studies have been ongoing to evaluate the use of tamoxifen as a preventive for women who do not have and have not had, but who are considered at high risk for, breast cancer. In the June 1998 issue of *Harvard Women's Health Watch,* a report from the Breast Cancer Prevention Trial is reviewed. Results of this trial showed a clear benefit for women at high risk for breast cancer in reducing breast cancer occurrence. In women older than 50 years of age, most of whom were postmenopausal, tamoxifen reduced the risk of the development of invasive breast cancer by 51% and noninvasive breast cancer by 30%. However, it also increased the risk of the development of premalignant overgrowth of the uterine lining, endometrial cancer, and blood clots in the veins and lungs. In women younger than 50 years of age, tamoxifen treatment reduced the risk of invasive cancer by 46% and noninvasive cancer by 73%. No risk to the uterus or increase in blood clots was observed in this age group ("Tamoxifen and Beyond," 1998). In tamoxifen trials conducted in England, fatalities due to hepatitis and liver failure were reported (DeMarco, 1996). Disturbing, but non–life-threatening, side effects of tamoxifen include hot flashes, mood swings, vaginal dryness, and weight gain (American Cancer Society, 1997).

Results of recent studies of tamoxifen use in women with breast cancer showed a protective effect for the first 5 years. Receiving tamoxifen for more than 5 years did not offer women any further protection and may actually have caused more cancers by stimulating rather than blocking non-estrogen receptors in breast tissue (Love & Lindsey, 1998).

Another SERM, called raloxifene hydrochloride (Evista), has been approved recently by the FDA for prevention of bone loss. (See chapter 13 for further discussion of Evista.) It reproduces many of tamoxifen's effects without stimulating growth of the uterine lining. The National Cancer Institute is scheduling new trials to compare raloxifene and tamoxifen. The development of a whole new class of these drugs can be expected in the near future.

A word of caution. Clearly, the use of drugs such as tamoxifen and raloxifene is still in its infancy. The long-term effects of these drugs are still unknown. Results of the recent study described earlier on use of tamoxifen for more than 5 years are providing clues that duration of use may be a crucial factor in the benefit:risk ratio of use of these drugs and remind health care providers that hormonal biochemistry is extremely complex and affects numerous organs and tissues. These new drugs have multiple and as yet unknown interactions in the human body, and they may have changing effects over time. Their use needs to be considered carefully and intelligently by each woman and her health care provider. Fear of cancer is an understandable but great deterrent to full consideration of all these issues. It is incumbent on the health care provider to recognize this and assist clients to become well informed about the pros and cons of all their treatment and prevention options. (Please see the resource guide, National Cancer Institute, for more information.)

New Areas of Investigation

Three new areas of investigation hold promise in breast cancer treatment:

1. **Sentinel lymph node biopsy:** With the sentinel lymph node biopsy, a radioactive tracer is injected into the region of the tumor (American Cancer Society, 1997). The dye will be taken by the lymphatic system to a lymph node. This is called the "sentinel node," and it is the lymph node most likely to contain metastasis. If no cancer is found in this node, the patient will avoid having to undergo more extensive lymph node surgery with its accompanying side effects, such as swelling of the arm (American Cancer Society, 1997).

2. **Monoclonal antibodies:** Monoclonal antibodies can be engineered to carry drugs or radiation directly to the tumor and may offer a way to treat very small metastases (American Cancer Society, 1997).

3. **Angiogenesis:** New drugs are being evaluated that may be useful in stopping the growth of breast cancer by interfering with the growth of new blood vessels by the cancer cells (American Cancer Society, 1997).

Complementary Therapies

According to Weed (1996), holistic medicine has much to offer in the way of therapy to assist the body, mind, and spirit through the process of breast cancer treatment. The immune system can be supported and enhanced naturally through use of diet and safe herbal remedies, as well as by having the client learn practices that reduce stress and restore balance to the body. These practices include visualization, meditation, journal writing, Qi-Gong, and tai chi (oriental movement exercises). Acupuncture, Chinese medicine, and homeopathy have much to offer to relieve symptoms resulting from surgery or therapy, as well as to support the body in its healing process. (Please refer to the resource guide for more information.)

BREAST RECONSTRUCTION AFTER MASTECTOMY

The decision to have, or not to have, breast reconstruction is very personal, and it is generated by a number of factors and emotions. As Latour (1993) describes, breast reconstruction involves more surgery and the pain and dangers inherent in major surgical procedures. On the other hand, it offers the potential benefit of much less alteration in appearance and body image.

Latour (1993) notes further that there are a number of different types of procedures, and skin may be taken from several different areas of the body. More than one surgery is usually required. Reconstruction can be done immediately along with the mastectomy, or it can be done as a separate surgical procedure.

Latour (1993) also points out that there are many emotional and lifestyle factors that make this decision one to be considered thoroughly and carefully by each woman. Talking with other women who have had the procedures done can be very helpful. There are a number of organizations that can help women facing this decision contact women who have gone through the process. (Please refer to the resource guide for more information.)

PSYCHOSOCIAL ASPECTS OF BREAST DISEASE AND CANCER

Only someone who has "been there" can truly understand the full impact of a diagnosis of breast cancer. At every stage of the process, from the first finding of a lump during SBE or during a routine physical examination, life is forever changed. Every resource a woman has will be called on in various ways as she works her way through the diagnostic process, makes decisions about treatment and possible breast reconstruction, experiences the surgery and adjuvant therapies, and faces the future with all its uncertainties. Women who face breast cancer truly go through a kind of initiation. They are called on to contact a depth in themselves that they may have never reached before. And with this can come a well of strength and self-acceptance.

Health care providers can be a source of support and advocacy for women who are diagnosed with breast cancer. Women should be encouraged to take the time they need to come to clarity about their decisions. They should be encouraged as well to seek other opinions or other providers if they do not feel comfortable with recommendations. There are a number of excellent books available, written by women who have gone through this process. There are organizations nationwide that can put women in contact with each other. The Internet is also a place to find resources and contact other women. (Please refer to the resource guide for more information.)

BREAST CANCER PREVENTION

Research on the role of estrogen and other hormones, diet, and exposure to environmental carcinogens such as pesticides—and thus the elimination or modification of these factors in women's lives—provides direction for preventive measures in breast cancer. Health care providers can glean important information from the research findings, as well as call on general recommendations and evolving knowledge, in teaching clients self-prevention of breast cancer.

Likely Targets To Address

Estrogen and the Hormone Equation

According to Kradjian (1994), breast cancer may have multiple causes and may follow the classic model of tumor growth that has been defined for cancer in general. From this model it is suggested that an initial genetic change or injury to the DNA at the cellular level occurs at some point in a woman's life. This may occur years before any cancer, perhaps through an environmental exposure. At some point, factors that promote the growth of these damaged cells begin a slow process of tumor formation.

As Kradjian (1994) points out, it is not known whether estrogen and other hormonally related growth factors play an indisputable role in breast cancer growth. He notes that approximately 70% of all breast cancers have estrogen receptors. Efforts at chemoprevention, primarily by using tamoxifen, have been directed at changing the body's hormonal environment by decreasing circulating estrogens or blocking their activity.

So what is known when the issue of estrogen's influence is considered further? Kradjian (1994) emphasizes that it is known that breast cancer is largely a hormone-dependent disease. Many of the risk factors for breast cancer listed earlier have in common an increased lifetime exposure to estrogen, whether through early menarche, late menopause, or having no children, which interrupts the monthly estrogen cycle. Thus, Kradjian notes, it makes sense that anything that increases estrogen in the body would increase cancer risk, and any intervention that decreases estrogen levels would provide a protective effect.

Diet

Although findings may be conflicting as well as confirmatory, much guiding information can be obtained from the research on diet and risk or incidence of breast cancer. The following statistics and research findings from general, cross-cultural, migration, and time-trend studies are gleaned from Kradjian (1994).

General Studies. Results of animal studies have linked high levels of dietary fat with increased incidence of breast cancer. The first scientist to note this did his research more than 75 years ago at what is now the Sloan Kettering Institute. Findings from numerous studies on fat and breast cancer include the following:

- Tumor growth increases when high levels of fat are consumed.

- Both dietary fat and total caloric intake (leading to obesity) have tumor-enhancing effects.

- Obese women tend to have higher levels of estrogen than their nonobese counterparts.

- Increases in dietary fiber protect against breast cancer in animals.

- High-fat diets are almost always low in fiber. Fiber is essential for helping the body excrete excess hormones.

- Intake of dietary fat is closely related to estrogen levels in a woman's body. Increasing fat intake increases estrogen levels; decreasing, decreases estrogen levels.

- DNA repair is impaired with high-fat diets.

- Dietary fat can suppress the immune system, especially the "killer cells" whose job is to seek out and destroy malignant cells and bacteria.

- Dietary fat promotes other types of cancer, such as colon, prostate, uterine, and ovarian cancer.

- High-fat diets alter the bacteria living in the colon, which usually help to eliminate excess estrogen. More estrogen is reabsorbed back into the blood stream rather than being excreted into the stool.

- Estrogen levels in stool samples obtained from women who eat meat are lower than those for women who are vegetarian; more estrogen is reabsorbed.

- Dramatic differences in estrogen metabolism have been found between women who are vegetarians and women who eat meat. Women who are vegetarians have decreased blood levels of estrogen and increased fecal excretion of estrogen.

- Women placed on a very low-fat (10% of total calories) diet show a 50% drop in blood estrogen levels.

Cross-Cultural Studies. In comparing breast cancer rates across cultures, the findings are consistent. Those whose populations generally have high fat intake have high breast cancer rates. Those with diets low in fat have low breast cancer rates.

Migration Studies. Some of the important studies linking dietary fat intake to breast cancer have focused on large population groups over time, observing changes in breast cancer rates when populations have migrated to other countries and changed their traditional eating and lifestyle patterns.

Migration studies were done with Japanese women who traditionally have a low incidence of breast cancer and eat a low-fat, high-fiber diet. When these women migrated to the United States and began to eat a diet higher in fat with lower fiber, their breast cancer rates quickly increased to those in the United States. The rate of breast cancer of the daughters was even higher, little different from any other woman in the adopted country. Results of these migration studies clearly point to environmental rather than genetic influences.

Studies have also been done on migration and dietary patterns within countries, and similar results have been found. In women who abandon traditional diets and move to urban areas, adopting more Westernized diets, the incidence of breast cancer is increased. In every study fat intake was the key. In China, fat intake is very low, with a range of 6%–24% of calories. Even at this very low range there was still a correlation between amount of breast cancer and fat intake.

Time-Trend Studies. Time-trend studies (i.e., studies in which a specific population is monitored over time) have revealed results consistent with those from the studies outlined earlier in this section. A good example is Japan, where traditional dietary patterns have changed dramatically since World War II. The Japanese have quadrupled their fat consumption over a 30-year period. Breast cancer incidence has risen accordingly, by 58% between 1975 and 1985 alone.

Some study findings seem to contradict this link between fat intake and breast cancer. A good example is the 1987 Harvard Nurses' Health Study, results of which showed that a drop in fat intake from 44% to 32% had minimal effect. On closer scrutiny of this study, it was revealed that it does not show that fat intake is not linked to breast cancer, as some critics claimed, but that the reduction in fat was too small to have an effect. Results of other studies have shown that protective effects occur if the fat intake is reduced to 20% or less of total calories (Kradjian, 1994).

In 1988, the U.S. Surgeon General released a report on the relationship between diet and health. The conclusion was that 60% of all cancers in American women were mostly or partially attributable to diet (Kradjian, 1994).

Kradjian (1994), in his book *Save Yourself from Breast Cancer,* reminds health care providers that it can never be conclusively proven that diet causes breast cancer, just as it cannot be conclusively proven that smoking cigarettes causes lung cancer. Matters of this complexity cannot be easily demonstrated. He makes this point to emphasize that the accumulated data point to a link between dietary fat and breast cancer, and it is time to stop waiting for scientific *proof* and start acting on what is already known.

Pesticides and Other Environmental Chemicals

The following information, statistics, and research findings on pesticides and other environmental chemicals are gleaned from DeMarco (1996).

A body of evidence is accumulating that links environmental toxins with breast cancer, although studies reveal conflicting results. Results of one study showed concentrations of specific pesticides were 50%–60% higher in the fatty tissues of women with breast cancer. In Israel where levels of pesticides in dairy products were reduced substantially by outlawing the use of pesticides such as DDT, the breast cancer death rate fell dramatically by an estimated 20%. The National Institute of Environmental Health Sciences is currently funding a large study measuring blood samples obtained from 15,000 women for pesticide residues to determine whether there is a correlation between pesticide exposure and breast cancer.

Pesticides generally accumulate in fatty tissue and therefore concentrate up the food chain. Hormones and other growth-promoting substances are fed to dairy cows and animals that are products in the meat and poultry industry. Consumption of these products by a woman would expose her to those chemicals. This may be one of the reasons why high-fat diets lead to increased incidence of breast cancer.

Greenpeace published a report in November 1992, the title of which—*Breast Cancer and the Environment: The Chlorine Connection*—heralds an important and neglected area of research. The environment may prove to be a missing link in the search for the causes of breast cancer.

General Preventive Measures

Included in the list below are recommendations for reducing cancer risk in general through dietary interventions, as well as measures specifically known to decrease breast cancer risk (Love & Lindsey, 1998):

- Diet rich in cruciferous vegetables, including broccoli, cauliflower, cabbage and brussel sprouts, and sprouted broccoli seeds

- Diet primarily of fruits, vegetables, grains, and beans, rather than a meat/dairy-based diet

- Foods rich in sources of carotenes, such as dark leafy greens and orange and yellow fruits and vegetables

- Diet high in foods rich in vitamin C, such as fresh fruits and vegetables

- Foods high in vitamin E, such as sunflower seeds and olive and flax oils

- Foods containing selenium, such as garlic, onions, and mushrooms

- Sufficient exposure to sunlight for vitamin D or consumption of foods rich in vitamin D, such as sardines and tuna

- Regular exercise

- Maintenance of normal weight for height and body type

- Minimal alcohol consumption

- No cigarette smoking

- Decreased consumption of animal products, which may contain hormones

- Low-fat diet

- Diet high in fiber, which helps eliminate excess estrogen

- Support for a strong immune system by getting regular exercise and adequate sleep; managing stress levels by having leisure time, supportive friends, laughter, and fun in life

- Avoiding processed foods, which contain chemicals

- Reduced exposure to environmental chemicals and electromagnetic fields

- Drinking lots of pure water

- Eating organic food if possible; washing food thoroughly before use

Evolving Interventions: Calcium Glucarate

Calcium glucarate is a naturally occurring substance that is currently under investigation by the National Cancer Institute at Memorial Sloan Kettering Cancer Center (Heerdt, Young & Borgen, 1995). Calcium glucarate occurs naturally in fruits and vegetables, and it has been shown in animal studies to have breast cancer preventive effects with no reported toxicity or deleterious side effects. It seems to inhibit tumor development by lowering estrogen levels as well as detoxifying environmental agents that may promote breast cancer.

Calcium glucarate is currently available as a nutritional supplement. This represents a possible breakthrough in breast cancer prevention (Heerdt, Young & Borgen, 1995). (Please see the resource guide for more information.)

CONCLUSION

Breast cancer is a problem worldwide, and it has reached epidemic proportions in both developed countries and developing nations. Health care providers can encourage women to practice early detection by doing breast self-examination, getting regular clinical breast examinations, and choosing judicious use of mammography and other diagnostic techniques. Clients can be supported in making changes in dietary and exercise habits and lifestyle that can have cancer-preventive effects. Health care providers can provide informed, compassionate care for women who are diagnosed with breast cancer.

CHAPTER 12

Questions 92–97

92. Normal breast tissue

    a. is smooth.

    b. is lumpy.

    c. does not change in texture during different phases of the menstrual cycle.

    d. changes in texture only after menopause.

93. A client came to your office after discovering a breast lump. After the examination she was advised to wait until after her next period. The lump was still there, so a mammogram was ordered. The mammogram showed nothing suspicious. The health care provider should

    a. let the client know that everything is fine.

    b. schedule her for another breast check in 3 months.

    c. advise the client that further evaluation is needed, and refer her to a specialist.

    d. schedule the client for another mammogram in 3 months.

94. Ultrasound can reveal whether a breast lump is

    a. fluid filled or solid.

    b. malignant.

    c. benign.

    d. potentially malignant.

95. Breast cancer that occurs before menopause tends to be

    a. slower growing than breast cancer that occurs after menopause.

    b. more aggressive than breast cancer that occurs after menopause.

    c. easier to detect than breast cancer that occurs after menopause.

    d. diagnosed at an earlier stage than breast cancer that occurs after menopause.

96. When is the best time to do breast self-examination?

    a. After menses

    b. Before menses

    c. It does not matter when

    d. While taking a shower

97. Breast self-examination includes which of the following maneuvers?

    a. Palpating under the arms for lymph nodes

    b. Raising the arms above the head to look for dimpling

    c. Using the pads of the fingers to feel for thickening or lumps

    d. All the above

CHAPTER 13

GROWING OLDER: MENOPAUSE AND BEYOND

"The most creative force in the world is the post-menopausal woman with zest."

—*Margaret Mead*

CHAPTER OBJECTIVE

After completing this chapter, the reader will be able to discuss the special health care needs of women growing older, with particular focus on the transition of menopause. The reader will also be able to discuss health care concerns and decisions about hormone replacement therapy, heart disease and osteoporosis. This chapter will also review self-care and health promotion.

LEARNING OBJECTIVES

After studying this chapter, the reader will be able to

1. define menopause and perimenopause.

2. describe the physiologic changes occurring during menopause.

3. discuss risk factors for osteoporosis.

4. identify risk factors for heart disease.

5. discuss some of the pros and cons of hormone replacement therapy.

6. identify self-care measures for a healthy menopause.

Key Words
- ERT
- HRT
- "Natural" progesterone
- Oral micronized progesterone
- Osteoporosis
- Progestin/progestogen

INTRODUCTION

Currently, menopause is perhaps the most talked about subject in women's health. This is in sharp contrast to recent history in which the subject was somewhat taboo. Growing numbers of women are entering the perimenopausal and postmenopausal age groups. This group of women is increasingly more educated and sophisticated, and they are questioning and seeking information to make informed choices about how to pass through menopause and beyond in the healthiest way possible.

Research on the physiology of menopause is still in its infancy. If the reader looks back over the previous chapters in this course, she or he cannot help but have a profound respect and sense of wonder about the complex physiology surrounding the interplay of hormones in the female body. Minute amounts of sex hormones have an astounding array of effects on the body, including effects on brain chemistry.

Some women's organizations and health care providers are concerned that menopause is becoming "medicalized," that it is being viewed as a disease process rather than as a natural part of aging (National Women's Health Network, 1995). This view tends to guide health practitioners in seeking drug regimens to treat or prevent disease. According to Love and Lindsey (1998), some sources are concerned that current recommendations involving hormone therapy are based on a very small body of evidence, in terms of taking into account both the myriad, subtle, and pervasive effects of tiny amounts of hormones and the long-term effects on women who may live 30–50 years beyond the time when these substances might be ingested. Others believe that the benefits outweigh the risks for most women (Stenchever, 1996). Results of studies to date have shown clear benefits for use of hormones, but not without risks (Love & Lindsey, 1998). It cannot be denied that hormone replacement therapy (HRT) is an experiment that women are participating in, with some definite and substantial benefits but no known outcome (Love & Lindsey, 1998).

Love and Lindsey (1998) note that women are wise to become well educated on the subject and be partners with their health care providers in the decision-making process. Gone are the days when women blindly followed the advice of their physicians. It is important for health care providers to help demystify—demedicalize, if you will—this process of menopause. Women are fully capable of understanding the issues and the controversies involved, so that they can make fully informed choices.

WHAT IS MENOPAUSE?

In the discussion on adolescence (see chapter 4), a process was described in which a young woman's body goes through what is essentially an *activation* of childbearing potential (Lichtman & Papera, 1990). In a similar fashion, menopause is a *process* that occurs over a number of years and marks the *completion* of childbearing potential (Lichtman & Papera, 1990). The ovaries, having become depleted of most of their egg supply, become progressively less sensitive to signals from the brain that stimulate the development of the menstrual cycle and ovulation. The complex coordination and synchronization between the brain and the ovaries progressively breaks down.

As with adolescence, notes Sifton (1994), this process is not well understood. He comments that the time when this process begins to happen varies among individuals and is somewhat influenced by genetics. This period usually begins at an age in the early to mid-40s range. Menstrual periods in American women cease on average around age 50 years. By age 52 years, 80% of women will no longer be menstruating. Lichtman and Papera (1990) comment that other factors can influence the time of menopause; disease, cigarette smoking, and surgical intervention can result in an early or premature menopause.

According to Lichtman and Papera (1990), the term *menopause* is defined by the medical community as cessation of menses for 1 year or more. The time preceding menopause is termed *perimenopause* or *the climacteric,* and it is marked by changes in the regularity of the menstrual cycle until periods cease altogether. Other changes continue to occur during the postmenopausal years as the entire body adjusts to a different hormonal environment.

Crawford (1996) notes that this whole transition period represents a profound change at every level. Physiologically, hormone levels shift and change and reach new balances, and the tissues and organs whose function is influenced by these hormones also change structurally and functionally.

There are shifts at mental and emotional levels, which are not well understood. Some of these shifts are physiologic, and some involve self-perception as women transition into a new phase of life.

As described by Love and Lindsey (1998), results of cross-cultural studies have shown clearly that the menopausal experience is very much influenced by the attitudes of the culture and community in which women reside. There has been a growing movement in the United States, spearheaded by the reaching of menopausal age of the baby-boom generation, in which attitudes toward menopause and aging altogether are beginning to shift. In many traditional cultures throughout the world, menopause is a time for women to take leadership roles in the culture, a time of being honored as one of the tribal members with an accumulation of wisdom. American women are calling on this broad cultural perspective to shift self-perceptions and create a positive cultural image of women in this stage of life.

What needs to be remembered about menopause is that it is a natural, intentional process, one that cannot be stopped. However, women do have control over how they go through the process. They can ease uncomfortable symptoms and minimize risks of chronic disease. As Susan Weed states in her book *Menopausal Years: The Wise Woman Way,* "the wise woman achieves menopause, it does not overcome her" (Weed, 1992, p. xxii). Many women describe a sense of well-being, hard-won individuality, and positive attitude toward life; that is, what Margaret Mead termed "post-menopausal zest!"

According to Sifton (1994), in 1900 the average age of menopause was 46 years. The average life expectancy was 51 years, although many women lived well beyond this age. In modern times, menopause does not mark the end of life, but rather a transition into another phase with a potential lifespan of another 30–50 years. Sifton comments further that it is the task of researchers to discover how the natural process of aging interacts with the hormonal changes of menopause, as well as how diet and lifestyle influence the aging process and the menopausal transition. Love and Lindsey (1998) state that much can be learned by studying other cultures, whose levels of osteoporosis and heart disease are much lower than in the American culture and whose women transition through menopause with fewer uncomfortable symptoms.

SIGNS AND SYMPTOMS OF MENOPAUSE AND NON-PHARMACEUTIC INTERVENTIONS

There are common signs and symptoms associated with menopause. In addition to standard regimens from the medical model to ease these manifestations, many nonpharmaceutic interventions are available to women.

Changes in the Menstrual Cycle

Stenchever (1996) describes the changes in the menstrual cycle as follows.

It is rare for a woman simply to stop bleeding. More commonly, menstrual periods become progressively less regular. They may occur closer together or farther apart and be heavier or more scanty. Midcycle spotting may occur. This is largely due to lack of ovulation. Lack of ovulation interrupts the production of progesterone, which acts to stabilize the uterine lining. The uterine lining builds up under the influence of estrogen, but ovulation does not occur. Thus no progesterone is produced. The lining is often sloughed off irregularly. Without ovulation a longer than usual release of estrogen may occur, which can overstimulate the growth of the uterine lining. When bleeding does occur it may be heavier or more prolonged. The lining may grow with irregular or thickened areas and may not slough off completely or evenly, causing menses to stop and start again.

Stenchever (1996) notes further that although irregular menses is a normal part of this process, any heavy bleeding should be investigated. Uterine fibroids—a frequent cause of increased bleeding—are common in women who are perimenopausal. Cervical or uterine cancer should be ruled out as a possible cause. If heavy bleeding is an ongoing problem and cancer has been ruled out, hormonal intervention in the form of low-dose oral contraceptives, progesterone alone, or some form of HRT may be suggested. If fibroids are the cause of heavy bleeding, surgical intervention may be advised. (See chapter 11 for information on abnormal uterine bleeding.)

Greenwood (1992) comments that it is important to remember that fertility declines during this period but does not disappear until menopause is complete. Menopause is signaled by a full year without menstruation. Birth control remains an important consideration during the perimenopausal period.

Shifts in Hormone Levels

During the perimenopausal period, hormone levels can be very erratic, with highs and lows occurring without the usual synchronicity. One common hormonal pattern that is seen when ovulation becomes unpredictable is an elevated level of estrogen throughout the cycle and low levels of progesterone during the second half of the cycle, when you would expect progesterone to be at its peak. Some women develop very low levels of estrogen as well. The ovaries are shutting down and losing their ability to manufacture large amounts of sex hormones. The feedback loops between the ovaries and the hypothalamus and pituitary glands are losing their synchronized pattern. It is progesterone that undergoes the most dramatic drop during menopause because its production depends upon ovulation and the development of the corpus luteum discussed earlier. Small amounts of estrogen continue to be produced by the ovaries up to ten years after periods have ceased. The body also has other ways of producing estrogen. The fat cells convert androgens produced by the adrenal glands to estrogens. Androgens are female forms of "male-type" hormones that are produced by the ovaries and the adrenal glands. Androgens are responsible for maintenance of muscle strength and sex drive. As estrogen and progesterone levels fall, the effects of these androgens often become relatively more pronounced. For example, these hormones can produce an increase in facial hair often noticed after menopause. For some women androgen levels (including testosterone) fall as well, producing symptoms of low libido, or decrease in muscle mass with relative increase in the amount of fat tissue (Love & Lindsey, 1998).

Changes in Skin and Hair

Sifton (1994) describes the following changes in skin and hair.

Lower levels of estrogen affect many tissues. Skin and mucous membranes in various parts of the body become drier. The fatty layer beneath the skin tends to shrink, resulting in a decrease in elasticity and moisture. Skin feels rougher, and the outer skin may be looser than the deeper layers, resulting in wrinkling. The skin produces less melanin, and it can burn more easily. The increasing predominance of androgens may cause a darker, thicker, more wiry hair to appear on the pubis, underarms, chest, lower abdomen, and back, and more facial hair may appear. The hair on the head may become drier, and pubic and axillary hair may thin.

Breast Changes

As noted by Sifton (1994), glandular tissues in the breasts shrink during the process of menopause. In addition, breasts may lose their fullness, flatten, and drop. Nipples may become smaller and flatter.

Vaginal Dryness

According to Crawford (1996), vaginal changes may occur during perimenopause or not occur until 5–10 years after menopause.

Crawford (1996) notes that the mucous membranes, which have been supported by stimulation of estrogen, become thin, drier, and more fragile. The vagina loses its rough texture and dark pink coloration and becomes smooth and pale. The vagina also shortens and narrows. There may be some itching or soreness. The vagina also lubricates more slowly, and there is less cervical mucus produced. Intercourse may become painful. There is a change in the normal vaginal flora, resulting in a decrease in the normal protective mechanisms of the vagina. There may also be an increase in urinary tract infections.

The following is a list of natural remedies, as well as diet and lifestyle factors, that can improve the symptoms associated with vaginal dryness:

- **Remain sexually active.** Results of studies have shown that sexual activity increases blood flow to the vagina, increases elasticity and lubrication of vaginal tissues, and maintains muscle tone (Sifton, 1994).

- **Experience orgasm.** Findings from a study of women who were postmenopausal showed that women who had an orgasm by any means, three or more times per month, were less likely to experience vaginal atrophy than those who had intercourse less than 10 times per year (Sifton, 1994).

- **Consume phytoestrogen-containing foods and herbs** (DeMarco, 1996). (See section on phytoestrogens later in this chapter.)

- **Apply vitamin E** topically to the vagina (DeMarco, 1996).

- **Take vitamin E supplements orally.** Supplementation can have an estrogenic effect (DeMarco, 1996). (Women who have hyper-tension should not supplement the diet with vitamin E.)

- **Supplement the diet with boron.** Supplementation increases estrogen levels (DeMarco, 1996).

- **Take vitamin C and bioflavonoids;** they increase estrogen levels (DeMarco, 1996).

If natural remedies and interventions do not resolve the signs and symptoms associated with vaginal dryness, various forms of estrogen cream are available by prescription (Crawford, 1996). As emphasized in an article in the July 1998 issue of *Women's Health Advocate Newsletter* ("Estrogen, the Estrogen Decision: Are Lower Doses Good Enough?," 1998), because these creams may be absorbed into the circulatory system, the woman should discuss the pros and cons of estrogen replacement therapy (ERT) and careful dosage recommendations with her health care practitioner. In addition, with very low doses blood levels of estrogen will not increase. DeMarco (1996) reports that a new estrogen-releasing vaginal ring is being developed and tested in Europe.

Hot Flashes

According to Stenchever (1996), one of the hallmarks of menopause is hot flashes. They are the most common symptom reported by women going through menopause, being experienced in some form by 50%–75% of women. Only 10%–15% of women find them debilitating.

Love and Lindsey (1998) note that in a number of non-Westernized cultures hot flashes either do not occur or are so minimal as to be barely noticed or enjoyed. Hot flashes lead women to seek medical advice more than any other symptom of menopause (Stenchever, 1996).

Stenchever (1996) reports that the cause of hot flashes is not well understood. However, they are related to hormone shifts, which affect the temperature-regulating centers in the hypothalamus. Low levels of estrogen alone are not responsible. It is thought that the presence of estrogen, followed by its withdrawal, triggers an imbalance in the body's temperature control center, which decreases the core body temperature. The body attempts to activate heat centers to readjust the body's thermostat.

According to Stenchever (1996), risk of developing hot flashes is increased in women who

- have a
  - strong family history of osteoporosis.
  - thin (ectomorphic) body type.
  - low calcium intake.
  - history of low estrogen levels early in life because of factors such as excessive exercise.
- consume an excessive amount of alcohol.
- smoke cigarettes.
- are inactive.

Sifton (1994) reports that the experience of a hot flash is very distinct. It may begin with a feeling of pressure in the head, followed by a warm feeling rising from the chest to the neck and face. The heat for some may be a very intense, hot, burning sensation. This is followed by sweating that can be profuse. The frequency of hot flashes can vary from 1–2 per week to 1–2 per hour. Average length for each is 4 minutes. Hot flashes may be accompanied by palpitations, weakness, fatigue, faintness, or dizziness.

Sifton (1994) notes further that hot flashes in and of themselves are completely harmless. However, when they occur at night they can cause a profound disruption in sleep, which can cause or exacerbate mood swings, fatigue, and memory loss.

Sifton (1994) states that for women who experience debilitating symptoms, intervention with hormones may be appropriate and is very effective in relieving hot flashes. Other nonhormonal medications may be advised, including clonidine

hydrochloride (Catapres®), naloxone hydrochloride (Narcan®), or pentazocine hydrochloride and naloxone hydrochloride (Talwin Nx®).

For women with milder symptoms, hot flashes may be relieved by a combination of natural interventions listed below (Love & Lindsey, 1998):

- Exercise regularly. Study findings show that women who exercise are less likely to experience hot flashes than their nonexercising counterparts.
- Avoid
  - smoking. Smokers have more hot flashes than nonsmokers.
  - fatty foods, sugar, and caffeine.
- Minimize intake of
  - hot drinks and spicy foods.
  - alcohol.
- Eat plenty of "cool" foods (i.e., foods that have a cooling, refreshing effect on the body), such as cabbage, cucumbers, and pineapple.
- Keep cool; dress in layers.
- Supplement the diet with vitamin E (unless the woman has hypertension), vitamin C, and bioflavonoids, all of which have estrogenic effects in the body.
- Take
  - B complex vitamins.
  - herbs that help with hot flashes: black cohosh, hibiscus, schizandra berries, lemon balm, linden, sage, and Siberian ginseng. Add the herb motherwort if palpitations are a problem.
- Increase consumption of
  - phytoestrogen-containing foods.
  - boron-containing foods.

According to Love and Lindsey (1998), black cohosh has been studied extensively in Europe and has been found to be very effective in relieving hot flashes, vaginal dryness, and depression. It carries with it no increased risk of either breast or uterine cancer. The recommended dosage is 20 mg twice per day.

According to DeMarco (1996), boron also has been found to have an estrogenic effect, as well as to decrease calcium loss in the urine. These effects were seen with supplementation of 3 mg of boron per day. DeMarco notes further that because boron can be toxic in large amounts and not enough research has been done with this mineral, the researcher who did the boron studies suggests that women eat foods high in boron, which include non-citrus fruits (apples, grapes, pears, cherries), leafy green vegetables (spinach, parsley, cabbage, broccoli, beet greens), and nuts and legumes. This should supply 2–6 mg of boron per day. Boron should not be used for its estrogenic effect in women with a history of breast cancer.

Sexuality

As reported by Stenchever (1996), study results have shown that sexual responsiveness reaches a peak for women in their late 30s and can remain on a high plateau into the 60s. Some women have an increased sexual desire after menopause. The fear of unwanted pregnancy often frees women to be much more sexually expressive and responsive than they were in their premenopausal years.

Stenchever (1996) notes further that Masters and Johnson studied sexuality in menopausal women and found a general reduction in the four phases of the sexual response cycle with increasing years after menopause. However, they found that women who maintained regular sexual activity experienced vaginal lubrication similar to that expected in women who were premenopausal, and these women continued to be capable of full sexual response and enjoyment.

According to DeMarco (1996), many women do, however, experience changes in libido and vaginal lubrication, discomfort during intercourse,

and changes in orgasmic response during menopause. By using lubricants such as Replens® or Astroglide®, which are specifically formulated as lubricants for menopause, women may be able to have more comfortable intercourse. Slower sex with more foreplay may provide more time for vaginal lubrication. For women who experience a large drop in sex drive, the use of ERT, often in the form of a cream, is generally helpful. According to Greenwood (1992), some practitioners prescribe a small amount of 1% testosterone cream applied to the clitoris and surrounding area, which is very effective in increasing sexual desire.

Stress Incontinence

As noted by Stenchever (1996), jogging, sneezing, coughing, laughing, or emotional distress resulting in loss of a small amount of urine from the bladder opening is termed *stress incontinence*. This is a common problem for women in menopause. Loss of estrogen supply to the estrogen-dependent tissues of the genitourinary tract results in a decrease in muscle tone and control in the bladder and urethra. This is more likely to occur in women who have given birth. For most women, Kegel exercises can be very effective in improving this condition, which is usually present in a mild form. To perform Kegel exercises (National Women's Health Network, 1995),

- contract the vaginal opening as if trying to stop the flow of urine.

- hold to the count of three; relax.

- repeat these maneuvers.

- or, alternatively, contract and relax quickly 5–10 times.

- do a total of 50–100 "Kegels" per day.

Stenchever (1996) reports further that regular sexual activity also improves tone and blood flow to this area. The use of a device such as a pessary, or surgical intervention, may be needed if incontinence is severe or due to prolapse of the uterus or bladder. This is a more common problem of the older woman who is postmenopausal, especially those who have had a number of children.

Other Symptoms

There are a number of other symptoms reported by women during the menopausal transition time (DeMarco, 1996):

- More than 50% of women experience joint pain.

- Migraine headaches may be experienced for the first time or worsen.

- Dry mouth occurs in up to 20% of women who are postmenopausal.

- Bloating, indigestion, and gas may occur.

- Changes in sleep patterns are very common, with insomnia either alone or as a result of hot flashes.

- Mood swings, forgetfulness, lack of concentration, and depression may occur, and these symptoms have multiple causes. (Results of studies have shown that estrogen influences the brain neurotransmitter serotonin, which influences mood. Findings from other studies have shown improved cognitive function with estrogen use [Smith & Hughes, 1998].)

- Weight gain is experienced. (Sedentary lifestyle and dietary habits probably contribute greatly.)

- Excessive bleeding can occur as well. (See chapter 11 for discussion.)

DeMarco (1996) notes that although there is no proof that these symptoms are related specifically to menopause, they may well be. Menopause may also be one piece of a larger puzzle.

Phytoestrogens

The following information on phytoestrogens is gleaned from Love and Lindsey (1998).

Results of cross-cultural studies have clearly shown that women in many traditional cultures experience menopause very differently, both emotionally and physically. Dietary practices have been proposed as one of the primary reasons for the lack of uncomfortable symptoms reported by many of these women.

There is a growing body of research identifying what are termed *phytoestrogens.* These substances are found naturally in whole plant foods and herbs, and their effects on the body are similar to those of endogenous hormones.

Hundreds of plants and herbs contain various forms of phytoestrogens. These include (Love & Lindsey, 1998):

- legumes, including peas and soy foods. (The most well documented have been soy products, including tofu and miso. Japanese women who have a diet high in soy products report few hot flashes.)

- flaxseed and flaxseed oil.

- cashews, peanuts, and almonds.

- oats.

- corn.

- wheat.

- apples.

- sage.

- hops.

- anise and fennel.

- licorice.

- red clover. (This can be used as an herb, or sprouts can be eaten.)

- alfalfa. (This can be used as a plant or seeds can be sprouted.)

- black cohosh. (The effectiveness of this herb in decreasing menopausal symptoms has been well documented by results from Western scientific studies.)

- dong quai.

- Siberian ginseng.

- garlic.

These substances are not converted to estrogen by the body, but they seem to fit into the estrogen receptor sites and act as very weak estrogens. During menopause when estrogen levels drop, these substances can act as a supplement by providing a weak estrogenic effect, thus reducing symptoms caused by lower estrogen levels. A few plants and foods do contain actual estrogens that are very similar to the types of estrogen the human body produces. These include pomegranates, dates, apples, oats, rice and barley (in trace amounts), green beans, licorice, and hops.

Herbs are medicine and should not be used casually. The herbs discussed in this course are generally safe and well tolerated. Although side effects can occur. For example both ginseng and licorice can elevate blood pressure. It is best to use herbs under the supervision of a qualified practitioner who can evaluate the specific herbs and health concerns of each individual.

CARDIOVASCULAR DISEASE

According to Love and Lindsey (1998), some health care providers and researchers are concerned that in the minds of the general public, heart disease and osteoporosis (discussed in next section) have been linked so firmly to menopause that many believe that menopause causes these serious illnesses. Although these illnesses generally occur with advancing age, by no means do all aging women get either heart disease or osteoporosis. Although estrogen replacement has clearly been shown to have protective effects against both cardiovascular disease and osteoporosis, a lack of estrogen alone does not cause these illnesses. Estrogen replacement alone cannot provide a cure.

As reported by Sifton (1994), heart disease is the No. 1 killer of older American women. One in

9 women age 45–64 years and 1 in 3 women older than 65 years has some form of heart disease. More than 500,000 women in the United States die of cardiovascular-related disease annually, twice the number that die of cancer.

As indicated in the report *Taking Hormones and Women's Health* (National Women's Health Network, 1995), in spite of these sobering statistics results of studies have shown that cardiovascular disease has actually been on the decline in the United States for the past 30 years, with rates in women decreasing more than 50% since 1963. A large percentage of this decline has been attributed directly to improvements in personal health care habits, such as diet and exercise.

The report *Taking Hormones and Women's Health* (National Women's Health Network, 1995) notes that cardiovascular disease is a chronic, degenerative disease. The exact mechanisms are not well understood, but research findings have shown that there is a deterioration in the elasticity of arterial vessels due to a laying down of deposits containing cholesterol and other compounds. This plaque formation may be due to attempts by the body to repair damage to the lining of blood vessels. Blood flow is slowed through these narrowed areas, and clots tend to form around the deposits, occluding blood vessels even further.

Risk Factors

There are several risk factors for cardiovascular disease, including the following (Love & Lindsey, 1998):

- Age
- Early menopause
- Family history
- Elevated serum cholesterol levels
- Diabetes
- Hypertension (often related to use of alcohol, cigarettes, excessive sodium, and obesity)

- Obesity

- Other risk factors, such as high-fat diet or sedentary and stressful lifestyles

Western diets seem to play a large role in cardiovascular disease. A number of the risk factors listed above can be eliminated or greatly reduced through simple diet and lifestyle changes, such as the following (Love & Lindsey, 1998):

- Eat a high-fiber, low-fat, and vegetable-based diet.

- Include the following specific foods or food products in the diet:

  — Legumes, whole grains, and fresh fruits and vegetables

  — Fish

  — Garlic, onions, and soy products

- Reduce consumption of

  — dairy products and other animal products.

  — caffeine, sugar, white flour products, and highly processed foods.

  — alcohol. (Red wine may be beneficial in small amounts.)

- Use fats and oils sparingly. (Olive oil is the heart healthiest of oils.)

- Correct nutritional deficiencies.

- Perform light-aerobic exercise regularly.

- Practice stress-reduction measures.

- Seek psychologic support as needed.

- Include leisure and fun in life events.

- Quit smoking.

Hormones and Heart Disease

The subject of HRT and heart disease risk and incidence is extremely broad and complex. Because heart disease is not well understood, the impact of medications that have multiple and complex biochemical effects in the body will take many years of careful study to clarify. In this section

some of the key studies will be discussed. This is a field of rapid change as new studies continue to be published that underscore the complexities involved in, as well as the limitations of different types of, scientific research.

According to Love and Lindsey (1998), estrogen seems to have a protective effect on the heart through mechanisms not fully understood. One of its known effects is its capacity for improving the metabolism of fats and cholesterol. Estrogen raises the "good" high-density lipoproteins (HDLs) associated with a decreased risk of heart disease while it lowers the "bad" low-density lipoproteins (LDLs), which are associated with an increased risk of heart disease. Estrogen also has protective effects on the arterial walls, acting as an antioxidant and thus preventing the oxidation of arterial wall deposits. In addition, estrogen has a direct dilating effect on the arteries. DeMarco (1996) notes that estrogen also decreases the levels of fibrinogen in the blood, a substance involved in the mechanism of blood clotting.

The problem with ERT alone, without a form of progesterone with the therapy, is that estrogen in the doses commonly prescribed promotes an overgrowth of the lining of the uterus, which increases the risk of uterine cancer (Love & Lindsey, 1998). The term for this overgrowth is *endometrial hyperplasia.* The July 1998 issue of *Women's Health Advocate Newsletter* describes a recent study done on the effects of taking lower doses of estrogen than those commonly prescribed by medical practitioners in the United States ("Estrogen, the Estrogen Decision: Are Lower Doses Good Enough?," 1998). Results of the study showed that lower doses of estrogen in the form of esterified estrogens (Estratab®) (0.3 mg) had a number of positive effects over the 2-year period of the study; that is,

- an increase in bone mineral density at the hip and spine, as well as in HDL levels.

- a decrease in LDL levels, as well as in the incidence of hot flashes and night sweats.

These positive effects occurred without inducing overgrowth of the uterine lining. The effects of estrogen on breast cancer risk remain unanswered as the study was conducted for only a 2-year period. Researchers caution that because of the short term nature of the study, longer term effects, both positive and negative, are unknown ("Estrogen, the Estrogen Decision: Are Lower Doses Good Enough?," 1998).

Currently, most health care providers who prescribe hormones are using a combination of estrogen and some form of progesterone, usually a synthetic progestin, for women with intact uteruses. Researchers have turned to determining the cardiovascular effects of the estrogen-progestin combinations. The PEPI study (Postmenopausal Estrogen/Progestin Interventions Trial), completed in 1994, was a 3-year study involving 875 healthy postmenopausal women (National Women's Health Network, 1995). This large study tested the effects of several combinations of estrogen and progestins. Also studied was a combination formula of estrogen with oral micronized progesterone. This is a form of progesterone used and studied more extensively in Europe. Its chemical structure is identical to the progesterone manufactured by the body, unlike the more commonly used progestins. Oral micronized progesterone has been found to have fewer negative side effects than the synthetic progestins (DeMarco, 1996). Results of the PEPI study showed that all combinations of estrogen and progestin/progesterone produced improvements in the HDL levels, as compared with findings with the placebo. Estrogen alone produced the best effect, but it caused endometrial hyperplasia. Estrogen used in combination with oral micronized progesterone produced a similar beneficial result as estrogen alone without the dangers of endometrial overgrowth. Estrogen plus the synthetic progestin had a lesser positive effect, indicating that the addition of a progestin to the estrogen regimen substantially interfered with the beneficial effect of estrogen used alone (National Women's Health Network, 1995).

The question remains as to whether increasing HDL levels in a woman ultimately reduces the chance of development of or death due to heart disease in that woman. Investigators with the Women's Health Initiative, a large clinical trial currently underway, hope to clarify this issue. This study will not be completed until the year 2007 (Love & Lindsey, 1998).

Results of a recent study reported in the August 19, 1998, issue of the *Journal of the American Medical Association* illustrate clearly just how complex and multifaceted this consideration of hormones and heart disease truly is. The study involved women with existing coronary heart disease, and the effects of HRT on further incidence of adverse cardiovascular events were evaluated. Results of the study revealed that a combination of estrogen plus progestin did not reduce the overall rate of coronary heart disease events in these postmenopausal women with established coronary disease during the first year of the study. Hormone replacement therapy increased the rate of thromboembolic events (blood clots), which could have accounted for this lack of positive effect as this would have a more immediate effect on cardiovascular disease than favorable changes in HDL levels. Improvement was found in adverse coronary events after several years of therapy (Hulley et al., 1998). The study raises a number of important questions about short- and long-term hormone effects, as well as questions about how these data might be applied to healthy women who are receiving hormones as preventive therapy.

To complicate the picture further, human behavior also influences the outcome of studies, making it difficult to reach clear conclusions.

Women who choose to take hormones tend to be healthier and more compliant with medication and health regimens, as well as have a more favorable coronary heart disease profile than women who do not (National Women's Health Network, 1995). More carefully designed, long-term research needs to be conducted to clarify these complex interrelationships.

Nonhormonal Drug Therapy for Heart Disease Prevention

There are a number of cholesterol-lowering medications on the market. They act by blocking either cholesterol absorption or the body's system for manufacturing cholesterol (Love & Lindsey, 1998):

- Cholestyramine (Questran®) and colestipol hydrochloride (Colestid®) inhibit fat absorption. These drugs decrease LDL levels and slightly increase HDL levels.

- Niacin supplementation has been proven to be effective in reducing LDL levels.

- Hydroxymethylglutaryl-coenzyme A reductase inhibitors are the newest class of cholesterol-lowering drugs, which act to prevent the body's manufacture of cholesterol. Results of studies have shown decreases in LDL levels, as well as a decrease in the rate of heart attacks.

- Gemfibrozil (Lopid®) is a recently developed drug that decreases high triglyceride levels and increases HDL levels.

- Aspirin does not lower cholesterol per se, but it prevents heart attacks by decreasing the blood's ability to clot. Even though aspirin is an over-the-counter medication, it should always be taken under the supervision of a physician or practitioner when used for this purpose, because it can have serious side effects with long-term use.

OSTEOPOROSIS

As referred to briefly in the section on cardiovascular disease, osteoporosis—like cardiovascular disease—is not caused or brought on by menopause. Like cardiovascular disease, osteoporosis can occur with advancing age, and estrogen therapy seems to have a protective influence on both osteoporosis and cardiovascular disease. However, women are not "doomed" to contract osteoporosis in association with menopause. Osteoporosis should be considered as a singular condition, one that is indeed seen in women during and after menopause, and a process to be viewed across the lifetime of a female, particularly from a preventive standpoint.

What Is Osteoporosis?

Osteoporosis is defined as thin or porous bone (Gaby, 1994). There are three major types of fractures that occur as a result of osteoporosis (Gaby, 1994):

1. **Spontaneous vertebral crush fracture:** With this type of fracture the vertebrae become so weak that one vertebra collapses under minimal stress of lifting or even because of the body's weight (see *Figure 13-1*). This causes a loss of height and kyphosis or Dowager's hump, the curvature of the upper back found in some older people (see *Figure 13-2*).

2. **Colles' fracture:** Colles' fracture occurs when a person breaks a fall by landing on a hand, causing fracture of the radius.

3. **Osteoporotic hip fracture:** The hip fracture related to osteoporotic processes is the most severe of these three types of fractures.

Tooth loss and periodontal disease are other aspects of osteoporosis (Gaby, 1994).

According to DeMarco (1996), in the United States approximately 25 million people are affected by osteoporosis. In addition, at least 1.2 million women suffer fractures every year as a result of

FIGURE 13-1
Hidden Fractures Plague One Woman in Three

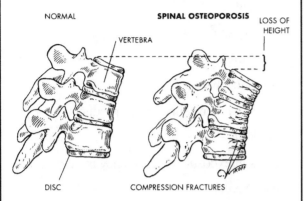

A persistent low backache, or sudden localized pain, could be a warning sign of compression fractures in the vertebrae of the spine. But for many, these breaks cause little pain, and may go undetected for years. For some, the only tip-off is a noticeable loss of height, which can reach as much as 8 inches.

Source: Sifton, D. W. (Ed.). (1994). *The PDR family guide to women's health and prescription drugs.* Montvale, NJ: Medical Economics Data Production Company.

FIGURE 13-2
No Need for "Dowager's Hump"

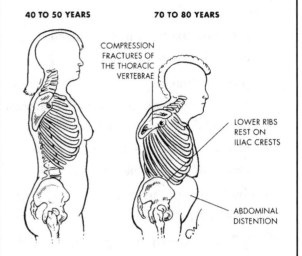

This unbecoming distortion of the spine is a direct result of osteoporosis and the spinal fractures that accompany it. Take measures to prevent osteoporosis now and you'll avoid this development in your later years.

Source: Sifton, D. W. (Ed.). (1994). *The PDR family guide to women's health and prescription drugs.* Montvale, NJ: Medical Economics Data Production Company.

osteoporosis. This usually occurs in women who are postmenopausal and in their 70s and beyond. DeMarco notes further that about 25% of White women who are postmenopausal have this disease. As many as 20% of those who suffer hip fractures die within 1 year, usually resulting from complications. Up to 50% of those with hip fractures end up in nursing homes.

What Causes Osteoporosis?

As reported by Gaby (1994), the possibility that osteoporosis is largely a disease of modern civilization is supported by results from cross-cultural studies. Those findings indicate that osteoporosis is more prevalent in modern societies than in developing countries.

Sifton (1994) notes that peak bone mass occurs around age 35 years in women, after which it begins a slow decline until menopause. At this time there is an acceleration in bone loss for a period of 8–10 years, after which the rate slows again. When estrogen is no longer abundant, bones dissolve more rapidly than they recalcify.

Gaby (1994) comments that other causes of osteoporosis include endocrine diseases, such as diabetes, overactive thyroid, and hyperparathyroidism; rheumatoid arthritis; and chronic lung disease. Gaby notes further that certain prescription drugs, including corticosteroids, anticoagulants, and some diuretics, as well as some over-the-counter aluminum-containing antacids, also contribute to bone loss.

Risk Factors

There are several risk factors for osteoporosis. Genetic and medical factors include the following (Love & Lindsey, 1998):

- Race. White women are at the highest risk, followed by Asian women; Black and Latina women have a lower risk.

- History of
  - previous fractures that occurred without any major trauma
  - poor absorption of calcium and other minerals or nutrients due to celiac disease; chronic diarrhea; low stomach acid (common in older people); surgical removal of part of stomach or intestines

- Family history of female osteoporosis or fractures (or both)

- Body build. Women who are small and slim and have small muscle mass are at more risk than women with other body builds.

- Early menopause (before age 40 years)

- Amenorrhea

- Never having gone through a pregnancy

- Anorexia

- Diabetes

- Liver disease

- Kidney disease with dialysis

- Lactose intolerance. Present in 60% of women with osteoporosis and in only 15% of the general population.

- Daily use of thyroid medication in amounts greater than 2 grains

- Use of
  - phenytoin sodium (Dilantin®). Dilantin interferes with the body's ability to absorb calcium.
  - aluminum-containing antacids
  - steroid medications

Risk factors related to lifestyle include the following (Love & Lindsey, 1998):

- Smoking

- Alcohol use

- Diet low in calcium

- Diet high in
  - salt
  - protein
  - caffeine
  - phosphates
  - sugar and refined flour products

- Lack of
  - sun exposure or deficiency in vitamin D
  - exercise

Hormones and Osteoporosis

According to Gaby (1994), estrogen is not the only hormone that has an important influence on the health of bone. Two other hormones produced by the ovary, progesterone and dehydroepiandrosterone (DHEA), influence bone metabolism as well. Testosterone (one of the male hormones also produced by women) may also play a role in bone health. In addition, Gaby notes that there is evidence that environmental pollution with heavy metals—such as aluminum, cadmium, lead, and tin—as well as from acid rain, may contribute to bone deterioration.

Physiology of Bone

The following discussion on the physiology of bone, including pertinent statistics and research findings on the topic, is gleaned from Gaby (1994).

Bone is a living tissue. It is involved constantly in a wide range of biochemical processes, which result in the constant breakdown and reformation of new bone. This process of remodeling replaces weakened areas with new, well-formed tissue.

Bone is composed of two types of bone cells and an intercellular matrix.

Osteoblasts: Osteoblasts are bone cells involved in the laying down of new bone.

Osteoclasts: Osteoclasts are bone cells involved in the breakdown or resorption of old or damaged bone tissue.

Intercellular matrix: The intercellular matrix is composed of organic compounds such as collagen and other proteins and inorganic components responsible for bone rigidity. Crystals are formed by minerals, including calcium phosphate, calcium carbonate, a small amount of magnesium, fluoride, and sulfate, as well as by other trace minerals. These crystalline structures are called hydroxyapatites.

Strength of bone is determined by not only the bone mass, but the integrity of the protein and crystal matrix. Another factor in bone strength is the efficiency of bone repair in response to mild trauma, which produces microfractures. Remodeling tends to occur along lines of stress, increasing the strength in those areas.

Health care providers are commonly taught that calcium is the major determinant of bone health. The information described above provides a broader picture of bone health beyond simply only how much calcium is present in the bone and body. Bone health and fracture prevention also involve

1. preventing loss of calcium and other minerals from bone.

2. maintaining soft tissue components around bone.

3. promoting efficiency of bone repair.

Measuring Bone Density

According to Sifton (1994), ordinary x-ray films do not detect osteoporosis until at least 30% of bone is already lost. A variety of x-ray and other techniques have been developed in recent years to measure bone density, and six of these are described below. They help identify women who are losing bone most rapidly and may be at risk for fractures. Risk is determined by comparing the findings with normal bone mass at age 35 years.

1. **Dual-energy x-ray absorptiometry (DEXA or DXA) or dual-photon absorptiometry (DPA):** The DEXA (or DXA) and DPA measure bone density in the vertebrae of the lower back and hip (Sifton, 1994). These tests are the most popular and accurate x-ray techniques used to measure bone density. They have the lowest dose of x-ray exposure of all currently used tests.

2. **Single photon absorptiometry (SPA):** The SPA measures bone density in the arm and heel. It is less expensive than, but not as helpful in predicting vertebrae or hip fractures as, other techniques (Sifton, 1994).

3. **Peripheral dual-energy x-ray absorptiometry (pDEXA or pDXA):** The pDEXA (or pDXA) measures bone density of the forearm. This test is inexpensive compared with the cost for the DEXA. Radiation exposure is minimal. (Contact the Foundation for Osteoporosis Research and Education [FORE] in the resource guide for more information.)

4. **Computed tomographic (CT) scan:** The CT scan surveys the same areas as those scanned with the absorptiometers described above, but a different technique is applied. This test uses much more radiation than the DEXA (or DXA) or DPA.

5. **Ultrasound:** Ultrasound of the heel is currently being offered as a bone density screening tool. No radiation is involved.

6. **Biochemical tests:** Measurements of levels of calcium and other products of bone breakdown in the urine are beginning to be used to evaluate rate of bone loss and response to treatment. The value of these studies awaits longer use in predicting osteoporosis and fracture rates (DeMarco, 1996).

Having a woman undergo a baseline test at the onset of menopause and again a year later may identify whether she tends to lose bone rapidly

(DeMarco, 1996). This can be used in making decisions about whether to use hormone therapy.

Diet and Bone Health

Although it is impossible to determine the precise effect of diet on bone health, there is at least circumstantial evidence that the standard American diet promotes the development of osteoporosis. Consider the following five diet elements:

1. **Sugar:** According to Gaby (1994), the average American ingests 139 pounds of refined sugar each year. He notes that results of some studies have shown that sugar intake was associated with large increases in calcium excretion in the urine. Because 99% of the body's calcium is stored in bone and the blood maintains a very narrow concentration range of calcium, when the body loses calcium it is likely to be from bone.

2. **Refined grains:** The nutrient-rich portions of grains have been removed through refinement, including vitamin B complex, calcium, magnesium, and zinc.

3. **Caffeine:** Caffeine in coffee, tea, and soft drinks, as well as similar substances in chocolate and some drugs, causes calcium to be excreted in the urine (Stenchever, 1996).

4. **Alcohol:** Excessive alcohol intake has been associated with increased osteoporosis risk (Stenchever, 1996).

5. **Protein, phosphorus, and sodium:** DeMarco (1996) notes that the typical American diet contains excessive amounts of protein, phosphorus, and sodium. Calcium is mobilized to neutralize the acidic byproducts and then excreted in the urine, causing loss of calcium from the body. Phosphorus is found in many soft drinks, and excess protein results from the high consumption of meat and dairy products in the American diet.

Gaby (1994) comments that osteoporosis prevention is another example of the benefits of a diet that is composed primarily of plant-based, unprocessed whole foods. Examples include legumes, fresh fruits and vegetables, whole grains, nuts, and seeds. These foods provide a rich supply of nutrients in the right proportions to be absorbed and used.

Nutrients Important in Bone Health

Gaby (1994) notes that there is an increasing body of research whose findings support the idea that a number of vitamins and minerals besides the well-known calcium play an important role in maintaining bone mass and preventing osteoporosis. Consider the following nine:

1. **Vitamin K:** According to Gaby (1994), vitamin K is also involved in bone metabolism. Its job is to attract calcium into the matrix to form bone—the process of bone mineralization and fracture healing. Vitamin K is made by normal intestinal bacteria, which are destroyed with antibiotic therapy. It is found in dark green leafy vegetables.

2. **Manganese:** Gaby (1994) notes that the highest concentration of manganese is found in bones and endocrine glands. He comments further that study findings show that manganese promotes calcification, and deficiencies in manganese levels have been found in people with osteoporosis. Sources of manganese include whole grains, nuts, seeds, leafy vegetables, and meat.

3. **Magnesium:** Gaby (1994) describes magnesium as an essential mineral involved in more than 50 different reactions in the body. As much as 50% of magnesium in the body is found in bone. Magnesium helps the body use calcium and vitamin D. Gaby reports further that magnesium deficiency is associated with abnormal formation of bone, resulting in decreased bone strength. Stress causes an

increase in magnesium excretion. Magnesium is found in whole grains, nuts, seeds, and green vegetables. Eighty percent of the magnesium is lost from white flour that is milled (Gaby, 1994).

4. **Boron:** According to DeMarco (1996), there is evidence that boron may play a role in bone health and hormone balance. Results of one study showed that boron supplementation decreased urinary calcium and magnesium excretion and increased serum estrogen levels to amounts equivalent to those given in HRT. Three milligrams of boron were used in the study. Boron supplementation also increased serum testosterone levels and may also enhance the conversion of vitamin D to its biologically active form. DeMarco reports that sources of boron include non-citrus fruits (apples, grapes, pears, cherries), leafy greens (spinach, parsley, cabbage, broccoli), nuts, and legumes. A diet high in these foods will provide a safe boron intake of 2–6 mg per day.

5. **Vitamin B^6:** Vitamin B^6 seems to be involved in bone matrix formation (Gaby, 1994). Sources of vitamin B^6 include whole grains, fish, chicken, nuts, watermelon, and tomatoes (Gaby, 1994).

6. **Zinc:** Study results show that zinc is essential for normal bone formation, enhancing the action of vitamin D (Gaby, 1994). In addition, it is required for normal DNA and protein synthesis in osteoblasts, osteoclasts, and bone matrix (Gaby, 1994).

7. **Vitamin C:** It is known, from the days of scurvy, that vitamin C is necessary for normal bone formation. It promotes the formation and cross-linking of some of the structural proteins found in bone (Gaby, 1994).

8. **Vitamin D:** Calcium metabolism and absorption depend on the presence of vitamin D. Exposing the skin to ultraviolet rays from the sun causes the cholesterol beneath the skin's surface to be converted to vitamin D, which is then stored in the liver until needed. Vitamin D increases the absorption of calcium by the intestines and promotes calcium uptake into the bone (Gaby, 1994).

With aging there is a decrease in synthesis of vitamin D by the skin. This problem is exacerbated by the common tendency with increasing age for people to decrease their exposure to sun (Stenchever, 1996). Sun exposure of as little as 10–15 minutes per day can have a positive impact on bone health by improving calcium absorption and use ("Vitamin D, Sunlight Redeemed? Reducing Osteoporosis and Cancer Risk," 1998).

Dietary sources of vitamin D include fish, eggs, liver, and dairy products (Gaby, 1994). The National Academy of Sciences (NAS) gives the following recommendations for vitamin D supplementation (Liebman, 1998b):

- Age 50 years or younger: 200 IU/day

- Age 51–70 years: 400 IU/day

- Older than 70 years: 600 IU/day

- Intake not to exceed 2,000 IU/day

9. **Calcium:** Calcium deficiency is only one of the factors predisposing toward osteoporosis in women, and not everyone with osteoporosis is deficient in calcium (Gaby, 1994). Calcium balance and metabolism in the body are complex and involve a number of factors, including ingestion, absorption, use, and excretion. In addition, calcium balance is modulated by hormone systems (Gaby, 1994). Adequate calcium intake for osteoporosis prevention should begin early in life when bone mass is reaching its peak. This occurs in the late teens to early 20s (Liebman, 1998a).

In August 1997, the NAS increased the recommended doses of calcium in response to concerns that most Americans are not getting enough calcium to prevent osteoporosis in the later years ("Are You Getting Enough Calcium?," 1998). The NAS made specific recommendations for each age group as follows:

- Age 9–18 years: 1,300 mg/day

- Age 19–50 years: 1,000 mg/day

- Age 51 years and older: 1,200 mg/day

The NAS also issued advice on maximum daily levels of intake at 2,500 mg/day. Risks of exceeding this limit include potential for calcium deposits in soft tissues, such as the kidneys and arteries, and impaired absorption of other vital minerals, such as iron, zinc, and manganese (Liebman, 1998b).

In considering calcium sources in the diet, most people are aware that dairy products are high in calcium, but many do not realize that the animal protein in these products can actually interfere with the body's ability to absorb the calcium. Other substances that can inhibit calcium absorption include those found in wheat bran, raw spinach, salt, caffeine, alcohol and tobacco, and fructose (found in many soft drinks) ("Are You Getting Enough Calcium?," 1998). Good sources of calcium include sardines, canned salmon, tofu, collard greens, broccoli, sesame seeds, tahini, and molasses. Soy milk and orange juice are now available with extra calcium added ("Are You Getting Enough Calcium?," 1998).

Absorption of calcium depends on adequate acidity in the stomach. Low stomach acid is a common problem and becomes more prevalent with increasing age. Suggestions for improving gastric acidity and thereby calcium absorption include the following (DeMarco, 1996):

- Eat slowly and chew well.

- Limit fluid intake with meals.

- Supplement dietary intake with

  — hydrochloric acid capsules (under the supervision of a health care provider).

  — digestive enzymes.

- Drink the juice of half a lemon in water or a teaspoon of apple cider vinegar in a glass of warm water 20 minutes before meals.

In considering among available calcium supplements, Sifton (1994) notes that the most absorbable forms of calcium on the market are calcium citrate, calcium citrate-maleate, and calcium aspartate. However, these forms tend to be more expensive than the more common calcium carbonate. Calcium carbonate is adequately absorbed by most people unless there is a problem with insufficient stomach acid, and it is affordable for most people as well ("Are You Getting Enough Calcium?," 1998). Dolomite or bone meal–based products should be avoided because they may contain lead and other toxic heavy metals ("Are You Getting Enough Calcium?," 1998). Antacids are not the best sources of calcium as they can cause other problems, including kidney stones, and aggravate other medical conditions. Some contain aluminum, which can cause the body to lose calcium (Sifton, 1994). If problems with constipation occur, a combined calcium-magnesium supplement should be taken. For best use, supplements should be taken in divided doses of no more than 500 mg of calcium with each meal (Sifton, 1994).

Controversy exists as to how effective calcium supplementation is in preventing osteoporosis (Stenchever, 1996). Results of some studies have shown that during the 5 years after menopause—when there is a phase of rapid bone loss of 1%–3% per year—bone loss did not respond to calcium supplementation. However, in the next 5-year period, calcium did help prevent further bone loss in women whose diets had been low in calcium (Stenchever, 1996). Findings in other studies have revealed that estrogen combined with calcium is more effective than either alone (Stenchever, 1996).

Exercise is also an important partner in bone health. (See discussion on this factor and osteoporosis next.) Results of recent studies show that exercise makes bones stronger only if calcium intake is greater than 1,000 mg per day. In addition, calcium intake made no difference unless the participants were moderately active ("Are You Getting Enough Calcium?," 1998). This is another arena in which more research needs to be done to clarify these complex interrelationships.

Exercise and Osteoporosis

Love and Lindsey (1998) have reported on some interesting research with exercise and osteoporosis. They note that results of studies of astronauts during their time in space have revealed accelerated rates of bone loss. Immobilization and bedrest have been found to increase bone loss. Findings from a number of studies have shown that bone mass is directly related to the amount of weight-bearing physical exercise an individual does. It has also been clearly demonstrated that women who engage in exercise programs can help prevent postmenopausal bone loss. The bone-building effect of exercise is due mainly to the repetitive physical stress applied to the bone. With weight-bearing exercise, pressure is placed on the bone either by the weight of the body or the force of muscular contraction. Examples of such exercise include running, walking, jumping on a trampoline, tennis, and weight lifting. An effective program involves regular exercise for 30 minutes, 3–4 times a week.

Drugs for Osteoporosis Prevention and Treatment

Estrogen

Results of studies have clearly shown that estrogen replacement slows bone loss by inhibiting the breakdown or resorption of bone (Stenchever, 1996) but does not build bone (Gaby, 1994). There is a lot of controversy about when to begin and how long to take estrogen for best effect. Study findings have shown that when estrogen is discontinued, accelerated bone loss resumes (Love & Lindsey, 1998). Love and Lindsey (1998) note that findings from a recent study of women age 60–98 years revealed that women who were currently receiving estrogen had the highest bone mineral density, but there was no significant difference between women who started receiving estrogen at menopause (receiving it for 20 years) and those who started receiving it after age 60 years (receiving estrogen for 9 years). In addition, Love and Lindsey note, past estrogen use, once discontinued, has little long-term effect on bone mass. Results of other studies, however, have shown that estrogen's protective effects did continue on after the hormone was stopped (Love & Lindsey, 1998). So once again, clarity on this subject awaits more long-term research.

Progesterone

Results of a small study with the use of progesterone showed that it binds to the osteoblasts and may stimulate bone formation (DeMarco, 1996). More research needs to be done to determine whether this effect can be repeated in long-term larger scale studies.

Calcitonin

Calcitonin is a synthetic version of a hormone secreted from the cells of the thyroid gland. It inhibits bone breakdown, as does estrogen. Calcitonin has only been tested in women who already have osteoporosis. It has been found to increase bone density by 5% when taken with calcium. Women (in the study) given only calcium had an increase in bone density of 2%. Long-term effectiveness has not been determined (Love & Lindsey, 1998). Calcitonin is expensive and has side effects, including facial flushing and nausea.

Calcitonin is available by injection or nasal spray. The nasal spray can be taken any time of the day. Nasal irritation is a potential side effect with the nasal spray. No known drug interactions have been found with calcitonin.

Bisphosphonates

Bisphosphonates are synthetic forms of a class of compounds found in the body. These compounds bind to the crystals in the bone matrix and inhibit bone resorption. Alendronate sodium (Fosamax®) and etidronate disodium (Didronel®) are two examples, and several other formulations are currently in development as well (Love & Lindsey, 1998):

1. **Fosamax:** Fosamax was approved in April 1997 for osteoporosis prevention on the basis of findings from two clinical trials, which are still ongoing. Study results showed reduction in hip fracture of 51% and wrist fracture of 44% with Fosamax therapy. In addition, study results have shown an increase in bone density. Safety with the use of Fosamax for more than 4 years has not been determined. Studies are ongoing (Love & Lindsey, 1998).

   Fosamax needs to be taken with water and in the morning, 30 minutes before food or other pills to prevent gastrointestinal problems (Love & Lindsey, 1998).

2. **Didronel:** Didronel was the first oral bisphosphonate available for use. It has been approved by the Food and Drug Administration (FDA) for uses other than osteoporosis. Although it has never been approved specifically for treatment or prevention of osteoporosis, it has been used for more than 7 years in the United States. In addition, it has been approved for this use in 17 other countries. Currently its use is recom-

mended if Fosamax cannot be tolerated (Love & Lindsey, 1998).

Calcitriol

Calcitriol® is a prescription drug that is the active form of vitamin D (which the body usually makes on its own). Overdoses can cause calcium-containing kidney stones, so dosage needs to be monitored carefully (DeMarco, 1996).

Fluoride

As Gaby (1994) notes, fluoride stimulates bone formation. He comments that use of fluoride is controversial because results of some studies indicate the quality of the new growth induced may not be high. Low doses of fluoride stimulate bone formation, but high doses can be toxic.

A new slow-release formulation of fluoride is available that is showing more effectiveness in decreasing fracture rates (Love & Lindsey, 1998). Ipriflavone, a new drug made from soybeans, has been approved in Italy and Japan for treatment of osteoporosis. Results of preliminary studies show that it may act to build bone. Side effects are minimal. More studies need to be done (Love & Lindsey, 1998).

HORMONE REPLACEMENT THERAPY: PROS AND CONS

The pros and cons associated with HRT are many. A look at the historical use of, current guidelines for, and risks of certain diseases with HRT can help women and their health care providers begin to sort through multiple data from multiple sources. The standard concerns with every drug therapy (e.g., contraindications and side effects) need to be addressed for HRT. New products are becoming available and deserve review in light of the continuum of controversy and confirmation centering around HRT.

An Historical Perspective

The National Women's Health Network (1995) has provided the following historical perspective on HRT.

The widespread use of prescribing estrogen began in the 1960s. It was touted as a wonder drug that allowed women to age more slowly. By 1975 conjugated estrogens (Premarin®), a popular form of estrogen, was one of the top most prescribed drugs in the United States. (Premarin is derived from the urine of pregnant mares. Animal rights activists have promoted awareness of the great cruelty to these animals and their offspring that is involved in the industry of producing Premarin.)

In 1975 two studies were published, results of which showed an increase in the rate of uterine cancer of 2–8 times for women receiving estrogen replacement. The risk is linked to dosage and amount of time estrogen is taken. This became a very political issue as women's organizations expressed concern that women were not given the information to be well informed of these risks. As this information became more widespread, use of estrogen in the United States declined. More studies were done, this time by using combinations of estrogen and a progestin (a synthetic form of progesterone). Results of studies with the use of this combination showed that the combination protected against precancerous changes of the uterine lining. On the basis of this information, a shift to prescribing combinations of estrogen and a progestin occurred.

By the late 1980s, results of several studies had shown that women who receive estrogen are less likely to have heart attacks than those who do not receive estrogen. Although the FDA refused to grant approval to the manufacturer for prescribing estrogen to healthy women as a heart disease preventive, many clinicians were recommending estrogen for this purpose. Without long-term data, the combination of estrogen and a progestin began

to be prescribed for this same purpose, even though the combination had not been in use long enough to evaluate its effect on heart disease. The PEPI study (mentioned briefly earlier in the chapter) was published in 1995. Its results showed that the most commonly used progestin, medroxyprogesterone acetate (Provera®), greatly interfered with the positive effect of estrogen alone on HDL levels. Natural progesterone (i.e., oral micronized progesterone), also used in the study, did not negate the positive effects of estrogen on HDL levels. A large study that is currently underway, The Women's Health Initiative, will evaluate the safety and effectiveness of estrogen, plus a estrogen/progestin combination given to healthy women. The study involves 25,000 women and extends for a 9-year period. Results will be available in the year 2007.

Current Guidelines

The National Women's Health Network (1995) notes in its booklet, *Taking Hormones and Women's Health: Choices, Risks, and Benefits,* that the decision about whether a woman should receive some form of hormone therapy is fraught with controversy and confusion. Physicians disagree on who should receive hormones, how long hormones should be taken, and what types and dosages of hormones should be used. According to the National Women's Health Network booklet, this is the first time in the history of medicine that a powerful drug, whose long-term effects are unknown, has been advised for large numbers of a healthy population for long-term use as a prevention for illness that large numbers would never experience without the intervention. At the same time, osteoporosis and heart disease are serious and potentially life-threatening illnesses that need to be addressed, and study results clearly have shown that hormone therapy lowers the risk of both these diseases (Stenchever, 1996).

The National Women's Health Network (1995) booklet states further that "menopause has become medicalized" (p. 13) and voices an objection to the commonly held view that normal menopause is "a deficiency disease" (p. 9), rather than a natural process. The Network goes on to take the position that "giving hormones to our entire population of midlife and older women to prevent bone loss and heart disease is the wrong way to approach these important problems. [It] take[s] the position that it is poor public health practice to attempt to prevent chronic disease conditions by using drugs of unknown safety and effectiveness on an entire population when lifestyle measures or other therapies may be more than adequate for many women" (p. 9).

Other researchers and clinicians believe that long-term therapy with hormones has benefits that far outweigh the risks involved for most women (Stenchever, 1996).

The following issues need to be considered in deciding whether hormones are an appropriate treatment (National Women's Health Network, 1995):

- The severity of menopausal symptoms, such as hot flashes and problems with the genitourinary tract
- Level of risk for
  — osteoporosis (as determined by family and personal medical history and bone density screening and other measurements of bone loss)
  — heart disease (as determined by family and personal history and results of laboratory tests)
  — breast and other reproductive cancers

Risks of HRT in Certain Diseases

The risks with HRT and breast cancer and gallbladder disease are described briefly next. The information, pertinent statistics, and research findings on breast cancer and gallbladder disease were gleaned from *Taking Hormones and Women's Health* (National Women's Health Network, 1995).

Breast Cancer

In 1991 the Centers for Disease Control published a summary of its review of 16 separate breast cancer studies. Findings revealed that breast cancer was increased by about 30% in women who received estrogen for 10 or more years.

A number of studies have been done with short-term estrogen use, findings from which show little increased breast cancer risk. However, in those studies in which large numbers of women had received estrogen longterm (8–10 years), an increased risk was found consistently. There have been only a few studies to date on the use of estrogen with a progestin (HRT) and breast cancer. Again, results of these studies show increased rates of breast cancer with long-term HRT.

Gallbladder Disease

The increased risk of gallbladder disease occurs with the use of oral hormone therapy because it contributes to the formation of cholesterone crystals in the bile duct, which supports the growth of gallstones. The risk is decreased with the use of the patch or cream form of hormone, which bypasses the liver and sends the hormones directly into the blood stream.

Estrogen and Alzheimer's Disease

The causes of Alzheimer's disease are not well understood. It seems that certain genes make some people's brain cells more susceptible to damage. However, exposure to biochemical or environmental factors may be needed to set the process in motion. Results of studies designed to look for ways to slow or prevent the process have shown that estrogen use greatly reduced the risk of developing Alzheimer's disease. The range of risk reduction was 30%–60%. Researchers suspect that estrogen protects the brain by acting as an antioxidant, cleaning up the toxic byproducts of oxidation that can damage cells. Estrogen is also involved in nerve cell repair. It may promote blood flow to the brain and help protect nerve cells from the damaging formation of protein plaques. Vitamin E has also been shown to have protective effects, as have nonsteroidal antiinflammatory drugs such as ibuprofen and the herb *Ginkgo biloba,* which has antioxidant and blood-thinning properties (Duke, 1998).

Specific Information for HRT

Contraindications to Estrogen

Contraindications to ERT include the following (Love & Lindsey, 1998):

- Known or suspected estrogen-dependent cancer
- Undiagnosed genital bleeding
- Active thrombophlebitis or thromboembolic disorder
- Active liver or gallbladder disease
- Known or suspected pregnancy

Side Effects

Estrogen: Side effects of estrogen include the following (Love & Lindsey, 1998):

- Increased risk of gallbladder disease
- Worsening of estrogen-dependent conditions, such as fibroids and endometriosis
- Breast pain
- Increase in fibrocystic breast problems
- Vaginal bleeding
- Hypertension
- Nausea and vomiting
- Headaches, jaundice, and fluid retention
- Impaired glucose tolerance

Progestins: Side effects of progestins include the following (Love & Lindsey, 1998):

- Blood clots

- Fluid retention
- Breast tenderness
- Jaundice
- Nausea
- Insomnia
- Depression
- Menstrual bleeding

Methods of Administration

The drugs used for HRT can be administered in the following six forms. Women who choose to take some form of estrogen without a progestin to avoid unpleasant side effects and bleeding need to have a yearly endometrial biopsy to test for uterine abnormalities (National Women's Health Network, 1995).

Pill

- The pill is the most frequently prescribed form (Stenchever, 1996).

- The most common prescription is a dose of 0.625 mg of conjugated estrogens with 5 mg of synthetic progesterone. This dose is considered effective in the prevention of osteoporosis and heart disease (Stenchever, 1996).

- With the use of progestin, 80%–90% of women have menstrual bleeding (Stenchever, 1996).

- Many possible dosage regimens exist, with the most common being estrogen daily and progesterone the first 14 days of each month, or estrogen days 1–25 and progestin days 15–25 (Sifton, 1994). Continuous daily dosage of both hormones may lower the dose of progestin needed, but 40%–60% of women still have some irregular bleeding during the first 6 months (Sifton, 1994). After 6 months, approximately 75% of women have no bleeding (Stenchever, 1996).

- Smaller doses may relieve symptoms but may not provide the protective effect for osteoporosis and heart disease (Sifton, 1994).

- Pills have one sixth the amount of estrogen and progestin as that in oral contraceptives (Sifton, 1994).

Injection

- With injection, the liver is bypassed (Sifton, 1994).

- Intramuscular injection is required once per month (Sifton, 1994).

- Blood hormone levels need to be monitored because it is more difficult to maintain steady levels with this form (Sifton, 1994).

Patch

- The patch is applied to the buttocks or the upper arm (Sifton, 1994).

- With the patch, the liver is bypassed. Thus the drug is absorbed directly into the blood stream (Sifton, 1994).

- Each patch lasts for several days (Sifton, 1994).

- The patch does not have some of the beneficial effects on HDL levels, as those associated with oral therapy (Sifton, 1994).

Implant

- An implant is placed surgically under the skin (National Women's Health Network, 1995).

- The implant lasts for several months. It has never been approved by the FDA, although it is used in other countries (National Women's Health Network, 1995).

- Hormone levels cannot be adjusted or controlled and thus overdose can occur easily (National Women's Health Network, 1995).

- The implant is not used much currently because of lack of control of side effects (National Women's Health Network, 1995).

Cream

- The cream can be applied to abdomen, thighs, or arms (Sifton, 1994).

- The cream needs to be applied carefully for correct dosing (Sifton, 1994).

- With the cream, the liver is bypassed (Sifton, 1994).

- The hormone is absorbed systemically (Sifton, 1994).

- With this form it is difficult to control blood hormone levels, so monitoring is needed (Sifton, 1994).

Vaginal Cream

- Vaginal cream is used to control symptoms of vaginal dryness and urinary symptoms (National Women's Health Network, 1995).

- Vaginal cream is absorbed systemically if the dosage is sufficient (National Women's Health Network, 1995).

New Drugs

There are several new drugs available in HRT. The following information, statistics, and pertinent research findings related to raloxifene are gleaned from Love and Lindsey (1998). Those on other forms of estrogen and oral micronized estrogen are gleaned from Gaby (1994). Those on progesterone are gleaned from Stenchever (1996) and DeMarco (1996). Finally, the information on Estratab has been taken from the article "Estrogen, the Estrogen Decision" (1998).

Raloxifene Hydrochloride (Evista®)

Raloxifene was approved by the FDA in 1997. This is one of a class of drugs known as selective estrogen receptor modulators (SERMs). (See also chapter 12.) The company that markets it claims it has all the benefits of older drugs like Premarin without any of the risks. The drug mimics estrogen's benefits in bone cells, but it does not stimulate tissues in the breast and uterus (Love & Lindsey, 1998).

In three large trials, findings revealed that use of raloxifene plus calcium increased bone density by 2%–3% when compared with calcium supplements alone. Studies of fracture prevention in women with osteoporosis are ongoing. Trials of effects on breast cancer and heart disease are also ongoing. Concerns have been raised that its approval was based on results from only a few short-term studies, none of which provided conclusive evidence that this new drug is as safe as purported (Love & Lindsey, 1998).

Raloxifene seems to reduce LDL, total cholesterol, and fibrinogen levels, but it does not raise HDL levels. There is no proof yet that raloxifene actually prevents bone fractures or heart attacks. Furthermore, because it seems to act like tamoxifen citrate on breast tissue, the concern is that with long-term use it may stimulate breast tissue. This has been the most recent finding with tamoxifen trials. Tamoxifen decreased the incidence of secondary cancers in women with breast cancer for 5 years, but it had the opposite effect after 10 years (Love & Lindsey, 1998). Study results show an increase in hot flashes with this drug (Love & Lindsey, 1998). There are many unanswered questions about this new medication (Love & Lindsey, 1998).

Other Forms of Estrogen

Estrogen is not a single substance but a class of compounds (Gaby, 1994). It exists in the female body in at least three forms. Estrone (E1) and estradiol (E2) are relatively potent estrogens; estriol is the weakest (E3). E1 and E2 are the strongest and most likely to promote cancer. These are the kinds of estrogen found in most drug formulas of estrogen. E3 is much less potent than the other two forms and has actually been shown to have anticancer activity. Because estriol is a weak estrogen, a higher dose than required with the other two

forms of estrogen may be needed to relieve menopausal symptoms (Gaby, 1994).

Estriol has been studied more extensively in Europe (Gaby, 1994). In the United States it has not been seriously investigated as an alternative to the commonly prescribed forms of estrogen. Results of preliminary studies have shown that estriol does not cause the proliferation of the uterine lining (endometrial hyperplasia) in doses high enough to control most menopausal symptoms, and it does not cause breakthrough bleeding (Gaby, 1994). These study results show that estriol may be an appropriate choice, with some of the beneficial effects of ERT and elimination of undesirable side effects such as the following (Gaby, 1994):

- Estriol may have a protective effect against breast cancer, as well as lower the risk of blood clots, as compared with these effects with other estrogens.

- Because estriol rarely causes bleeding its use would reduce the need for invasive evaluation of bleeding for possible disease.

- Estriol has been available for years in Europe, so a body of clinical practice is available for evaluation.

- Estriol may not be protective for osteoporosis or heart disease.

A triestrogen cream, containing all three forms of estrogen, has been developed and is currently available in the United States. (See resource guide.)

Oral Micronized Estrogen

Oral micronized estrogen has the same structure as estrogen naturally produced by the body. This is being studied as an alternative to currently used estrogen formulations (Gaby, 1994).

Low-Dose Estrogen

A 0.3-mg formulation of Estratab has been on the market for years, but it has been approved recently by the FDA for its bone-building effects. The results of the latest study on this drug were discussed earlier. Those results showed bone building and beneficial effects on lipids without overgrowth of the uterine lining ("Estrogen, the Estrogen Decision: Are Lower Doses Good Enough?," 1998).

Other Forms of Progesterone

Oral micronized progesterone is a form of progesterone that has the same structure as the progesterone produced by the body. Unlike with synthetic progestins, results of studies thus far have shown that the beneficial effects produced by estrogen on cholesterol and lipid levels are not adversely affected by the addition of oral micronized progesterone, whereas synthetic progestins seem to interfere with the beneficial effects of estrogen (Stenchever, 1996). Findings also indicate that natural progesterone produces minimal side effects, as compared to those with synthetic progestins (DeMarco, 1996).

CONCLUSION

It is evident from this discussion that an ever-expanding array of drug therapies is becoming available to women entering menopause. New combinations and dosage recommendations of hormones are being researched, as are nonhormonal drugs, which have benefits for heart and bone health. The important roles played by diet, exercise, and lifestyle and the beneficial pharmaceutic properties of specific foods and herbs are being more widely recognized and more rigorously researched.

In the United States today there are more than 35 million women age 50 years and older (Stenchever, 1996). It is critical that the issues surrounding menopause and aging be well researched and clarified, so that women can have clear guidelines for therapeutic intervention if it is needed. At the same time, women and health care providers alike can learn from the experiences of other cultures, that have a much lower incidence of heart disease and breast cancer and experience few of the symptoms that have come to be recognized as hallmarks of menopause.

There is no cure for menopause. Menopause is not a disease, but a natural, inevitable life-positive transition. The experience of this generation of menopausal women, as well as the research that has been generated from the collective interest and need for information, will inform women in years to come. In the meantime, women and their health care providers need to stay well informed and consider carefully the benefits, risks, and long-term effects of therapeutic options, creating an individualized plan of care that is minimally invasive and provides protection and enhancement of each woman's health as she ages.

CHAPTER 13
Questions 98–100

98. Estrogen replacement therapy alone has been shown to decrease the risk of all but which of the following conditions or diseases:

    a. Alzheimer's disease.

    b. Heart disease.

    c. Uterine cancer.

    d. Osteoporosis.

99. Oral micronized progesterone

    a. is identical to human progesterone.

    b. is a synthetic form of progesterone.

    c. interferes with estrogens protective effects on the heart.

    d. has more side effects than progestins.

100. The best way to establish bone density is by

    a. taking a special type of x-ray film.

    b. obtaining and analyzing a 24-hour urine sample.

    c. analyzing components of the blood.

    d. taking a bone marrow biopsy.

This concludes the final examination. An answer key will be sent with your certificate so that you can determine which of your answers were correct and incorrect.

CHAPTER 14

CHALLENGES TO WOMEN'S HEALTH

CHAPTER OBJECTIVE

After completing this chapter, the reader will be able to recognize the prevalence in the environment of chemicals and pollutants called estrogen "mimics." The reader will also be able to recognize the obsession in American culture with a very narrow and confining standard of beauty that is giving rise to an epidemic of low self-esteem among women of all ages.

LEARNING OBJECTIVES

After studying this chapter, the reader will be able to

1. identify challenges facing women in American society.

2. describe the emerging problem of environmental "estrogens" and their potential adverse impact.

3. discuss the impact of media images of beauty on women's self-esteem.

Key Words

- Chronic fatigue syndrome
- Estrogen "mimics"
- TMJ pain dysfunction syndrome

INTRODUCTION

This chapter concludes the consideration of health concerns facing women. Beginning with the discussion of the Fourth Worldwide Conference on Women in Beijing (Lee, Estes, & Close, 1997) in chapter 1, many personal as well as societal issues that have an impact on women's health have been highlighted. In this final chapter, special attention is given to two concerns that are quietly undermining the health of women: estrogen "mimics" in the environment and the standards of beauty that lead to low self-esteem.

According to Lee and associates (1997), in the past several decades great progress has been made in the field of women's health. Women now have more control over their health and decision making for their families and children than ever before. Women's options for birth control have expanded, and they have more control over pregnancy options and more self-determination and equality in other areas of their lives. Health research that targets women is blossoming. Complementary health care options are becoming more acceptable and available.

At the same time, Lee and colleagues (1997) note, women face serious challenges. Socioeconomic status remains the primary barrier to education, access to health care, and self-determination. Women most in need are often those whose options and access are limited. In addition, there are a large number of women who are working in low-paying jobs under unhealthy conditions. This trend will continue as more women both immigrate to the United States from other countries and enter the work force to support their families. Occupational exposures and hazards are increasingly having an impact on women's health. Smoking, drug abuse, exposure to sexually transmitted infection, domestic violence, and rape are current issues that cross economic strata. Ever-increasing levels of stress contribute to disorders common to women, such as headaches, menstrual problems, temporomandibular joint (TMJ) pain dysfunction syndrome, depression, and chronic fatigue syndrome.

ENVIRONMENTAL HAZARDS

The following discussion, as well as pertinent statistics and research findings, on environmental hazards and women's health is gleaned from Raloff (1994).

Over the past 15 years, research findings have unmasked a number of environmental "hormones." These are chemicals and pollutants that disrupt biologic processes, often mimicking the effects of naturally produced hormones. Many of these chemicals seem to mimic estrogen in their effects.

There is an ever-growing list of these chemical pollutants; among these are pesticides (some of which have been banned in the United States) that are still being used in other parts of the world. They tend to persist in the environment because they are soluble in fat. Therefore they accumulate in animal and human fatty tissue. Other chemicals include DDT, DDE, PCBs, dioxin from the bleaching of paper products, some ingredients in plastics, and some of the breakdown products of common household detergents.

The hormonal activity of these chemicals usually bears little relationship to their intended function. These chemicals may be contributing to an increased risk of cancer of the reproductive system in women. Prenatal exposure, during the development of the embryo, may disrupt the processes that establish male or female gender. Results of animal studies are beginning to indicate that far smaller exposures are needed to trigger these reproductive effects than to induce cancer.

Concerns about environmental "hormones" first made the news with studies about the effects of DDT on the thinning of eggshells in sea gulls. In addition to the eggshell effects, many of the offspring did not survive. Among those that did it was discovered that the males had female sexual organs. Males also exhibited a disinterest in mating, and females began to share nests. Findings from more recent studies on alligators living in a polluted lake in Florida showed that 80%–95% of eggs failed to hatch. Many of those that survived died within 2 weeks. The female alligators who did survive had twice the normal amount of estrogen in their blood, and males had almost no testosterone. The sex organs were also feminized. Many other studies have been conducted on other animal species, all with similar results.

Toxic pollutant concentrations in the environment are low enough that they seldom kill most adult animals or human beings. The concern is that the adults may look healthy, but they have been reproductively impaired by their exposure to these chemicals to such a degree that essentially the species is destined to extinction. For the human population, research in the future may uncover links between environmental "estrogens" and decreasing fertility in men and women, reproductive cancers, and a host of diseases whose cause is not well understood but is thought to be related to altered hormone levels. Such diseases or tumors include premenstrual syndrome, endometriosis, and fibroids.

To summarize Raloff's comments on environmental hazards and women's health, there is great cause for concern. This is an area of health care that is not as yet widely discussed, nor well researched. Health care providers need to become more educated about this issue and discuss it with their colleagues and clients. The good news is that there is something that can be done. Members of the health profession need to make their voices heard. (Please see the resource guide for more information.)

EPIDEMIC OF LOW SELF-ESTEEM

Emerging as a new epidemic in American society is the obsessive concern for youth and thinness. Resulting from these obsessions are disorders that affect women of all ages, and especially young women, including anorexia, bulimia, depression, and more subtle forms of altered body image and low self-esteem.

According to an article in the September 1997 issue of *Full Voice* ("The Body and Self-Esteem," 1997), the whole idealized beauty nonsense that is everywhere in the media is destroying the very people that it is meant to celebrate. When women were surveyed, 70% tended to feel depressed, guilty, and shameful after looking through pictures of models in magazines. Of this same group, 70%–90% reported dissatisfaction with some aspect of their bodies. A limiting and limited beauty ideal that cramps the individual inside each woman stunts her personal growth. Forty-eight million American women are dieting at any one time.

Comments From Young Women About Beauty

Comments such as the following provide insight into the effects of "beauty standards" on youth in American culture ("The Body and Self-Esteem," 1997):

Jacqueline, 17 years old:

"I try to like myself for what I am but I

open a magazine and immediately compare myself with those perfect models."

Or, another 16-year-old:

"Sometimes I wish supermodels didn't exist and body shape didn't matter because then you wouldn't have to keep up."

Or, a 14-year-old:

"Why can't we have healthy role models of all sizes, so it's fair to everyone? Why does everyone have this Beauty Thing? It's like a curse and eventually wrecks people's lives."

Some Comments From Women About Beauty and Growing Older

The following comments provide interesting and thoughtful perspectives on aging and can assist health care providers who work with women older than 40 years of age ("The Body and Self-Esteem," 1997):

"I'm happy with the way I look. I've earned every wrinkle, every scar. The best thing about getting older is the freedom to say, This is what I am, this is what I do."

Or,

"Wrinkles don't worry me—what worries me most about aging is the idea of being invisible, undesirable."

Or,

"I've met some very beautiful people, but then you start talking to them and after a few minutes, they're no longer beautiful. Likewise, I know plain people who become beautiful as you talk to them. That is the power of character."

Psychologists who work with women and body image say that body hatred and obsession with appearance is really about deep-seated feelings of inadequacy. The body becomes the battlefield for self-doubts. In addition, women are constantly bombarded with media images of perfection. They are constantly comparing themselves to other women. Body image may have little to do with a woman's actual appearance ("Body Image: The Last Frontier of Women's Rights?," 1997).

According to the article "Body as Battlefield" (1997), therapy is often aimed at reeducating women, by having them notice when they have a "bad body thought" and look at what incident, feeling, or situation was disturbing. Bad body thoughts are always a detour; they are never about the body. However, women are trained to make a detour to the body, rather than to think about the actual issue. Women have to stop buying into the idea that the only nice body is a nonthreatening girl's body, rather than a woman's body. Roundness is part of femininity.

Health care providers may find the following suggestions helpful in working with female clients to improve their relationship with their body ("Body as Battlefield," 1997):

- Focus on
  — enjoying movement.
  — healthy eating habits.
- Limit your exposure to the mass media.
- Find new role models.
- Give your friends and daughters praise for parts of themselves other than their appearance.
- Explore what underlies your "bad body thoughts."

The following provides hope and direction for all womankind ("The Body and Self-Esteem," 1997):

"Somewhere in time, our society decided that how a person looked was more important than who that person was. When that time was, no one knows, but we can remember the time we started to put it right."

CONCLUSION

As is clear from reading the material throughout this course, there seem to be more questions than answers about many women's health issues. In addition, general health-promotion measures throughout history have had a powerful impact on women's health. Thousands of women's lives have been saved by basic improvements such as simple handwashing.

Efforts to clean up the water supply and establish proper sewage disposal were primarily responsible for the major health improvements in the past century. Although these solutions seem obvious now, many of women's own health issues elude them. Someday, perhaps these answers will be evident as well. Perhaps women are blind to simplicity in this age of complexity. Perhaps they are waiting for scientists to tell them what they already intuitively know.

Human beings are in a very real sense drowning in their own waste. They are destroying themselves. They have to work on a broad scale to clean up the environment, improve economic conditions, and make health care available to all. At the same time, change must occur on a personal level by people adopting a healthy diet, exercise, and work habits. The tides may begin to turn, and health care providers are an important part of this process.

It has been the intention of this course to provide current information about women's health issues, as well as to spark your interest, raise questions for your consideration, and encourage you to continue to educate yourself and others.

GLOSSARY

Adjuvant: Cancer treatment that is not the primary form of treatment for removal of cancerous tissue. It is instead a systemic treatment that is initiated after surgery to prevent return of the cancer by killing cells that may have traveled elsewhere in the body.

Agglutination: Clumping together. An abnormal sign in evaluation of sperm function that could indicate an immune response.

Amenorrhea: Absence of menstruation.

Anovulatory cycle: Menstrual cycle in which no egg is released from the ovary.

Artificial menopause: A condition brought on by surgical removal of the ovaries, radiation, or chemotherapy, which renders the ovaries non-functional.

Aspiration: Withdrawal by gentle suction.

Assisted hatching: A micromanipulation technique used in assisted reproductive technology interventions in which a hole is made in the outer covering of the egg to assist the sperm to penetrate and fertilize.

Assisted reproductive technologies (ARTs): The various new technologies for assisting infertile couples to conceive.

Asymptomatic: Absence of symptoms in the presence of a disease.

Atherosclerosis: Build up of fatty plaque on the walls of an artery, stiffening the artery and reducing blood flow.

Basal body temperature (BBT) charting:

Purpose: To verify ovulation and determine adequacy of the luteal phase of the menstrual cycle.

Procedure: Body temperature must be taken before arising and at the same time every morning. It is best to use a special basal body temperature thermometer that has the appropriate range spread for easy reading. Also to be recorded are days of menstrual flow, discharge, mucus, illness, nights up late or less than 6 hours of sleep, and sexual intercourse (SIC). Recordings are made for 2–6 months while other tests are being done.

Results: Charting reveals whether the couple's timing of SIC is optimal. Standard recommendation is SIC 2 days before ovulation is expected and every 2 days, until 2–4 days have passed after the increase in basal body temperature.

Basal thermometer: Specially calibrated instrument to measure body temperature in relation to ovulation.

Benign: Noncancerous.

Bimanual examination: Part of the standard examination of the female pelvic organs in which the examiner inserts two fingers into the vagina, with the opposing hand on the abdomen. In this way the ovaries and uterus are palpated for any abnormalities.

Biopsy: A procedure to remove a small piece of tissue for microscopic analysis by a specialist.

Bone density screening: Measurement of bone mass by using low-dose x-ray procedures.

Breast self-examination (SBE): Monthly examination advised for all adult women in which women examine their breasts for any changes by using both visual inspection and palpation.

Carcinoma: Cancer of the tissue that covers body surfaces, both internal and external.

Carcinoma in situ: Carcinoma that has not yet invaded surrounding tissue.

Cervicitis: Inflammation of the cervix caused by infection, injury, or irritation.

Cervicography: Diagnostic technique in which photographs are taken of the cervix.

Cholesterol: A substance that is manufactured by the liver, as well as derived from animal fat. Hormones, such as estrogen and progesterone, are made from cholesterol. It is also a part of cell membranes. Cholesterol is transported through the blood stream attached to lipoproteins.

Chronic fatigue syndrome: A constellation of symptoms characterized by debilitating fatigue and flu-like symptoms. The cause is not well understood but thought to be multifactorial.

Climacteric: The period, which can last from months to years, when the menstrual cycle of women becomes irregular, hormone levels fluctuate and eventually decrease, and periods cease altogether.

Clinical breast examination (CBE): A breast examination performed by a licensed professional trained to do breast examinations.

Clitoris: A small, pea-sized, hooded erectile structure located on the vulva above the vagina. It is the anatomic homologue of the penis in the male and highly responsive to sexual stimulation.

Colposcopy: Technique for viewing the cervix under magnification, making it possible to see structures not visible to the naked eye. Used to evaluate the cervix and vagina.

Columnar epithelium: Glandular tissue of the cervix that is composed of tall, narrow cells.

Congenital: Existing at or dating from birth, but not due to heredity.

Conization of the cervix: A surgical procedure in which a part of the cervix surrounding the cervical canal is removed.

Corpus luteum: A structure formed after ovulation by the remaining tissue of the follicle. Its main function is secretion of progesterone, which prepares the uterine lining for implantation by a fertilized embryo. The corpus luteum helps support the developing embryo, or it disintegrates if no fertilization has occurred.

Cryopreservation: Use of a medium, usually liquid nitrogen, to store something in a frozen state. Refers to preservation of embryos in assisted reproductive technology.

Cryosurgery: Use of a cold source to freeze abnormal tissue.

Cryotherapy: A treatment that involves freezing of abnormal tissue. Cryotherapy is commonly used to remove abnormal cervical cells as well as genital warts from the vagina and external genitalia.

Depo-Provera: A synthetic progesterone (medroxyprogesterone acetate) used as an injectable method of birth control.

Diethylstilbestrol (DES): A synthetic estrogen that was once given to women early in pregnancy to prevent miscarriage. It was taken off the market because of its multiple effects on the offspring of women who took it, including increased risk of a rare type of vaginal cancer and increased rates of infertility in male and female offspring.

Dysmenorrhea: Painful menstrual cramps.

Dyspareunia: Pain with sexual intercourse.

Dysplasia: Abnormal cell growth that can be a pre-cancerous condition.

Dysuria: Painful urination.

Ectopic pregnancy: A pregnancy that implants and develops outside the uterus, most often in the fallopian tube. This can be life threatening and requires immediate intervention.

Embryo: Fertilized egg. The developing organism is an embryo usually after approximately 1 week of development through the eighth week.

Emergency contraception pill (ECP, MAP): Also known as the morning after pill. It is used to deter pregnancy in case of an accidental method failure or unprotected intercourse. Specific birth control pill formulations are used to interrupt fertilization and implantation.

Endocervical canal: Canal that runs down the center of the cervix and opens into the vagina on one side and into the uterus on the other.

Endometrial biopsy: A test done to sample the uterine lining. Used in infertility evaluation for evidence that ovulation has occurred. Also used to diagnose abnormalities of the uterine lining such as uterine cancer.

Procedure: Usually done about 10 days after a rise in basal body temperature. A small cannula is inserted through the cervical canal into the uterus where a sample of the lining is gathered by suction or curettage. Mild to moderate cramping can be expected. Use of a nonsteroidal anti-inflammatory drug beforehand is helpful. A vasovagal response may occur, in which case having the patient elevate the legs and take time to come to an upright position will usually abate the response. Nausea and vomiting or fainting may occur if the reaction is more pronounced.

Endometrial hyperplasia: Abnormally rapid and extensive growth of the uterine lining.

Endometrioma: Implant of endometrial tissue outside the uterus, found in endometriosis.

Endometrium: Inner lining of the uterus that responds to the cyclic influence of hormones during the menstrual cycle.

Endorphins: Hormones found in the brain that give a sensation of well-being and affect pain perception and emotion.

Environmental "estrogens": Pollutants and household and industrial chemicals that are hormone mimics. Study findings (Raloff, 1994) are showing profound disruption of normal sexual maturation in a number of different exposed animal populations, and potential links to hormone-mediated cancers are suspected.

Enzyme: A protein that is needed for specific chemical reactions in the body, but it is not changed by the reaction and therefore can be used again.

Epithelial cells: Cells that make up the type of tissue that covers the surfaces of the body and its internal organs.

Estrogen: Group of similar hormones that produce the effect of stimulating maturation of egg follicles, leading to ovulation. There are three forms of estrogen found in the human body: estradiol, estriol, and estrone. Synthetic forms are used in formulations of the birth control pill and standard hormone replacement therapy.

Estrogen "mimics": Used to describe chemicals, such as pesticides and some household and industrial chemicals, that bind with estrogen receptor sites in tissue, causing disruption of the normal hormonal environment.

Estrogen replacement therapy (ERT): Use of a form of the hormone estrogen to create a state of hormone balance in a woman who has stopped menstruating, similar to her hormonal state before menopause. Use of estrogen alone in women who still have their uteruses increases the risk of uterine cancer.

False negative: Failure of a test to detect an existing abnormality.

False positive: Indication of abnormality when none exists.

Fibroadenoma: A benign tumor containing glandular and fibrous elements commonly found in the breast.

Fibrocystic breast disease: This is not really a disease but a condition in which fluid-filled cysts enlarge in conjunction with the second half of the menstrual cycle, causing discomfort and swelling of the breasts.

Fine needle aspiration: Technique for evaluating breast masses thought to be fluid filled (cysts) by attempting to remove fluid with a fine needle.

Folic acid: One of the B vitamins, which is involved in normal cell growth.

Follicle: Group of tissues in the ovary that develop around an immature egg and are responsible for producing hormones and growth-promoting factors. Rupture of the follicle from the ovary is ovulation.

Follicle-stimulating hormone (FSH): Hormone produced by the pituitary gland and targeting the ovary. This hormone promotes growth of ovarian follicles.

Fomite: An object, such as clothing or towels, that can provide a location for transmission of infection.

Galactorrhea: Spontaneous discharge of milk from the breasts not associated with breast-feeding and caused by a hormone imbalance.

Gamete: A reproductive cell (egg or sperm).

Gamete intrafallopian transfer (GIFT): Transfer of a retrieved egg, along with prepared sperm, into the fallopian tube of the woman.

Gland: Organized group of cells that secretes substances such as hormones.

Gonadotropin: Substance produced by the pituitary gland that stimulates the gonads (ovaries or testes).

Gonadotropin releasing hormone (Gn-RH): Hormone produced by the hypothalamus that stimulates the pituitary gland to release gonadotropins.

High-density lipoprotein (HDL): A protein that carries fats and cholesterol through the blood stream. Referred to as "good cholesterol" because it transports cholesterol out of tissues and allows it to be excreted.

Hormone: Glandular secretion that controls the activity of tissues and organs.

Hormone replacement therapy (HRT): Use of an estrogen and progestin to replace hormones no longer produced by the ovary after menopause.

Human chorionic gonadotropin (HCG): Hormone secreted in the urine and into the blood stream of pregnant women. Its detection is the basis of both urine and serum pregnancy tests.

Hypothalamus: Part of the brain that regulates a number of different body processes, including body temperature; appetite; thirst; and hormonal stimulation to the ovaries, thyroid gland, and adrenal glands by way of its action on the pituitary gland.

Hysterosalpingogram:

Purpose: Indirect visualization of the reproductive tract of the woman. It can be used to achieve patency of a blocked tube.

Procedure: Radiopaque iodine-based dye is injected through the cervix and follows the normal pathway into the uterus, fallopian tubes, and abdominal cavity. It should be scheduled for the first half of the menstrual cycle. It can be a very uncomfortable procedure, especially if the tubes are blocked. Vasovagal reactions may occur after the dye is injected. This is an outpatient procedure.

Results: It reveals abnormalities of the internal configuration of the uterus, such as fibroids or bicornate uterus. It also determines patency of the tubes, and it can sometimes clear an obstruction.

Hysteroscopy: A procedure in which contrast medium, usually iodine based, is used to distend the uterine cavity. Visualization of the structures is possible by using the hysteroscope, a lighted scope that is inserted through the cervix into the uterus. With hysteroscopy, one can perform a simple biopsy or remove a small polyp in the office setting. It can also be used for more complex operative procedures on the uterine lining, such as electrocautery, laser, and fibroid removal. These would be done in the operating room. Mild to moderate cramping often accompanies hysteroscopy.

Insemination: Introduction of semen into the female reproductive tract.

In situ: Used in this course in reference to carcinoma in situ. An early stage of cancer that is confined to the immediate area in which it began. In breast cancer it means that the cancer remains confined to the ducts or lobules and has not invaded the surrounding fatty tissue or spread to other organs.

Integrated medical therapies: A general term that refers to the combined use of Western medical therapeutics and other healing modalities, such as Chinese medicine, Western herbology, and massage.

Intracytoplasmic sperm injection (ICSI): A micromanipulation technique used during assisted reproductive technology interventions in which a single sperm is injected into the egg, bypassing the egg's outer coating.

In vitro: "In glass" or outside the human body, usually referring to fertilization of an egg in assisted reproductive technologies.

In vitro fertilization/embryo transfer (IVF/ET): The oldest of the assisted reproductive technologies. Eggs are harvested from the ovary through the vaginal wall, placed in a laboratory environment, and fertilized. Then the fertilized eggs are transferred to the uterus for implantation.

Kegel exercises: Exercises done to strengthen the muscles of the pelvic floor and control urination.

Laparoscopy: Surgical procedure in which a fiberoptic scope and instruments are inserted through a small incision near the umbilicus to view pelvic structures and remove abnormal tissue. It is also used as one method of evaluating the fallopian tubes.

Laparotomy: Abdominal surgery.

Laser: An electrosurgical instrument in which electricity is converted to light, which is concentrated and thereby produces heat. The light of a laser is ordinary light that has been controlled and organized to emit one wavelength. The light travels through space in a beam, which can be finely focused to intensify its effects. Laser light can be used to cut, vaporize, coagulate, or fulgurate (superficial charring of surface) tissue. Heat is created when the tissue absorbs the radiation.

Lesion: Any abnormal tissue.

Low-density lipoprotein (LDL): A protein that carries cholesterol and tends to promote deposits on arterial walls. Known as "bad cholesterol."

Luteinizing hormone (LH): One of the hormones secreted by the pituitary gland that is essential to development of the ovarian follicle and ovulation.

Lymph nodes: Glands of the lymphatic system that supply white blood cells to the general circulation and filter out bacteria and foreign particles from the lymph fluid.

Malignant: Cancerous.

Mammotome: A new breast biopsy technique that uses a tiny hollow needle probe guided to the abnormal area with the help of computer images or ultrasound. The needle uses a vacuum to withdraw tissue, which is removed by means of a high-speed cutter. A larger sample of tissue can be obtained than with the current core needle biopsy method, increasing the accuracy of the diagnosis.

Medical abortion: Use of drugs to induce abortion, rather than a surgical termination of pregnancy.

Menarche: Initiation of menstrual cycles with the first menstrual period.

Metastasis: Spread of cancer from the original site (referred to as the primary cancer) to a lymph node or distant organ.

Microcalcifications: Calcium deposits, often found in clusters by means of a mammogram. They are neither cancer nor tumors. They can be the result of aging and are very common. Certain patterns of calcifications are associated with breast cancer.

Micromanipulation: Procedure to manipulate the tiny sperm or egg to improve chances of fertilization.

Minilaparotomy: Female sterilization procedure in which the fallopian tubes are cauterized or blocked through a small abdominal incision.

National Survey of Family Growth: A large survey conducted by the U.S. Department of Health and Human Services, National Center for Health Statistics and the Centers for Disease Control and Prevention determining trends in the U.S. population. The study was used to assess a number of reproductive factors, including age at first intercourse, age at first menstruation, voluntary vs. involuntary first intercourse, relationship of marriage to first intercourse, number of sexual partners according to age for different populations, use of birth control methods at first intercourse, and type of contraception used.

"Natural" progesterone: A manufactured form of progesterone derived from plant sources, whose chemical structure is identical to that of the progesterone produced by the female body.

Node negative: Results of the biopsy of lymph nodes reveal that the lymph nodes are free of cancer. This is an indication that the cancer is less likely to recur.

Node positive: Results of the biopsy of lymph nodes reveal that cancer has spread to the lymph nodes under the arm on the same side as the original tumor.

Oocyte: Developing ovum or egg.

Open biopsy: Surgical removal of all or a portion of an abnormal breast mass with the client under general anesthesia.

Oral micronized progesterone: A specially formulated type of progesterone, which has the same structure as the progesterone produced by women. The particles are very finely ground. This form of progesterone is better absorbed into the blood stream than other oral forms of progesterone.

Os: Opening of the cervical canal.

Osteoblasts: Bone cells that are responsible for laying down new bone.

Osteoclasts: Bone cells that are responsible for breaking down old bone in a process called remodeling.

Osteoporosis: A condition in which a large amount of bone mass is lost, leading to brittle, porous bone that can be easily fractured.

Ovarian follicle: (*See* Follicle.)

Over-the-counter (OTC) drugs: Medications sold without the need for a prescription.

Pelvic inflammatory disease (PID): A serious infection of the reproductive organs, often caused by infection with sexual pathogens. Tissue destruction can occur without symptoms. Infertility is a major long-term consequence.

Perimenopause: A period preceding menopause when menses becomes more and more irregular (also termed climacteric).

Piaget: A researcher who made major contributions to the field of childhood cognitive development, describing maturation of cognitive abilities by stages from infancy to adulthood.

Pituitary desensitization: Drugs are used during assisted reproductive technology interventions to suppress the release of hormones from the pituitary gland, which would result in ovulation, before all the multiple eggs are matured.

Pituitary gland: Structure at the base of the brain that receives instructions by means of hormones from the hypothalamus and sends hormonal messages to a number of glands and organs, including the ovaries.

Postcoital test (PCT): Part of infertility workup that is used to evaluate aspects of sperm function and cervical mucus.

Procedure: The test needs to be timed carefully with the immediate preovulatory phase. The basal body temperature should not yet show an increase. Sexual intercourse should have taken place at home either the night before or morning of examination. A sample of mucus from the exocervix and endocervix is obtained with a small syringe during a pelvic examination. Evaluation under the microscope reveals the type of mucus present and the number and motility of sperm. A normal sperm count is a minimum of 5–10 motile sperm per high-power field. Conducive mucus should be present.

Results: If the mucus is favorable and the semen analysis reveals normal findings, more specialized testing is needed to determine sperm-mucus incompatibilities or sperm capacitation problems.

Premenstrual syndrome or premenstrual tension (PMS/PMT): Collection of symptoms that occur during the second phase of the menstrual cycle and improve with the onset of menses. Causes are not well understood.

Primary tumor: Original site of a cancerous tumor.

Prodromal symptom: An early sign of an outbreak of disease. It most typically refers to the itching or skin sensitivity that often precedes an outbreak of herpes.

Progestin/progestogen: Synthetic forms of the naturally occurring hormone progesterone, which is produced by the ovaries. Used in hormone replacement therapies and hormonal birth control methods.

Prostaglandin inhibitors: A group of drugs, used to treat inflammatory diseases, that inhibit synthesis and activity of prostaglandins. These drugs have been approved by the Food and Drug Administration for treatment of menstrual pain. These drugs do have side effects. Although many are over-the-counter drugs, they should be used intelligently and monitored by the client and health care practitioner. Ibuprofen (Motrin), indomethacin (Indocin), and mefenamic acid (Ponstel) are all prostaglandin inhibitors.

Prostaglandins: Local substances produced by the tissues and found in many parts of the body. Prostaglandins play an important role in menstrual cramps. They may cause vasodilation and pain in breast tissue. They also play a role in body water content, appetite, and body temperature.

Receptors: Part of the molecular structure of a cell. Substances circulating in the blood stream whose molecular "shape" matches the receptor's shape can bind to the cell membrane and activate reactions in the cell. This is the process whereby hormones produce their effects. Certain tumors also have hormone receptors that recognize estrogen or progesterone. If a tumor has receptor sites for hormones, this information is used in decision making about treatment options.

Refractory period: That period after orgasm in which another orgasm cannot occur. This period varies between men and women, and it can change with age and other factors.

Safer sex: A commonly used way of acknowledging that there is no such thing as totally safe sex. Safer sex describes practices designed to minimize transfer of any body fluids between partners.

Semen evaluation: At least two semen samples are collected on separate days by masturbation. Each sample should be collected after abstaining from ejaculation for a minimum of 48 hours but not longer than 3–4 days. The ejaculate should be collected in a sterile container, and should be examined within one hour of collection. Analysis involves a complex array of tests that evaluate many aspects of sperm health including sperm count, motility, shape, clumping, presence of bacteria antibodies or other elements, and biochemical analysis.

Sexually transmitted infection or sexually transmitted disease (STI/STD): Sexually transmitted infection is the newer term and is replacing the term sexually transmitted disease. This infection is spread primarily by intimate contact between partners, through either skin-to-skin or bodily fluid contact.

Sonogram: Also called ultrasound, a procedure that uses sound waves to form an image of internal structures. Hollow or fluid-filled structures appear black, and more solid structures are white.

Sonohysterography: A procedure in which saline is inserted into the uterine cavity, distending the cavity. Ultrasound is then used to outline structures, such as polyps, submucous myomas, and adhesions.

Speculum: Instrument used during a pelvic examination to allow visualization of the cervix and vaginal lining by holding the vaginal walls apart.

Sperm penetration assay (SPA): Part of a semen evaluation for male factor infertility that tests the ability of sperm to shed its protein coating and release enzymes that are needed to penetrate the coating of the egg.

Squamocolumnar junction: Area on the cervix in which the squamous tissue of the outer aspects of the cervix and the glandular tissue arising in the cervical canal meet. This area is characterized by rapid cell turnover and is a common site for cancerous or precancerous cells to arise.

Squamous epithelium: Epithelial cells cover internal and external surfaces of the body. Squamous epithelial cells are flat, platelike cells. They are one of two types of cells that make up the cervix. Squamous cells cover the outer surface of the cervix.

Squamous metaplasia: A normal process of cell growth and replacement in which the squamous tissue slowly replaces the glandular tissue that arises in the cervical canal.

Squamous tissue: A type of tissue that lines many internal and external body surfaces. It is a smooth, flat, and nonglandular type of tissue.

Staging: A system of defining how widespread a cancer is by using information learned through diagnostic techniques. This information is used to determine appropriate treatment.

Steroid: A group name for chemicals that have a particular molecular configuration and contain cholesterol as part of their structure. A number of hormones, including the sex hormones, are steroids.

Stress incontinence: The inability to hold urine, which can develop as a result of relaxation of pelvic floor muscle support. Pressure from sneezing, laughing, or jogging can result in loss of urine.

Surrogate: A substitute.

Temporomandibular joint (TMJ) pain dysfunction syndrome: The temporomandibular joint is the junction of the jaw and the skull. Usually related to stress, dysfunction of this joint has been linked to headaches and ear pain.

Thromboembolic disease: A disorder in which blood clots can travel to various organs, causing blockage of the circulatory system. Sites of blockage can include the heart (myocardial infarction), the brain (stroke), the lungs (pulmonary embolism), or other organs.

Transformation zone: Another term for the squamocolumnar junction.

Transvaginal: Through the vagina, referring to the current methods of retrieving eggs from the ovary. This route is also being used for hysterectomy.

Tubal embryo transfer (TET): A variation of the gamete intrafallopian transfer (GIFT) procedure in which the egg is fertilized before being placed in the fallopian tube.

Tubal patency: Unobstructed fallopian tubes.

Tubal reanastomosis: A surgical procedure in which the cut ends of the fallopian tubes are brought together to reverse a previous sterilization.

Ultrasound: Use of high-frequency sound waves to obtain images of internal structures. Used in conjunction with other diagnostic and surgical procedures to guide probes and instruments. Used for diagnosis of breast disease, as well as for diagnosis of pelvic reproductive abnormalities, and to assist in monitoring women undergoing assisted reproductive technologies. (*See* Sonogram.)

Vacuum aspiration: Removal of tissue by the creation of negative pressure through the removal of air.

Vaginismus: Painful, unintentional muscle spasms in the thighs, pelvis, and vagina that lead to constriction of the pelvic muscles, often making sexual intercourse or a pelvic examination impossible. Usually occurs when a woman senses that something is about to penetrate the vagina and often is associated with prior emotional or physical trauma.

Vas deferens (ductus deferens): Tube in the male reproductive system through which sperm pass from the testes to the ejaculatory duct and then into the urethra.

Vasectomy: Surgical removal or blockage of the duct that carries semen, resulting in male sterilization.

Zygote: Term for an early fertilized egg before implantation.

Zygote intrafallopian transfer (ZIFT): An assisted reproductive technology technique in which fertilization of the egg is accomplished before transfer to the fallopian tube. The ZIFT is the same assisted reproductive technology technique as the tubal embryo transfer (TET).

RESOURCE GUIDE

AND RECOMMENDED READING LIST

BIRTH CONTROL/ SEXUALLY TRANSMITTED INFECTIONS/ABNORMAL PAP SMEAR FINDINGS

AIDS Clinical Trials Information Service
1-800-874-2572
P.O. Box 6421, Rockville, MD 20849-6421
http://www.actis.org

The Alan Guttmacher Institute
(Research, Policy Analysis & Public Education)
(212) 248-1111
120 Wall St., New York, NY 10005
http://www.agi-usa.org

American Foundation for AIDS Research
(AmFAR)
(212) 682-7440
733 Third Ave., 12th Floor, New York, NY 10017
http://www.amfar.org

American Liver Foundation
1-800-GO LIVER (1-800-465-4837)
1425 Pompton Ave., Cedar Grove, NJ 07009
http://www.liverfoundation.org

American Social Health Association (ASHA)
Newsletters on human papillomavirus and herpes:
HPV News, The Helper
Hotline 1-800-230-6039

ASHA/HPV
P. O. Box 13827
Research Triangle Park, NC 27709-3827
http://www.ashastd.org

Centers for Disease Control and Prevention
(CDC) National AIDS Hotline
1-800-342-AIDS (1-800-342-2437) (English)
1-800-344-SIDA (1-800-344-7432) (Spanish)
P. O. Box 13827
Research Triangle Park, NC 27709-3827

Centers for Disease Control (CDC) National
Sexually Transmitted Diseases (STD) Hotline
1-800-227-8922

Hepatitis Foundation International
1-800-891-0707
30 Sunrise Ter., Cedar Grove, NJ 07009-1423
http://www.hepfi.org

National Cervical Cancer Coalition (NCCC)
(818) 909-3849
16501 Sherman Way, Ste. 110
Van Nuys, CA 91406
http://www.nccc-online.org

National Network of Libraries of Medicine
(Access to online databases on HIV and other topics)
1-800-338-7657
http://www.nnlm.nlm.nih.gov

**Project Inform (Information, Inspiration, and
Advocacy for People Living with HIV/AIDS)**
1-800-822-7422
205 13th St., No. 2001, San Francisco, CA 94103
http://www.projinf.org

Other Resources:

Hatcher, R. A., Trussell, J., Stewart, F. H., Cates,
W., Stewart, G. K., Guest, F. & Kowal, D.
(Eds.). (1998). *Contraceptive technology* (17th
ed.). New York: Ardent Media.
Kass-Annese, B. & Danzer, H. (1992). *The fertility
awareness handbook: The natural guide to
avoiding or achieving pregnancy* (6th ed.).
Alameda, CA: Hunter House.

BODY IMAGE/SELF-ESTEEM/EATING DISORDERS

The Body and Self-Esteem
Full Voice, Issue I
http://www.the-body-shop.com/fullvoice/index.html

The Body Shop
1-800-BODY-SHOP (1-800-263-7467)
106 Iron Mountain Rd., Mine Hill, NJ 07803-2300
http:www.bodyshop.com

National Center for Overcoming Overeating
(212) 875-0442
P. O. Box 1257, Old Chelsea Stn.
New York, NY 10113-0920
http://www.overcomingovereating.com

Other Resources:

Freedman, R. J. (1988). *Bodylove: Learning to like
our looks—and ourselves.* New York: Harper &
Row.

Hirschmann, J. R. & Munter, C. H. (1995). *When
women stop hating their bodies: Freeing yourself from food and weight obsession.* New
York: Fawcett Columbine.
Rodin, J. (1992). *Body traps: Breaking the binds
that keep you from feeling good about your
body.* New York: William Morrow.

BREAST CANCER

American Cancer Society
1-800-ACS-2345 (1-800-227-2345)
http://www.cancer.org

Breast Cancer Action
1-877-278-6722, (415) 243-9301
55 New Montgomery St., Ste. 323
San Francisco, CA 94105
http://www.bcaction.org

**Cancer Information Service, National Cancer
Institute**
1-800-4-CANCER (1-800-422-6237)
31 Center Dr., MSC 2580, Bldg. 31, Rm. 10A16
Bethesda, MD 20892-2580
http://198.77.70.14

MammaCare®
(Breast models and teaching tools)
1-800-626-2273
930 NW 8th Ave., Gainesville, FL 32601
P. O. Box 15748, Gainesville, FL 32602
http://www.mammacare.com

**National Alliance of Breast Cancer Organizations
(NABCO)**
1-800-80NABCO (1-800-806-2226)
9 E. 37th St., 10th Floor, New York, NY 10016
http://www.nabco.org

National Breast Cancer Coalition (NBCC)
(202) 296-7477
1707 L St., NW, Ste. 1060, Washington, DC 20036
http://www.natlbcc.org

National Cancer Institute
See Cancer Information Service, National Cancer
  Institute

National Coalition for Cancer Survivorship
1-888-650-9127
1010 Wayne Ave., Ste. 505
Silver Spring, MD 20910-5600
http://www.cansearch.org

Susan G. Komen Breast Cancer Foundation
1-800-462-9273
5005 LBJ Freeway, Ste. 370, Dallas, TX 75244
http://www.breastcancerinfo.com

Y-ME National Breast Cancer Organization
Hotline: 1-800-221-2141 (English)
    1-800-986-9505 (Spanish)
212 W. Van Buren, 5th Floor
Chicago, IL 60607-3907
http://www.y-me.org

Contact for research trials on calcium glucarate:

Dr. A. S. Heerdt
Breast Service
Memorial Sloan-Kettering Cancer Center
1275 York Ave., New York, NY 10021

Other Resources:

Kradjian, R. M. (1994). *Save yourself from breast
  cancer.* New York: Berkley Books.
Latour, K. (1993). *The breast cancer companion:
  From diagnosis through treatment to recovery—Everything you need to know for every
  step along the way.* New York: W. Morrow.

Love, S. M. & Lindsey, K. (1990). *Dr. Susan
  Love's breast book.* Reading, MA: Addison-
  Wesley.
Mayer, M. (1997). *Holding tight, letting go: Living
  with metastatic breast cancer.* Sebastopol, CA:
  O'Reilly.
Weed, S. S. (1996). *Breast cancer? Breast health!:
  The wise woman way.* Woodstock, NY: Ash
  Tree.

ENVIRONMENTAL POLLUTANTS AND ESTROGEN "MIMICS"

Greenpeace
1-800-326-0959
564 Mission St. or P. O. Box 416
San Francisco, CA 94105
http://www.greenpeaceusa.org
http://www.greenpeace.org *(for international
  organization)*

Pesticide Education Center
(415) 391-8511
P. O. Box 420870, San Francisco, CA 94142-0870
e-mail: pec@igc.apc.org
http://www.igc.apc.org/pesticides

Other Resource:

Sherman, J. (1994). *Chemical exposure and disease (The professional and layperson's guide
  to understanding cause and effect).* Princeton,
  NJ: Princeton Scientific. P.O. Box 2155,
  Princeton, NJ 08543.

GENERAL INFORMATION ON WOMEN'S HEALTH ISSUES

Alzheimer's Disease Education and Referral (ADEAR) Center
1-800-438-4380
ADEAR Center
P. O. Box 8250, Silver Spring, MD 20907-8250
http://www.alzheimers.org/adear

Center for Women Policy Studies
- The National Resource Center for Women and AIDS
- Women Health Decision Making Project
- The Law and Pregnancy—Women's Reproductive Rights
(202) 872-1770
1211 Connecticut Ave., NW, Ste. 312
Washington, DC 20036

Communicore
(360) 378-4248
P. O. Box 2389, Friday Harbor, WA 98250
http://www.communicore.com

Dr. Christiane Northrup's Health Wisdom for Women (*Newsletter*)
1-800-211-8561
To order write to: Health Wisdom for Women
P.O. Box 60042, Potomac, MD 20854

Endometriosis Association, Inc.
1-800-426-2END (1-800-426-2363)
(414) 355-2200
8585 N. 76th Pl., Milwaukee, WI 53223
http://www.endometriosisassn.org

Hysterectomy Educational Resources and Services Foundation
(610) 667-7757
422 Bryn Mawr Ave., Bala Cynwyd, PA 19004
http://www.aoa.dhhs.gov/aoa/dir/113.html

National Women's Health Network
(202) 347-1140
514 10th St., NW, Ste. 400
Washington, DC 20004

National Women's Health Resource Center
(202) 537-4015
5255 Loughboro Rd., NW, Washington, DC 20016
http://www.healthywomen.org

Ovarian Cancer National Alliance
(202) 452-5910
P.O. Box 33107, Washington, DC 20033-0107
http://www.ovariancancer.org/index.html

Women's Health Advocate Newsletter
1-800-829-5876
P.O. Box 420235, Palm Coast, FL 32142-0235

Women's Health Interactive
(970) 282-9437
P. O. Box 271276, Fort Collins, CO 80527-1276
http://www.womens-health.com

For a review of the 1995 Fourth Worldwide Conference on Women in Beijing and Healthy People 2000 Goals:

Lee, P. R., Estes, C. L., & Close, L. (Eds.). (1997). *The nation's health* (5th ed.). Boston: Jones & Bartlett.

Other Resources:

Boston Women's Health Book Collective. (1992). *The new our bodies, ourselves: A book by and for women.* New York: Simon & Schuster.

Boston Women's Health Book Collective. (1998). *Our bodies, ourselves for the new century: A book by and for women.* New York: Touchstone, Simon & Schuster.

DeMarco, C. (1996, July). *Take charge of your body: Women's health advisor* (rev. 6th ed.). Winlaw, Canada: Well Woman Press.

Payer, L. (1987). *How to avoid a hysterectomy: An indispensable guide to exploring all your options—before you consent to a hysterectomy.* New York: Pantheon Books.

INFERTILITY

Behavioral Medicine Infertility Program

(One of series of Special Programs sponsored by the Behavioral Medicine Medical Department at Beth Israel Deaconess Medical Center)

(617) 632-9529

W/Lowry Medical Office Bldg. 1-A

http://www.bih.harvard.edu/medcenter/about-bidmc/med-depts/special/sp-infertile.html

Also contact: Beth Israel Deaconess Medical Center

(617) 667-7000

330 Brookline Ave., Boston, MA 02215

Centers for Disease Control and Prevention

1995 Assisted Reproductive Technology Success Rates, National Summary and Fertility Clinic Reports

http://www.cdc.gov/nccdphp/drh/arts/

Internet Health Resources Company

(925) 284-9362

1133 Garden Ln., Lafayette, CA 94549

http://www.ihr.com/ihr

Reproductive Science Center® of the Bay Area Fertility & Gynecology Medical Group, Inc.

(510) 867-1800

3160 Crow Canyon Rd., Ste. 150

San Ramon, CA 94583

http://www.ihr.com/bafertil

RESOLVE

(617) 623-0744

1310 Broadway, Somerville, MA 02144-1779

http://www.resolve.org

Other Resources:

Kass-Annese, B. & Danzer, H. (1992). *The fertility awareness handbook: The natural guide to avoiding or achieving pregnancy* (6th ed.). Alameda, CA: Hunter House.

Wallmark, L. S. (1997). *Infertility: The tapestry guide.* Ringoes, NJ: Tapestry Books. http://www.tapestrybooks.com/catalog/moreinfo/tapin.html

INTEGRATIVE/ COMPLEMENTARY MEDICINE

Chinese Medicine:

To find a practitioner near you:

National Acupuncture and Oriental Medicine Alliance

(253) 851-6896

14637 Starr Rd., SE, Olalla, WA 98359

http://www.acuall.org

National Certification Commission for Acupuncture and Oriental Medicine (NCCAOM)

(703) 548-9004

11 Canal Center Plaza, Ste. 300

Alexandria, VA 22314

http://www.nccaom.org

Dr. Andrew Weil's Clinic on the Internet

http://www.drweil.com

Dr. Andrew Weil's Self-Healing *(Newsletter)*
1-888-3DR-WEIL
Write to: Self-Healing
P. O. Box 2057, Marion, OH 43305-2057

News from the Herbal Village
1-800-437-2257
Nature's Herbs
600 E. Quality Dr., American Fork, UT 84003
http://www.naturesherbs.com/nh

Other Resources:

Fuchs, N. K. & Winograd, K. (1985). *The nutrition detective: A woman's guide to treating your health problems through the foods you eat.* Los Angeles: Jeremy P. Tarcher.

Gladstar, R. (1993). *Herbal healing for women: Simple home remedies for women of all ages.* New York: Simon & Schuster.

Hoffmann, D. (1996). *The complete illustrated holistic herbal: A safe and practical guide to making and using herbal remedies.* Rockport, MA: Elemental Books.

Keville, K. & Korn, P. (1996). *Herbs for health and healing: A drug-free guide to prevention and cure.* Emmaus, PA: Rodale Press.

Lark, S. (1984). *Premenstrual syndrome self-help book: A woman's guide to feeling good all month.* Los Altos, CA: PMS Self-Help Center.

McIntyre, A. (1995). *The complete woman's herbal: A manual of healing herbs and nutrition for personal well-being and family care.* New York: Henry Holt.

LESBIAN HEALTH

Lesbian Connection
(A free international forum of news for, by, and about Lesbians and ideas published six times per year.)
(517) 371-5257
Elsie Publishing Institute
P. O. Box 811, East Lansing, MI 48826
e-mail: ElsiePub@aol.com

Other Resource:

Hepburn, C. & Gutierrez, B. (1988). *Alive & well: A Lesbian health guide.* Freedom, CA: Crossing Press.

MENOPAUSE

Women's International Pharmacy
(Natural hormone therapy prescriptions and research articles about natural hormones)
1-800-279-5708
5708 Monona Dr., Madison, WI 53716-3152
13925 W. Meeker Blvd., Ste. 13
Sun City West, AZ 85375
http://www.wipws.com

Other Resources:

Crawford, A. M. (1996). *The herbal menopause book.* Freedom, CA: Crossing Press.

Greenwood, S. (1992). *Menopause, naturally: Preparing for the second half of life* (updated ed.). Volcano, CA: Volcano Press.

Kamen, B. (1993). *Hormone replacement therapy, yes or no?: How to make an informed decision about estrogen, progesterone & other strategies for dealing with PMS, menopause & osteoporosis—A new solution to the estrogen replacement therapy dilemma.* Novato, CA: Nutrition Encounter.

Lark, S. (1992). *The menopause self-help book: A woman's guide to feeling wonderful for the second half of her life.* Berkeley, CA: Celestial Arts.

Lee, J. (1995). *Natural progesterone: The multiple roles of a remarkable hormone.* Sebastopol, CA: B.B.L. Write to: B.B.L. Publishing, P. O. Box 2068, Sebastopol, CA 95473.

National Women's Health Network. (1995). *Taking hormones and women's health: Choices, risks, and benefits* (4th ed.). Washington, DC: Author.

Weed, S. (1992). *Menopausal years: The wise woman way.* Woodstock, NY: Ash Tree.

OSTEOPOROSIS

Foundation for Osteoporosis Research and Education (FORE)

1-888-266-3015

300 27th St., Ste. 103, Oakland, CA 94612

http://www.fore.org

National Osteoporosis Foundation

1150 17th St., NW, Ste. 500

Washington, DC 20036-4603

Other Resources:

Appleton, N. (1991). *Healthy bones: What you should know about osteoporosis.* Garden City Park, NY: Avery.

Gaby, A. (1994). *Preventing and reversing osteoporosis: Every woman's essential guide.* Rocklin, CA: Prima.

Kamen, B. (1992). *Startling new facts about osteoporosis: Why calcium alone does not prevent bone disease—How to select a calcium supplement* (rev. ed., 2nd printing). Novato, CA: Nutrition Encounter.

TEEN-AGERS

Ward, L. (1997). *Choosing—A novel for teenage girls.* Austin, TX: Plain View Press.

1-800-878-3605

To order, write to: Plain View Press

P. O. Box 33311, Austin, TX 78764

http://www.eden.com/~sbpvp/choose.html

TIPS ON INTERNET RESOURCES

- Check the date of information or data you find on the Internet. Some may be outdated, especially for fast-changing research topics, such as human papillomavirus, hormone replacement therapy, or abnormal Pap smear findings.

- Be aware that some sites have more reliable information than others. Some sites are "juried" by organizations to control content; others are not.

- Surf at your own risk. Be discriminating about the information you receive, and confirm it with a health practitioner. Look at other sites for confirmation as well.

In addition to the Internet sites listed previously in this guide, some sites for good quality information include the following:

- **U.S. National Library of Medicine**
  Internet Grateful Med v2.6
  http://igm.nlm.nih.gov/

- **Mayo Clinic Health Oasis**
  http://www.mayohealth.org

- **Division of STD Prevention, Centers for Disease Control and Prevention (CDC)**
  http://www.cdc.gov/nchstp/dstd/dstdp.html

BIBLIOGRAPHY

Abma, J., Driscoll, A. & Moore, K. (1998, January/February). Young women's degree of control over first intercourse: An exploratory analysis. *Family Planning Perspectives, 30,* 12–18.

Abnormal uterine bleeding, treatment options. (1998, June). *National Women's Health Report, 20,* 1, 2, 4, 5.

Addressing the issue of undetected abnormalities on Pap smears. (1997, June). *Early Detection, Issues and Advances in Cervical Cancer Screening, 1,* 1, 5.[1]

American Cancer Society. (1997, March). *Breast cancer* (pp. 1–35). Atlanta, GA: Available from the American Cancer Society's Cancer Information Database, 1-800-ACS-2345.

Are you getting enough calcium? (1998, September). *Dr. Andrew Weil's Self-Healing,* 4, 5.

Begley, S. (1997, February 24). The mammogram War. *Newsweek, CXXIX,* 55–58.

Body as battlefield. (1997, December). *Women's Health Advocate Newsletter,* 4, 5, 6.

Body image: The last frontier of women's rights. (1997, December). *Women's Health Advocate Newsletter,* 4, 4, 6.

The body and self-esteem. (1997, September). *Full Voice, I.* Mine Hill, NJ: The Body Shop. Available: The Body Shop, 106 Iron Mountain Rd., Mine Hill, NJ 07803; 1-800-BODY-SHOP; http://www.the-body-shop.com

Bone marrow transplants: Theory, hope, and hype—Gambling with breast cancer. (1997, December). *Women's Health Advocate Newsletter,* 4, 1, 2, 8.

Bonfiglio, T. A., Inhorn, S., Krieger, P. A., Sedlacek, T. V., Sheets, E. E. & Solomon, D. (1996, August). Cervical cancer screening: Today and tomorrow—Proceedings of a clinical roundtable. *Supplement to OB-Gyn News and Family Practice News,* 1–7, 9–16.

Boston Women's Health Book Collective. (1992). *The new our bodies, ourselves: A book by and for women.* New York: Simon & Schuster.

Brenner, B. A. (1997, April/May). Fiddling while Rome burns: The latest mammogram controversy. *Breast Cancer Action,* 2, 10.

Centers for Disease Control and Prevention, Division of STD Prevention. (1997). *Assisted Reproductive Technology Success Rates, National Summary and Fertility Clinic Reports.* [Available Online: http://www.cdc.gov/nccdphp/drh/art97/index.htm].

Centers for Disease Control and Prevention, Division of STD Prevention. (1997, September). *Sexually transmitted disease surveillance, 1996* [Online]. U.S. Department of Health and Human Services, Public Health Service. Atlanta, GA: Centers for Disease Control and Prevention. Available: http://wonder.cdc.gov/ wonder/STD/Title4000.html.

Cervical cancer risk factors. (1997, June). *Women's Health Forum: Discussions in Pap Smear Screening, 1,* 1.

[1]Available: Communicore, P. O. Box 2389, Friday Harbor, WA 98250; http://www.communicore.com

Chandra, A. & Stephen, E. H. (1998, January/February). Impaired fecundity in the United States: 1982–1995. *Family Planning Perspectives, 30,* 34–42.

Cowley, G. (1997, February 24). Beyond the mammogram. *Newsweek, CXXIX,* 59.

Crawford, A. M. (1996). *The herbal menopause book.* Freedom, CA: Crossing Press.

Crouch, J. (1978). *Functional human anatomy* (3rd ed.). Philadelphia: Lea & Febiger.

Degen, C. & Wilkinson, K. (1998, April/May). "Breakthrough" gene test: How helpful is it? *Breast Cancer Action Newsletter,* 1.

DeMarco, C. (1996, July). *Take charge of your body: Women's health advisor* (rev. 6th ed.). Winlaw, Canada: Well Woman Press.

Depo-Provera and bone density: What should you tell teen users? (1998, January). *Contraceptive Technology Update, 19,* 1–3.

Did you know? (1997, June). *Women's Health Forum: Discussions in Pap Smear Screening, 1,* 2.

Does the pill help spread HIV? (1998, January/February). *Family Planning Perspectives, 30,* 3.

Duke, J. (1998, March). Alzheimer's. *News From the Herbal Village,* 1–15.

Emerson, E. (1997, November). Study examines non-invasive way to detect cancer of the breast [Online]. Available: http://www.usc.edu/hsc/info/pr/1vol3/329/parisky.html.

Estrogen, the estrogen decision: Are lower doses good enough? (1998, July). *Women's Health Advocate Newsletter, 5,* 1, 6.

The female condom: Clinical research—An overview (compilation of more than 40 clinical studies on the female condom). (1997, February). Abstracts available: The Female Health Company, 875 N. Michigan Ave., No. 3660, Chicago, IL 60611.

Fibroid surgery alternative. (1998, April). *Women's Health Advocate Newsletter, 5,* 6.

Fibroids and abnormal uterine bleeding. (1998, June). *National Women's Health Report, 20,* 5.

Finer, L. B. & Zabin, L. S. (1998, January/February). Does the timing of the first family planning visit still matter? *Family Planning Perspectives, 30,* 30–33, 42.

Frequently asked questions about infertility [Online]. (1996). Available: Infertility, Gynecology, & Obstetrics (IGO) Medical Group of San Diego, Inc., http://www.ihr.com/igo/index.html.

Fuchs, N. K. & Winograd, K. (1985). *The nutrition detective: A woman's guide to treating your health problems through the foods you eat.* Los Angeles: Jeremy P. Tarcher.

Gaby, A. (1994). *Preventing and reversing osteoporosis: Every woman's essential guide.* Rocklin, CA: Prima.

Gladstar, R. (1993). *Herbal healing for women: Simple home remedies for women of all ages.* New York: Simon & Schuster.

Greenpeace. (1992). *Breast cancer and the environment: The chlorine connection.* Chicago: Author.

Greenwood, S. (1992). *Menopause, naturally: Preparing for the second half of life* (updated ed.). Volcano, CA: Volcano Press.

Hatcher, R. (1998, January). Ten common questions on emergency contraception. *Contraceptive Technology Update, 19,* 6, 11, 12.

Hatcher, R. A., Trussell, J., Stewart, F. H., Cates, W., Stewart, G. K., Guest, F. & Kowal, D. (Eds.). (1998). *Contraceptive technology (17th ed.).* New York: Ardent Media.

Hatcher, R. A., Trussell, J., Stuart, F., Stewart, G. K., Kowal, D., Guest, F., Cates, W., Jr. & Policar, M. S. (1994). *Contraceptive technology (16th ed.).* New York: Irvington.

Hawkins, J. W., Roberto, D. M. & Stanley-Haney, J. L. (1993). *Protocols for nurse practitioners in gynecologic settings.* New York: Tiresias Press.

Heerdt, A. S., Young, C. W. & Borgen, P. I. (1995). Calcium glucarate as a chemopreventive agent in breast cancer. *Israel Journal of Medical Sciences, 31,* 101–105.

Henshaw, S. K. (1998, January/February). Unintended pregnancy in the United States. *Family Planning Perspectives, 30,* 24–29.

Hepatitis A and B: Should you be immunized? (1998, April). *Dr. Andrew Weil's Self-Healing,* 7.

Hepatitis C, the silent epidemic: Who's at risk. (1998, July). *Women's Health Advocate Newsletter, 5,* 2, 3.

Hepatitis C: Testing for a "stealth virus." (1998, April). *Dr. Andrew Weil's Self-Healing,* 6.

Herpes the silent epidemic: One in three women now affected. (1988, March). *Women's Health Advocate Newsletter, 5,* 1, 2.

HPV: Myths and misconceptions. (1998, Spring). *HPV News, 8,* 1, 3, 4–7.

Hulley, S., Grady, D., Bush, T., Furberg, C., Herrington, D., Riggs, B. & Vittinghoff, E. (1998, August 19). Randomized trial of estrogen plus progestin for secondary prevention of coronary heart disease in postmenopausal women. *Journal of the American Medical Association, 280,* 605–613.

Human papillomavirus—An initiator of cervical cancer. (1997). *Early Detection, Issues and Advances in Cervical Cancer Screening, 1,* 1, 6.[1]

Kass-Annese, B. & Danzer, H. (1992). *The fertility awareness handbook: The natural guide to avoiding or achieving pregnancy* (6th ed.). Alameda, CA: Hunter House.

Kelsey, B. & Freeman, S. (1997, November). Identifying and treating pelvic inflammatory disease. *American Journal of Nursing Supplement,* 17–22.

Keville, K. & Korn, P. (1996). *Herbs for health and healing: A drug-free guide to prevention and cure.* Emmaus, PA: Rodale Press.

Keye, D. S. & Keye, W. R., Jr. (1998, July). Premenstrual syndrome: Diagnosis and treatment. *Physician Assistant, 22,* 30, 32, 37, 38, 40, 43, 44, 47, 48.

Kozier, B., Erb, G., Blais, K. & Wilkinson, J. M. (1995). *Fundamentals of nursing: Concepts, process and practice* (5th ed.). Redwood City, CA: Addison-Wesley.

Kradjian, R. M. (1994). *Save yourself from breast cancer.* New York: Berkley Books.

Lark, S. (1984). *Premenstrual syndrome self-help book: A woman's guide to feeling good all month.* Los Altos, CA: PMS Self-Help Center.

Latour, K. (1993). *The breast cancer companion: From diagnosis through treatment to recovery—Everything you need to know for every step along the way.* New York: W. Morrow.

Lee, P. R., Estes, C. L. & Close, L. (Eds.). (1997). *The nation's health* (5th ed.). Boston: Jones & Bartlett.

Leeper, M. A. & Stein, Z. (1998). The female condom: Cause and effect of protection. Paper from the Proceedings of the 1998 World AIDS Conference, Geneva, Switzerland, June 1998. Available: The Female Health Company, 875 N. Michigan Ave., No. 3660, Chicago, IL 60618.

Lichtman, R. & Papera, S. (1990). *Gynecology: Well-woman care.* Norwalk, CT: Appleton & Lange.

Liebman, B. (1998a, April). Avoiding the fracture zone, calcium: Why get more? *Nutrition Action Health Letter, 25,* 3–5.

Liebman, B. (1998b, April). Calcium supplements: The way to go? *Nutrition Action Health Letter, 25,* 5–7.

Love, S. M. & Lindsey, K. (1998). *Dr. Susan Love's hormone book: Making informed choices about menopause.* New York: Time Books.

Mammotome biopsies: More accurate, less invasive. (1997, October). *National Women's Health Report, 19,* 7.

Marchiondo, K. (1998, March). A new look at urinary tract infections. *American Journal of Nursing, 98,* 34–39.

McIntyre, A. (1995). *The complete woman's herbal: A manual of healing herbs and nutrition for personal well-being and family care.* New York: Henry Holt.

Medical abortion: Safe, effective, and legal in Britain. (1992, January). *British Medical Journal, 304,* 195–196.

Monohan, K. (1997, November/December). Mastectomies...and alternatives. *The Network News,* 3–4.

National Cancer Institute. (1998, September 15). Screening mammograms. *Cancer Facts,* 1–6.

National Women's Health Network. (1995). *Taking hormones and women's health: Choices, risks, and benefits.* Washington, DC: Author.

Natural help for hepatitis. (1998, April). *Dr. Andrew Weil's Self-Healing,* 1, 6, 7.

New hope for infertility. (1997, December). *Dr. Andrew Weil's Self-Healing,* 1, 6, 7.

New year, new option: Cyclo-Provera awaits word. (1998, January). *Contraceptive Technology Update, 19,* 1–3.

Northrup, C. (1994). *Women's bodies, women's wisdom.* New York: Bantam Books.

The older woman and cervical cancer. (1997, June). *Early Detection, Issues and Advances in Cervical Cancer Screening, 1,* 3.[1]

The Pap smear: Success in cervical cancer screening. (1997, June). *Women's Health Forum: Discussions in Pap Smear Screening, 1,* 1, 2.

Parker, P. D. (1994). Premenstrual syndrome. *American Family Physician, 50,* 1309–1317.

Physicians' desk reference (52nd ed.). (1998). Montvale, NJ: Medical Economics.

Raloff, J. (1994, January 8). The gender benders. *Science News, 145,* 24–27.

Reproductive Science Center of the Bay Area Fertility & Gynecology Medical Group, Inc. (1995). *Clomiphine Citrate (Clomid) (Serophene).* [Available Online: http://www.ihr.bafertil/articles/clomiphe.html].

Reproductive Science Center of the Bay Area Fertility & Gynecology Medical Group, Inc. (1995). *Overview of Assisted Reproductive Technologies.* [Available Online: http://www.ihr.bafertil/assistre.html].

Reproductive Science Center of the Bay Area Fertility & Gynecology Medical Group, Inc. (1996). *IVF with ICSI.* [Available Online: http://www.ihr.bafertil/articles/azoosper.htm].

Reproductive Science Center of the Bay Area Fertility & Gynecology Medical Group, Inc. (1998). *Gonal F/Follistim Gonadotropins.* [Available Online: http://www.ihr.bafertil/articles/gonalf.html].

Reproductive Science Center of the Bay Area Fertility & Gynecology Medical Group, Inc. (1998). *Pergonal and Metrodin.* [Available Online: http://www.ihr.bafertil/articles/pergmetr.html].

Reproductive Science Center of the Bay Area Fertility & Gynecology Medical Group, Inc. (1995/1996). *Assisted Hatching.* [Available Online: http://www.ihr.bafertil/articles/assistha.html].

REALITY® female condom. (1997). Chicago: The Female Health Company. Brochure available: The Female Health Company, 875 N. Michigan Ave., No. 3660, Chicago, IL 60618.

Schaff, E. A., Eisinger, S. H., Franks, P. & Kim, S. S. (1996, March). Methotrexate and misoprostol for early abortion. *Family Medicine, 28,* 198–203.

Schuster, M. A., Bell, R. M., Berry, S. H. & Kanouse, D. E. (1998, March-April). Impact of a high school condom availability program on sexual attitudes and behaviors. *Family Planning Perspectives, 30,* 67–72, 88.

Seibert, D. C. & McMullen, P. (1996, November). How to manage the patient with an abnormal Pap smear. *American Journal of Nursing Supplement,* 17–23.

Should women be informed of screening options? (1997, June). *Early Detection, Issues and Advances in Cervical Cancer Screening, 1,* 2–4.[1]

Sifton, D. W. (Ed.). (1994). *The PDR family guide to women's health and prescription drugs.* Montvale, NJ: Medical Economics Data Production.

Silvestre, L., Dubois, C., Renault, M., Rezvani, Y., Baulieu, E.-E. & Ulmann, A. (1990, March). Voluntary interruption of pregnancy with mifepristone (RU486) and a prostaglandin analogue: A large-scale French experience. *New England Journal of Medicine, 322,* 645–648.

Smith, A. & Hughes, P. L. (1998, April). The estrogen dilemma. *American Journal of Nursing, 98,* 17–20.

Stenchever, M. (1996). *Office gynecology* (2nd ed.). St. Louis, MO: Mosby–Year Book.

Tamoxifen and beyond. (1998, June). *Harvard Women's Health Watch, V,* 1.

Vaccine update. (1997, Winter). *HPV News, 7,* 1, 3, 4–6.

Vitamin D, sunlight redeemed? Reducing osteoporosis and cancer risk. (1998, February). *Women's Health Advocate Newsletter, 4,* 1, 8.

Warts, frustrating but common, experts say. (1997, Winter). *HPV News, 7,* 8, 9.

Weckstein, L. N. (1996). Treating the infertile woman over 40 [Online]. Available: Reproductive Science Center of the Bay Area Fertility & Gynecology Medical Group, Inc., http://www.ihr.com/bafertil/index.html.

Weed, S. (1992). *Menopausal years: The wise woman way.* Woodstock, NY: Ash Tree.

Weed, S. (1996). *Breast cancer? Breast health!: The wise woman way.* Woodstock, NY: Ash Tree.

When physicians assure confidentiality, teenagers are willing to talk openly. (1998, January/February). *Family Planning Perspectives, 30,* 52.

Winegardner, M. F. (1998, February). The atypical Pap smear: New concerns. *The Clinical Advisor for Physicians Assistants, 1,* 26–31.

INDEX

PRETEST KEY

1.	C	Chapter 1
2.	D	Chapter 2
3.	B	Chapter 2
4.	C	Chapter 2
5.	B	Chapter 3
6.	D	Chapter 3
7.	B	Chapter 4
8.	C	Chapter 4
9.	A	Chapter 5
10.	C	Chapter 5
11.	A	Chapter 5
12.	D	Chapter 6
13.	A	Chapter 6
14.	A	Chapter 7
15.	C	Chapter 7
16.	A	Chapter 7
17.	C	Chapter 8
18.	C	Chapter 8
19.	B	Chapter 9
20.	D	Chapter 10
21.	B	Chapter 11
22.	A	Chapter 12
23.	B	Chapter 12
24.	B	Chapter 13
25.	A	Chapter 13